Diffusion MRI of the Breast

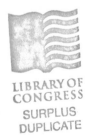

Diffusion MRI of the Breast

Mami Iima, MD, PhD
Assistant Professor, Department of Diagnostic Imaging and Nuclear Medicine
Kyoto University Graduate School of Medicine
Institute for Advancement of Clinical and Translational Science (iACT)
Kyoto University Hospital
Kyoto, Japan

Savannah C. Partridge, PhD
Professor, Departments of Radiology and Bioengineering
Research Director, Breast Imaging
University of Washington School of Medicine
Associate Director of Cancer Imaging
Seattle Cancer Care Alliance
Seattle, Washington, USA

Denis Le Bihan, MD, PhD
Founding Director, NeuroSpin
Joliot Institute
Department of Fundamental Research
CEA-Saclay, Paris-Saclay University, Gif-sur-Yvette, France

Visiting Professor of Kyoto University Graduate School of Medicine
Kyoto Prefectural University of Medicine and the Japan National Institute for Physiological Sciences
Okazaki, Japan

ELSEVIER

ELSEVIER

1600 John F. Kennedy Blvd.
Ste 1800
Philadelphia, PA 19103-2899

DIFFUSION MRI OF THE BREAST   ISBN: 978-0-323-79702-3

Content Strategist: Melanie Tucker
Content Development Specialist: Ranjana Sharma
Publishing Services Manager: Deepthi Unni
Project Manager: Sindhuraj Thulasingam
Design Direction: Amy Buxton

Printed in India

Last digit is the print number: 9   8   7   6   5   4   3   2   1

List of Contributors

Nita Amornsiripanitch, MD
Brigham and Women's Hospital
Harvard Medical School, Boston
Massachusetts, United States

Debbie Anaby, PhD
Head, Microstructural Imaging Lab
Diagnostic and Imaging Department
Sheba Medical Center
Tel HaShomer, Ramat Gan, Israel

Margarita Arango-Lievano, PhD
Solutions Owner Clinical Solutions
Olea Medical
La Ciotat, France

Pascal A. T. Baltzer, MD
Assoc. Prof. Priv.-Doz. Dr.
Department of Biomedical Imaging and
    Image-Guided Therapy
Medical University of Vienna
Vienna, Austria

Tone Frost Bathen, PhD
Department of Circulation and Medical Imaging
    Norwegian University of Science and Technology
    (NTNU) Trondheim, Norway

Ethan Henry Bauer, BM
Research Assistant Radiology Sheba
    Medical Center
Ramat Gan, Israel

Gabrielle C. Baxter, PhD
Research Associate
Department of Radiology
University of Cambridge
Cambridge, United Kingdom

Ersin Bayram, PhD
Director
Body & Oncology MRI GE Healthcare
Houston Texas, United States

Thomas Benkert, PhD
Employer
MR Application Predevelopment
Siemens Healthcare GmbH,
Erlangen, Germany

Petra Bildhauer
SHS DI MR DL AR ACQ Siemens Healthineers,
Erlangen, Germany

Almir Bitencourt, MD, PhD
Radiologist
Imaging
A. C. Camargo Cancer Center
São Paulo, Brazil;
Radiologist
Breast Imaging
DASA
São Paulo, Brazil

Timothé Boutelier, PhD
Senior researcher
Research and Innovation
Olea Medical, La Ciotat, France

Lucile Brun, MS
Research Engineer Department of Research and
    Innovation Olea Medical
La Ciotat, France

Brianna Bucciarelli, MSc
Clinical & Scientific Research Engineer
Clinical Affairs
Olea Medical
La Ciotat, France

Sophie Campana, PhD
Research Engineer
Clinical Affairs Olea Medical,
La Ciotat, France

Thomas L. Chenevert, PhD
Professor Department of Radiology
    University of Michigan
Ann Arbor Michigan, United States

Bruce L. Daniel, MD
Professor
Radiology
Stanford University, Stanford
California, United States;
Professor, by courtesy
Bioengineering
Stanford University, Stanford
California, United States

Adam J. Davis, MD
Chief Medical Officer
Olea Medical
La Ciotat, France

Sarah Eskreis-Winkler, MD, PhD
Radiology
Memorial Sloan Kettering Cancer Center
New York, United States

Florence Feret, MRT
Product Owner Products Olea Medical
La Ciotat, France

Edna Furman-Haran, PhD
Head of MRI Unit
Life Sciences Core Facilities
The Weizmann Institute of Science
Rehovot, Israel

Liesbeth Geerts, PhD
Global Director Clinical Science
MR Clinical Science
Philips, Best, Netherlands

Peter Gibbs, PhD
Dr Radiology Memorial Sloan
Kettering Cancer Center
New York, United States

Fiona J. Gilbert, MD, FRCR, FRCP
Professor of Radiology
Department of Radiology
University of Cambridge
Cambridge, United Kingdom

Robert Grimm, PhD
MR Application Predevelopment
SHS DI MR DL ONCO
Siemens Healthcare
Erlangen, Germany

Brian A. Hargreaves, PhD
Professor
Radiology and (by courtesy) Bioengineering
    and Electrical Engineering
Stanford University, Stanford
California, United States

Laura Heacock, MS, MD
Clinical Associate Professor of Radiology
Breast Imaging Section
NYU Langone Health, New York
New York, United States

Aurélia Hermoso
Application Specialist
Abys Medical
La Rochelle, France

Maya Honda, MD, PhD
Department of Diagnostic Radiology
Kansai Electric Power Hospital, Osaka, Japan;
Visiting Researcher
Department of Diagnostic Imaging and Nuclear
    Medicine, Kyoto University Graduate School of
    Medicine, Kyoto, Japan

Nola M. Hylton, PhD
Professor
Radiology and Biomedical Imaging
University of California
San Francisco, California, United States

Mami Iima, MD, PhD
Assistant Professor
Department of Diagnostic Imaging and Nuclear
    Medicine, Kyoto University Graduate School of
    Medicine, and Department of Clinical Innovative
    Medicine, Institute for Advancement of Clinical
    and Translational Science, Kyoto University
    Hospital, Kyoto, Japan
Institute for Advancement of Clinical and
    Translational Science (iACT)
Kyoto University Hospital
Japan

Neil Peter Jerome, MChem, MA, PhD
Department of Circulation and Medical Imaging
Norwegian University of Science and Technology
   (NTNU)
Trondheim, Norway

Masako Kataoka, MD, PhD
Lecturer
Department of Diagnostic Imaging and Nuclear
   Medicine
Kyoto University Graduate School of Medicine
Kyoto, Japan

Toshiki Kazama, MD, PhD
Associate Professor
Diagnostic Radiology
Tokai University School of Medicine
Isehara, Japan

Miho Kita, MD, PhD
Chief Department of Radiology Fuchu Hospital
Izumi City, Osaka, Japan

Thomas Kwee, MD, PhD
Department of Radiology
University Medical Center Groningen
Groningen, Netherlands

Denis Le Bihan, MD, PhD
Founding Director, NeuroSpin, CEA-Saclay,
   Paris-Saclay University, Gif-sur-Yvette, France
Member of the Institute of France
Visiting Professor
Kyoto University Graduate School of Medicine
Kyoto Prefectural University of Medicine and the
   Japan National Institute for Physiological Sciences
Okazaki, Japan

Wen Li, PhD
Assistant Professional Researcher
Radiology & Biomedical Imaging
University of California
San Francisco, California, United States

Wei Liu, PhD
Senior Key Expert
Department of Digital
Siemens Shenzhen Magnetic Resonance Ltd
Shenzhen, Guang Dong, China

Roberto Lo Gullo, MD
Department of Radiology, Breast Imaging Service
Memorial Sloan Kettering Cancer Center
New York, United States

Dariya Malyarenko, PhD
Associate Research Scientist
Radiology
University of Michigan
Ann Arbor, Michigan, United States

Ritse Mann, MD, PhD
Breast and Interventional Radiologist Medical
   Imaging Radboudumc
Nijmegen Netherlands;
Breast Radiologist
Radiology The Netherlands Cancer Institute,
Amsterdam, Netherlands

Jessica A. McKay, PhD
Postdoctoral Fellow
Department of Radiology
Stanford University, Stanford
California, United States

Anca Mitulescu, PhD
Vice President of Clinical Affairs
Clinical Affairs
Olea Medical
La Ciotat, France

Woo Kyung Moon, MD, PhD
Professor
Radiology
Seoul National University Hospital
Seoul, Republic of Korea

Catherine J. Moran, PhD
Senior Research Scientist
Department of Radiology Stanford University
Stanford California, United States

Linda Moy, MD
Professor
Radiology
NYU Grossman School of Medicine
New York, New York, United States

Jaladhar Neelavalli, PhD
Senior Clinical Scientist
Clinical Science
Philips Healthcare
Bengaluru, Karnataka, India

Noam Nissan, MD, PhD
Senior Radiologist
Radiology Sheba Medical Center
Ramat Gan, Israel

Savannah C. Partridge, PhD
Professor
Departments of Radiology and Bioengineering
Research Director, Breast Imaging
University of Washington School of Medicine
Associate Director of Cancer Imaging
Fred Hutchinson Cancer Center
Seattle, Washington, United States

Andrew J. Patterson, PhD, MBA
Radiology
University of Cambridge
Cambridge, United Kingdom

Johannes M. Peeters, PhD
Clinical Scientist MR Clinical Science
Philips, Best, Netherlands

Katja Pinker, MD, PhD
Professor of Radiology
Radiology
Memorial Sloan Kettering Cancer Center
New York, New York, United States

Beatriu Reig, MD, MPH
Assistant Professor
The Department of Radiology
New York University Grossman School of
    Medicine
New York, New York, United States

Ilse Rubie, B
Clinical Application Specialist MR
BIU MR
Philips, Best, Netherlands

Ann Shimakawa, MS
Applications Engineer
MR Applications & Workflow
GE Healthcare, 333 Ravenswood Ave
Menlo Park California United States

Hee Jung Shin, PhD
Professor
Department of Radiology and Research Institute of
    Radiology
Asan Medical Center
University of Ulsan
Seoul, Republic of Korea

Eric E. Sigmund, BS, MS, PhD
Associate Professor (Research)
Radiology
NYU Langone Health
New York, New York, United States

Miri Sklair-Levy, MD
Director Breast Imaging Unit
Meirav Center
Radiology Department
Sheba, Tel-HaShomer, Israel

Taro Takahara, MD, PhD
Professor
Biomedical Engineering
Tokai University School of Engineering
Isehara, Kanagawa, Japan

Sunitha B. Thakur, MSc, PhD
Associate Attending Member
Medical Physics
Memorial Sloan Kettering Cancer Center
New York, New York, United States;
Attending Member
Radiology
Memorial Sloan Kettering Cancer Center
New York, New York, United States

Gregor Thoermer, PhD
Department Head
Magnetic Resonance Oncology Predevelopment
Siemens Healthcare GmbH
Erlangen, Germany

Elisabeth Weiland, PhD
SHS DI MR DL
Siemens Healthcare GmbH
Erlangen, Germany

Lisa J. Wilmes, PhD
Specialist
Radiology and Biomedical Imaging
University of California San Francisco
San Francisco, California, United States

Ramona Woitek, MD, PhD
Senior Research Associate
Department of Radiology
University of Cambridge
Cambridge, United Kingdom

Foreword

Diffusion-weighted imaging (DWI) provides structural and functional information that complements the excellent anatomical detail rendered by magnetic resonance imaging (MRI). There is common agreement that DWI is able to provide image contrast that is sensitive to microstructural and cellular remodeling. Since 1997, when Englander addressed the possibility of applying DWI to the human breast, several studies have shown that this technique is highly useful in the detection and characterization of breast lesions, as well as in the assessment of response to therapy. Moreover, it is a safe technique, it can be performed in a short period of time (2–4 minutes), and it does not employ ionizing radiation, nor does it require the use of contrast media, avoiding the drawbacks associated with these agents. Another major advantage of DWI is that the apparent diffusion coefficient (ADC) derived from it provides quantitative information of the underlying pathophysiological mechanisms, establishing DWI as a promising imaging biomarker. As a result, a growing number of centers are incorporating DWI into clinical breast MRI protocols.

However, DWI acquisition protocols must be optimized to reduce artifacts and achieve adequate signal-to-noise ratio (SNR). Furthermore, the ensuing signal analysis and feature extraction from each voxel necessary to yield the tissue properties also suffers from variability. Indeed, there are different interpretation approaches in the published literature, all of which place a limit on its widespread clinical use and incorporation into the Breast Imaging Reporting and Data System (BI-RADS).

In March 2017 the European Society of Breast Imaging (EUSOBI) supported the creation of an international working group (the "Breast DWI Club") to address the challenges that the clinical implementation of the technique poses. The primary goals of the EUSOBI International DWI Working Group are to issue consensus statements and define standards that promote the integration of DWI into clinical practice, to develop a standardized quality assurance protocol that endorses multicentric studies, and to find agreement on optimal methods for image analysis and interpretation. Clinical breast MRI experts, MRI physicists, and major vendor representatives from 25 sites in 16 countries, gathered to work over the ensuing months and published a consensus and mission statement in 2019.[1] This joint effort proposed basic requirements for routine clinical application of breast DWI, established a common ground for the future objectives of expanding the technical recommendations of DWI protocols and developing of methods for quality control, and encouraged research into more sophisticated DWI methods.

It is a great privilege for me to introduce this book, devoted to the current and future clinical applications of diffusion MRI of the breast. The editors and the authors, all well-recognized experts in the field, have assembled a body of knowledge on breast DWI that will be of immense help to breast and general radiologists, as well as radiology technologists and breast care clinicians who seek to expand their knowledge on breast imaging biomarkers. The book is divided into five sections. The first chapter deals with the basics of DWI, a necessary introduction to understand and use DWI in clinical practice. Chapters 2 to 7 provide an in-depth discussion of the clinical applications of breast imaging, namely the position of DWI in respect to other modalities, the use of DWI in the diagnosis of suspicious lesions with a multiparametric protocol, the use of DWI as an imaging biomarker of prognosis and response prediction, the clinical implementation of DWI in the diagnosis of the most common lesions, the potential use of DWI as a stand-alone approach, and the biological validation of DWI (the influence of the hormonal status on ADC measurements). Chapters 8 to 12 deal with the challenges of DWI and advanced techniques (intravoxel incoherent motion [IVIM], non-Gaussian diffusion, diffusion tensor imaging [DTI], and other novel techniques), as well as with radiomics and artificial intelligence. Chapters 13 and 14 provide a practical approach to clinical interpretation and quality assurance issues, and Chapters 15 to 18 or appendix shows the different vendor approaches in breast DWI packages.

This book is clearly a steadfast continuation and a necessary companion to the EUSOBI International DWI Working Group endeavor, and I am sure that it will further set the foundations for the integration and advancement of DWI as a crucial breast imaging biomarker in clinical practice.

Julia Camps-Herrero
Chief of Breast Health in Ribera
Valencia, Spain;
EUSOBI past-President
Vienna, Austria

REFERENCE

1. Baltzer P, Mann RM, Iima M, et al. Diffusion-weighted imaging of the breast—a consensus and mission statement from the EUSOBI International Breast Diffusion—Weighted Imaging Working Group. *Eur Radiol*. 2020;30(3):1436–1450.

Table of Contents

Foreword,   x
Julia Camps-Herrero

1. **General Principles and Challenges of Diffusion MRI,**   1
   Denis Le Bihan, Mami Iima, and Savannah C. Partridge

2. **Conventional Breast Imaging,**   18
   Ritse Mann

3. **Overview of Breast DWI: Diagnosis of Suspicious Lesions Using DWI in Combination With Standard MRI,**   40
   Pascal A. T. Baltzer

4. **Biomarkers, Prognosis, and Prediction Factors,**   49
   Beatriu Reig, Linda Moy, Eric E. Sigmund, and Laura Heacock

5. **Disease and Treatment Monitoring,**   71
   Wen Li, David C. Newitt, Savannah C. Partridge, and Nola M. Hylton

6. **Diffusion MRI as a Stand-Alone Unenhanced Approach for Breast Imaging and Screening,**   86
   Hee Jung Shin, Woo Kyung Moon, Nita Amornsiripanitch, and Savannah C. Partridge

7. **DWI and Breast Physiology Status,**   108
   Noam Nissan, Debbie Anaby, Ethan Bauer, and Miri Sklair-Levy

8. **IVIM and Non-Gaussian DWI of the Breast,**   116
   Mami Iima, Sunitha B. Thakur, Neil Peter Jerome, Maya Honda, Masako Kataoka, Tone Frost Bathen, and Eric E. Sigmund

9. **Diffusion Tensor Imaging (DTI) of the Breast,**   144
   Eric E. Sigmund, Edna Furman-Haran, Pascal A. T. Baltzer, and Savannah C. Partridge

10. **Artificial Intelligence—Enhanced Breast MRI and DWI: Current Status and Future Applications,**   162
    Katja Pinker, Roberto Lo Gullo, Sarah Eskreis-Winkler, Almir Bitencourt, Peter Gibbs, and Sunitha B. Thakur

11. **Diffusion-Weighted Whole Body Imaging With Background Body Signal Suppression (DWIBS),**   176
    Taro Takahara, Toshiki Kazama, Miho Kita, and Thomas Kwee

12. **High-Resolution Diffusion-Weighted Breast MRI Acquisition,**   186
    Brian A. Hargreaves, Catherine J. Moran, and Jessica A. McKay, and Bruce L. Daniel

13. **Clinical Interpretation of Diffusion MRI, ROI Assessment, Common Errors, Pitfalls and Artifacts, Challenges in Acquisition,**   203
    Gabrielle C. Baxter, Ramona Woitek, Andrew J. Patterson, and Fiona J. Gilbert

14. **Multiplatform Standardization of Breast DWI Protocols: Quality Control and Test Objects,**   220
    Dariya Malyarenko, Lisa J. Wilmes, and Thomas L. Chenevert

15. **Routine and Advanced Breast DWI Techniques and Processing: The Siemens Healthineers Perspective,**   244
    Gregor Thoermer, Petra Bildhauer, Thomas Benkert, Wei Liu, Robert Grimm, and Elisabeth Weiland

16. **Breast Diffusion MRI Acquisition and Processing Techniques: The GE Healthcare Perspective,**   251
    Ann Shimakawa and Ersin Bayram

17. **Breast DWI Techniques and Processing: The Philips Perspective,**   256
    Johannes M. Peeters, Ilse Rubie, Jaladhar Neelavalli, and Liesbeth Geerts

18. **Diffusion-Weighted Imaging (DWI) for Breast Lesion Characterization: The Olea Medical Perspective and the Utilization of Olea Sphere Software,**   264
    Margarita Arango-Lievano, Timothé Boutelier, Lucile Brun, Brianna Bucciarelli, Sophie Campana, Adam J. Davis, Florence Feret, Aurélia Hermoso, and Anca Mitulescu

Index,   271

Chapter 1

General Principles and Challenges of Diffusion MRI

Denis Le Bihan, MD, PhD, Mami Iima, MD, PhD, and Savannah C. Partridge, PhD

The concept of diffusion magnetic resonance imaging (MRI) emerged in the mid-1980s, together with the first images of water molecular diffusion in the human brain,[1,2] as a way to probe tissue structure. Since then, diffusion MRI has become a pillar of modern clinical imaging. Diffusion MRI is both a method and a powerful concept, because diffusing water molecules provide unique information on the tissue microscopic architecture. Diffusion MRI has initially been used to investigate neurological disorders, aided by amenable conditions of relatively immobile and high T2 signal of the brain. However, further work has shown that diffusion MRI could work in the body as well,[3] and applications are now rapidly expanding in oncology[4,5] for the detection of malignant lesions and metastases and for monitoring therapy. Water diffusion is significantly decreased in most malignant tissues, and diffusion MRI, which does not require any tracer injection, is rapidly becoming a modality of choice to detect, characterize, or even grade malignant lesions, especially in the prostate and the breast.

Basic Diffusion MRI, Diffusion-Weighted Imaging (DWI), and the Classic Apparent Diffusion Coefficient (ADC)

Molecular diffusion refers to the random translational motion of molecules (also called Brownian motion), a physical process that results from the thermal energy carried by these molecules, which was well characterized by Einstein.[6] In a free medium, during a given time interval, molecular displacements obey a 3D Gaussian distribution (Fig. 1.1): molecules travel randomly in space over a distance that is statistically well described by a diffusion coefficient (D). This coefficient depends only on the size (mass) of the molecules, the temperature, and the nature (viscosity) of the medium. For example, in the case of "free" water molecules self-diffusing in water at body temperature (37°C), the diffusion coefficient is 3×10^{-3} mm^2/s, which, based on Einstein's mean displacement equation,[6] translates to a mean diffusion distance of 17 μm during 50 ms along one direction (Fig. 1.1). Diffusion MRI is thus deeply rooted in the concept that, during their diffusion-driven displacements, molecules probe tissue structure at a *microscopic* scale well beyond the usual *millimetric* image resolution. During typical diffusion imaging times of about 50 to 100 ms, water molecules move in tissues on average over distances around 1 to 15 μm, bouncing, crossing, or interacting with many tissue components, such as cell membranes, fibers, or macromolecules. (The diffusion of other metabolites can also be detected with diffusion MR spectroscopy.) Because of the tortuous movement of water molecules around those obstacles (i.e., "hindered" diffusion; see Fig. 1.1), the actual diffusion distance is reduced compared with free water (see Fig. 1.1), and the displacement distribution is no longer Gaussian (the shrinkage of the distribution is characterized by a parameter called "kurtosis"). In other words, over very short times, diffusion reflects the local intrinsic viscosity, whereas at longer diffusion times the effects of the obstacles become predominant. Hence, the noninvasive observation of the water diffusion-driven displacement distributions in vivo provides unique clues to the fine structural features and geometrical organization of cells in tissues and to changes in those features with physiological or pathological states.

IMAGING DIFFUSION WITH MRI

Although early water diffusion measurements were made in biological tissues using nuclear magnetic

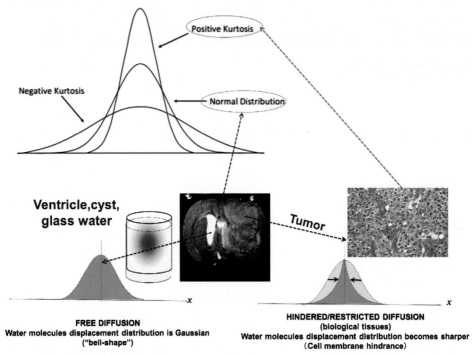

Fig. 1.1 Free versus hindered diffusion. In pure-water, free-diffusion environments (e.g., cerebrospinal fluid in brain ventricles), the diffusion-driven displacement of water molecules is a normal distribution (Gaussian). At body temperature of ~37°C, about 32% of the molecules have explored at least 17μm, whereas only 5% of them have traveled over distances greater than 34μm. However, in tissues, displacements are hindered or restricted by cell membranes and other obstacles, and the distribution becomes sharper. The deviation from a Gaussian distribution can be quantified by a mathematical parameter called kurtosis.

resonance in the 1960s and 1970s, it was not until the mid-1980s that the basic principles of diffusion MRI were laid out.[1,2] By combining MRI principles with those introduced earlier in nuclear magnetic resonance physics and chemistry to encode molecular diffusion effects,[1] it became possible for the first time to obtain local measurements of water diffusion in vivo in the human brain.[2] Contrast underlying standard MRI results from the water hydrogen nuclei (proton) density and the "relaxation times," called T1 and T2, which characterize how fast water magnetization returns to equilibrium after the perturbation induced by the MRI radiofrequency pulse and which roughly depend on the tissue chemical nature. MRI signals can be sensitized to diffusion through the application of a pair of sharp magnetic field gradient pulses, the duration and the separation of which can be adjusted to achieve a specific level of diffusion sensitization. In an otherwise homogeneous field, the first pulse

magnetically labels hydrogen nuclei carried by water molecules according to their spatial location, as for a short time the magnetic field slowly varies along the magnetic field gradient pulse direction (Fig. 1.2). As a result, those nuclei dephase linearly according to their location along this direction. The second pulse is introduced slightly later to exactly rephase nuclei that have not moved. Any nuclei that have changed location due to their diffusion between the two pulses will maintain some degree of phase shift depending on the net nuclei displacement history that occurred during the time interval (or "diffusion time") between the two pulses. Considering now a population comprising a considerably large number of diffusing water molecules, the overall effect is that the corresponding hydrogen nuclei will experience various phase shifts reflecting the statistical displacement distribution of this population (i.e., the overall diffusion process). This phase distribution contributes to a decrease in

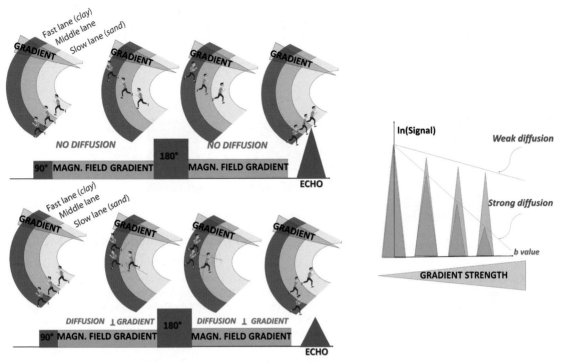

Fig. 1.2 Principles of diffusion encoding. The basic magnetic resonance imaging (MRI) sequence for diffusion MRI is the spin echo with two radio-frequency (RF) pulses, 90 and 180 degrees. Spatially encoding magnetic field gradient pulses are inserted between the RF pulses: where the magnetic field is high, spins precess more rapidly and vice versa, as in a stadium where runners have different speeds depending on the nature of the lane surface. At the time of the 180 degree pulse (which occurs at half the echo time [TE], TE/2) the phase of the spins is reversed (runners reverse direction). In the absence of diffusion (runners remain in their lane, preserving their speed) spins are perfectly rephased at TE, forming the echo signal *(top left)*. In the presence of diffusion, spins change location during the sequence (runners change lanes), so that their speed changes over the sequence (slow runners may increase their speed or vice versa), which results in some dephasing at the time of the echo (for the components of the displacements perpendicular to the gradient direction), leading to a signal attenuation *(bottom left)*. One can see *(right)* that this attenuation depends on two parameters: the strength of the gradient pulses (characterized by the so-called *b* value, the attenuation increases with the *b* value), and the diffusion effect (high or fast diffusion leads to greater attenuation).

the amplitude of the MRI signal compared with that which would be obtained from a population of perfectly stationary nuclei in a perfectly homogeneous field. This signal attenuation is precisely and quantitatively linked to the amplitude of the displacement distribution: fast (slow) diffusion results in a large (small) distribution and a large (small) signal attenuation. Of course, the effect also depends on the intensity of the magnetic field gradient pulses used for this diffusion encoding.

In practice, almost any MRI technique can be sensitized to diffusion by inserting the adequate magnetic field gradient pulses, but the most commonly used in clinical practice is the spin-echo sequence

(as illustrated in Fig. 1.2). Other sequences, namely, oscillating gradient spin echo (OGSE) and stimulated echo (STEAM) sequences may also be used to access very short or very long diffusion times, respectively. By acquiring data with various gradient pulse amplitudes, one obtains images with different degrees of diffusion sensitivity (see Fig. 1.2). The degree of sensitivity to diffusion is described by the so-called *b* value (usually in s/mm^2; typical values are around 1000 s/mm^2), which was introduced to take into account the intensity and time profile of the gradient pulses used both for diffusion encoding and MRI spatial encoding.[1,2] The overall effect of diffusion in the presence of those gradient pulses is

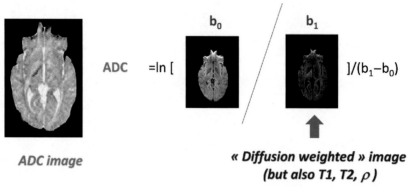

$$S/So = exp\ (-b.ADC)$$

ADC image

« Diffusion weighted » image
(but also T1, T2, ρ)

Fig. 1.3 ADC map calculation from diffusion-weighted images. Images acquired with the diffusion magnetic resonance (MRI) sequence are "weighted" by diffusion (to a degree dependent on the *b* value) but also remain weighted according to the parameters of the spin-echo sequence (i.e., spin density, T1 depending on the repetition time [TR], and T2 depending on echo time [TE]). To remove nondiffusion effects, diffusion-weighted images acquired with two different *b* values, b_0 and b_1, are divided according to Eq. (1), as the effects of the nondiffusion parameters are the same at both *b* values and cancel out. Contrast in the resulting image, called the apparent diffusion coefficient (ADC) map, reflects pure (Gaussian) diffusion effects altered due to the diffusion hindrance in tissues.

a signal attenuation, and the MRI signal becomes diffusion weighted, hence the term "diffusion-weighted imaging" (DWI). The signal attenuation is more pronounced when using large *b* values and when diffusion is fast. Finally, it is important to notice that only the displacement (diffusion) component along the gradient direction is detectable.

ADC

Contrast in these images depends on diffusion, but also on other MRI parameters, such as the water relaxation times T1 and T2, which could lead to well-known artifacts, such as the "T2-shine-through" effect, as lesions with a high T2 signal (e.g., necrosis, cysts) may retain a relatively high signal level at high *b* values. Hence, these images are often numerically combined to determine, using a global diffusion model, a quantitative estimate of the diffusion coefficient in each image location. The resulting images are maps of the diffusion process and can be visualized using a quantitative scale (Fig. 1.3).

The most basic model is that of the ADC[2]:

$$ADC = \ln[S(b_0) - S(b_1)]/(b_1 - b_0) \qquad [1]$$

where $S(b_0)$ and $S(b_1)$ are the signals (in a voxel or a region-of-interest, ROI) acquired at the *b* values b_0 and b_1, respectively.

An important point to consider, however, is that Einstein's equation, which serves as the basis for diffusion MRI, was established for "free" (Gaussian) diffusion, as can be found in a glass of water. In biological tissues, however, diffusion is no longer free, as we have seen (see Fig. 1.1). This is indeed what has made diffusion MRI so exquisitely sensitive to tissue structure in various pathological or physiological conditions. As the molecular displacement distribution deviates from a Gaussian law, the diffusion effect on the MRI signal is no longer adequately described by Einstein's equation. Furthermore, the overall signal observed in a diffusion MRI image volume element (voxel, often larger than 2mm in size for common breast diffusion MRI) results from the integration, on a statistical basis, of all the *microscopic* displacement distributions of the water molecules present in this voxel.

For those reasons, as a departure from earlier biological diffusion studies where efforts were made to depict the true diffusion process, the ADC concept was introduced[2,7] to portray the complex diffusion

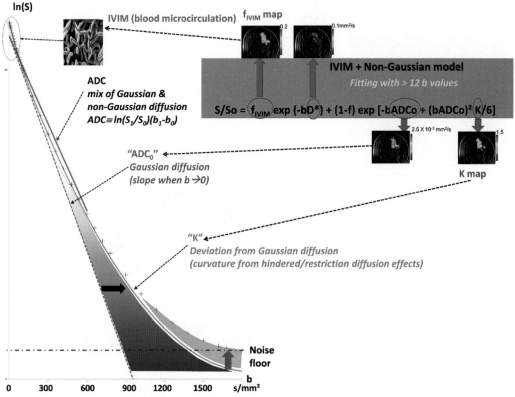

Fig. 1.4 Diffusion signal attenuation. In the presence of "free" (Gaussian) diffusion, the signal attenuation is expected to decrease linearly when the *b* value increases (straight line in a log plot), the slope of which is the diffusion coefficient. In practice, the attenuation is seen as curved in biological tissues. Three domains can be identified. At very low *b* values, the deviation from a straight line results from blood microcirculation (b) in the pseudorandomly oriented capillary segments within the capillary network (intravoxel incoherent motion [IVIM] effect). At high *b* values, the curvature originated from non-Gaussian diffusion effects resulting from the interaction of diffusing molecules with microscopic tissue features (hindrance and restriction). In the intermediate regime, the attenuation curve is closer to a straight line (with the apparent diffusion coefficient [ADC] as the slope), as expected from the basic (monoexponential) diffusion model.

A popular model that considers IVIM, Gaussian, and non-Gaussian diffusion relies on the revision of the original IVIM model (Eq. 2), replacing the monoexponential diffusion component with the kurtosis non-Gaussian diffusion term. Besides f_{IVIM} and D^*, the whole model introduces two more parameters, K (kurtosis) and ADC_0, which is the virtual ADC value at b = 0 (Gaussian diffusion term). By acquiring data at multiple *b* values, one can fit signals in each image voxel to the model equation to generate parametric images of ADC_0, K, and f_{IVIM}, each reflecting different features of lesions. In this example (invasive ductal carcinoma [IDC]), ADC_0 is low (below 1.2×10^{-3} mm^2/s) and K is high (above 0.8) in the tumor, reflecting diffusion hindrance by cell proliferation, whereas f_{IVIM} is high (around 0.1), reflecting neovascularization. The model may also need to be corrected for noise floor effects (see also Fig. 1.11). (Clinical images Courtesy Kyoto University, Radiology Department, Breast Imaging group.)

processes that occur in a biological tissue on a voxel scale using the *microscopic, free diffusion physical* model. In clinical diffusion MRI, the physical diffusion coefficient (D) is replaced by a *global, statistical* parameter, the ADC. This parametrization allows us to bridge the gap between the two scales without the need to use sophisticated models. Indeed, this simple ADC has been an incredibly robust and powerful parameter, which has been largely used across all clinical applications of diffusion MRI[5,8] since its debut.

BEYOND THE ADC: ADVANCED DIFFUSION MRI

Looking at the signal decay with the *b* value, one immediately sees that the attenuation is not linear but presents a marked curvature, especially at the extremities (Fig. 1.4), at the beginning of the curve (very small

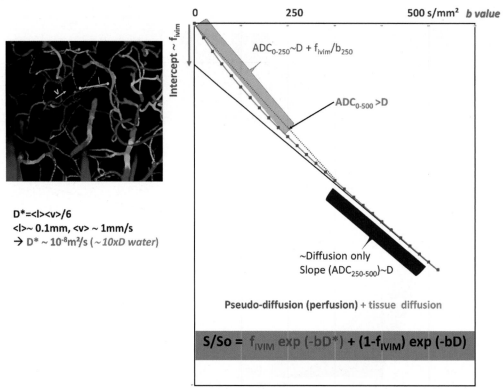

Fig. 1.5 IVIM effect. *Left:* The movement of flowing blood water in capillaries can be considered as a pseudodiffusion process. If <l> is the mean length of capillary segments randomly oriented in space and <v> the mean blood velocity, the associated pseudodiffusion coefficient, D^*, is simply <l><v>/6, which comes around 10^{-8} m²/s, about 10 times the diffusion coefficient of water. *Right:* The perfusion-driven intravoxel incoherent motion (IVIM) effect appears as a deviation on top of the diffusion-driven signal decay. If the flowing fraction, f_{IVIM}, is small, the apparent diffusion coefficient (ADC) calculated from low *b* values (e.g., here 0 and 250 s/mm²) is just the sum of the tissue diffusion coefficient D and f_{IVIM}/b. At higher *b* values (e.g., here 250 and 500 s/mm²), the ADC reflects genuine diffusion only (which we refer to as "D" here, as a simplification). In a simple approach, the flowing blood fraction can be obtained from only three *b* values (here 0, 250, and 500 s/mm²) from $ADC_{250-500}$ and ADC_{0-250}. Note that fIVIM is also the intercept of the diffusion attenuation curve extrapolated to b = 0.

b values), and when *b* values become large (beyond 800 s/mm²). This curvature provides important clues on the underlying tissue properties that can be elucidated by going beyond the classic ADC model. We provide here a short description of the general principles underlying such advanced applications, which will be developed in more detail in the third section of this book.

Diffusion MRI at Very Low *b* Values: IVIM and Perfusion

The ADC concept was introduced to encompass all types of incoherent motions present within each image voxel (hence the abbreviation IVIM for intravoxel

incoherent motion), which could contribute to the signal attenuation observed with diffusion MRI. Beyond molecular diffusion, blood microcirculation in the capillary networks (perfusion) also contributes.[7] Indeed, the flow of blood in large vessels passing through voxels can be seen as coherent (hence not affecting diffusion-weighted images), whereas the flow of blood water in randomly oriented capillaries (at voxel level) mimics a random walk ("pseudodiffusion"),[7] which results in a signal attenuation in the presence of the diffusion-encoding gradient pulses. This apparent motion randomness for perfusion results from the geometry of the microvessel network where blood circulates, under the hypothesis that the microvascular network can be modeled by a series of straight segments randomly oriented in space with a uniform angular coverage (4π solid angle) within each voxel. Here, randomness thus results from the *collective* motion of blood water molecules in the network, flowing from one capillary segment to the next, in addition to the individual diffusion movement of blood water molecules. This *collective* movement has been described as a *pseudodiffusion* process where average displacements, l, would now correspond to the mean capillary segment length and the mean velocity, v, would be that of blood in the vessels[7] (Fig. 1.5). In the presence of blood microcirculation the overall MRI signal attenuation, S(b)/S(0), becomes the sum of two exponentials (biexponential decay),[7] one for tissue diffusion and one for the blood compartment (assuming water exchange between blood and tissues is negligible during the encoding time, a hypothesis that has not yet been deeply investigated):

$$S(b)/S0 = f_{IVIM}\exp[-b(D^* + D_{blood})] \\ + (1 - f_{IVIM})\exp(-bD) \qquad [2]$$

where f_{IVIM} is the flowing blood fraction (sometimes also called fp, or even simply f), D^* the pseudodiffusion coefficient ascribed to blood random microcirculation, D the water diffusion coefficient in the tissue, and D_{blood} the water diffusion coefficient in blood (as diffusion of individual water molecules also occurs in blood).

The effect (curvature of the tissue diffusion driven monoexponential signal decay) is seen at low b values only, because the pseudodiffusion coefficient (D^*) associated with blood flow is higher than the water diffusion coefficient and decays faster with the b value. Furthermore, because the fraction of the flowing blood is usually small (a few percent) compared with the overall tissue water content, the perfusion-driven IVIM signature appears mainly at very low b values. In the breast, f_{IVIM} values as high as 20% (malignant tumors) are not uncommon, whereas D may be on the order of 0.001 mm²/s, so that the IVIM component can still exist for b values as high as 400 s/mm² and may quickly become negligible with higher b values. Indeed, the one order of magnitude or so difference between true diffusion and pseudodiffusion allows

them to be separated. When f_{IVIM} is small, one has ADC~D + f_{IVIM}/b, and f_{IVIM} simply appears as the (negative) intercept of the diffusion component of the signal decay in log plots with b values.[7] However, fitting signal decays with Eq. (2) provides a better estimation of both f_{IVIM} and D^*.

It should be noted here that tissue and blood contribute to S(0) with different T_2 and T_1-weightings, which means that f_{IVIM} values might be misestimated, depending on echo time (TE) and the field strength B0, as well as the tissue voxel content (e.g., local blood oxygen level), which is an issue when comparing literature results. Furthermore, the model described by Eq. (2) assumes that blood changes direction along the capillary segments several times during the measurement time (typically around 50 ms). Other variants have been proposed to account for other situations (slow flow and/or long segments or short diffusion times).[7,9] Please also refer to Section C about those important issues.

The idea to use diffusion and IVIM MRI to obtain images of perfusion was groundbreaking[10] yet very controversial at the beginning, and it took more than 20 years before the concept was applied in clinical practice. Indeed, IVIM MRI has experienced a remarkable revival for applications throughout the body,[5,9,11] especially in the field of cancer imaging (Fig. 1.6). A key feature of IVIM diffusion MRI is that it does not involve contrast agents, and it may serve as an interesting alternative to perfusion MRI in some patients with contraindications for contrast agents, patients with renal failure at risk for nephrogenic systemic fibrosis (NSF),[12,13] or to avoid possible gadolinium deposits[14] in tissues in the case of repeated injections. Still, deeper insight into the IVIM concept and a clear understanding of associated strengths and limitations are necessary to fully garner the benefits of the method in the clinical setting. Specifically, the relationship of IVIM parameters (D^* and f_{IVIM}) with blood volume and blood flow estimates using other approaches needs to be clarified. Separation of perfusion from diffusion requires high signal-to-noise ratios, and there are some technical challenges to overcome, such artifacts from other bulk flow phenomena. Active transport resulting from glandular secretion (e.g., breast ducts) may also be challenging to separate from microcapillary perfusion. One also has to keep in mind that IVIM imaging

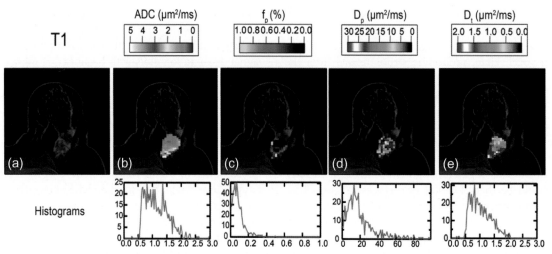

Fig. 1.6 Example of IVIM imaging in breast cancer. Intravoxel incoherent motion (IVIM) magnetic resonance image (MRI) of an invasive lobular carcinoma (ILC) lesion. (A) Postcontrast T1-weighted image, providing background for overlaid (B) apparent diffusion coefficient (ADC), (C) perfusion fraction (fp), (D) pseudodiffusivity (Dp), and (E) tissue diffusivity (Dt) parametric maps. Full lesion volume histograms for each parameter are shown under the corresponding panels. The lesion shows high central cell density (low ADC, Dt) and high peripheral vascularity (high fp), in agreement with the appearance in T1 postcontrast imaging (A). (Reprinted with permission from Partridge SC, Nissan N, Rahbar H, Kitsch AE, Sigmund EE Diffusion-weighted breast MRI: clinical applications and emerging techniques. *J Magn Reson Imaging*. 2016;45:337–355.)

has a differential sensitivity to vessel sizes according to the range of b values that are used.

Diffusion in Space and Time in Tissues: Free, Hindered, and Restricted Diffusion

Another important feature is that diffusion, compared with other parameters such as T1 or T2, is a genuine physical process occurring in tissues on its own, not linked to MRI (MRI is merely a tool to investigate it), as opposed to T1 or T2, which are only defined in the MRI context and depend heavily, for instance, on field strength and MRI sequences. In contrast, the results of diffusion MRI, such as the ADC, should be in principle equivalent across centers using different MRI systems or sequence parameters. Unfortunately, this is true only to some extent: Problems may arise because diffusion in tissues is not free. With free (Gaussian) diffusion the ADC remains the same whichever set of b values is used to measure it; only the accuracy of the ADC estimates will change with the b values. In this case one may find the optimal b value that provides the highest contrast-to-noise ratio, that is, enough signal attenuation (and diffusion encoding) while maintaining a sufficient signal level. In the brain, the optimal b value for brain tissue is about 1000 s/mm², whereas it is lower in the breast,[15] around 800 s/mm². However, using those b values one deprives oneself of the potentially valuable clinical information encoded in non-Gaussian diffusion provided by higher b values. When diffusion is non-Gaussian, the degree of diffusion related signal attenuation decreases as the b value increases (Fig. 1.7); in other words, the ADC value decreases when high b values are used.[16] It is thus mandatory to indicate which b values have been used to acquire data if one wishes to make meaningful comparisons across literature.

The b Dimension: Non-Gaussian Diffusion ADC_0, sADC, and Kurtosis

Such non-Gaussian diffusion effects become visible, however, only when using high b values, which is now possible thanks to progress made in gradient hardware. Although achievable b values in the mid-1980s were in the range of 100 s/mm², they extended to around 1000 s/mm² in the 1990s to easily reach 3000 s/mm² today, or even higher with some prototype gradient systems or preclinical systems where gradient amplitudes of 1000 mT/m are not uncommon (compared with 30–80 mT in clinical systems). Using such high b values the ADC concept (also often referred to as the

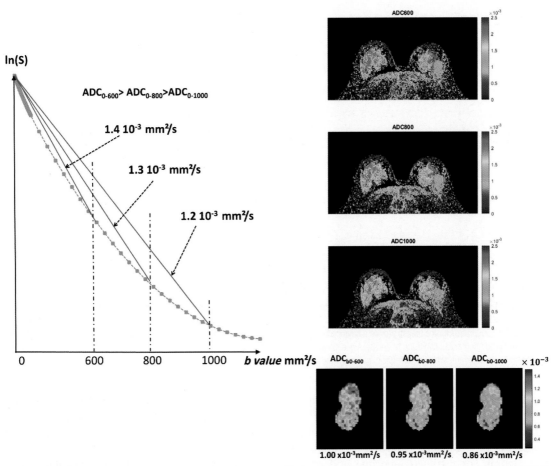

Fig. 1.7 Effect of the *b* value on the ADC. *Left:* Because of non-Gaussian diffusion, the log-plot of signal attenuation versus *b* values is curved. Consequently, the apparent diffusion coefficient (ADC), which is calculated from two points (representing the virtual slope of the attenuation between those two *b* values) depends on the choice of pairs of *b* values, becoming smaller when the highest *b* value increases. *Right:* This effect is readily observed in breast tissue and is important to consider as lesion type classification based on ADC threshold values will highly depend on the *b* values, hence the need for standardization. (Reprinted with permission from Iima M, Partridge SC, Le Bihan D Six DWI questions you always wanted to know but were afraid to ask: clinical relevance for breast diffusion MRI. *Eur Radiol.* 2020;30:2561–2570.)

monoexponential model) reaches its limitation, as it cannot accommodate a proper account of the curvature of the signal attenuation (in semilog coordinates), which becomes apparent at high *b* values (see Fig. 1.4). Indeed, some extremely valuable information on tissue structure can be found in this curvature,[8] and several models have been suggested to *empirically* handle this non-Gaussian behavior, such as the polynomial or kurtosis model[17] (also called diffusion kurtosis imaging [DKI],[18] the biexponential model,[19] the statistical model,[20] the stretched exponential model,[21] and others[22,23]; see also the third Section of this book).

With such models, new parameters have emerged beyond the ADC, such as the kurtosis for DKI, which have shown great potential to characterize pathological or physiological conditions,[24] although they only give empirical information on the degree of diffusion non-Gaussianity and nothing specific on tissue features (see Fig. 1.4). These models have been used to evaluate cerebral infarction,[25] liver fibrosis,[26] and tumor characterization.[27,28] Other models have been designed not just to describe the signal decay with *b* values mathematically, but to provide more insightful, explanatory information on the tissue features,

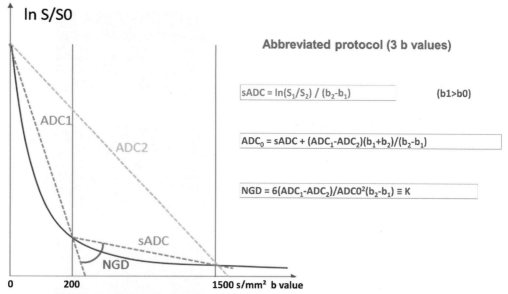

Fig. 1.8 Abbreviated diffusion-weighted imaging (DWI) protocol. When acquisition time is a premium, and only small sets of ***b*** values can be acquired, useful information can still be obtained on Gaussian and non-Gaussian diffusion. The shifted ADC (sADC) calculated from two carefully chosen ("key") ***b*** values b_1 and b_2 (200 and 1500 s/mm² for the breast) provide a balanced mix of Gaussian and non-Gaussian diffusion effects. ADC_0 values (Gaussian diffusion) can be derived from sADC and ADCs calculated using b_1 and b_2. A non-Gaussian diffusion (NGD) index can then be derived from ADC_0, ADC_1, and ADC_2. NGD is formally equivalent to the kurtosis parameter in the absence of perfusion-related intravoxel incoherent motion (IVIM) effects.

but mainly in the brain (e.g., the neurite orientation dispersion and density imaging [NODDI] model[29] for neurite density). However, those extremely refined models require strong assumptions on the underlying tissue structure, sophisticated modeling and analysis, and still must be validated across the full range of clinical conditions. It is understandable that clinicians might be puzzled by this array of diffusion models and the variety of ways to process the diffusion-weighted images they require. However, clinically relevant images can be derived from "parametric maps" produced by combining images acquired with a range of *b* values according to the relevant physical models using one's preferred software, either in-house or provided by vendors. Such maps often allow one, in particular, to assess lesion heterogeneity.

The use of such advanced models also often requires the acquisition of large data sets with multiple *b* values, which significantly increases acquisition times, a premium in clinical practice. Providing images have a good quality, especially in terms of signal-to-noise ratio (SNR), it is possible to get useful information on the Gaussian diffusion part of the DWI signal: ADC_0

(ADC values extrapolated when *b* approaches 0) and a non-Gaussian diffusion index (NGD, formally equal to the kurtosis [K]) from sets of only three *b* values (so-called abbreviated diffusion MRI protocol; Fig. 1.8). The shifted ADC (sADC),[5] which is calculated from shifted key *b* values (200 and 1500 s/mm² for the breast, instead of 0 and 800 s/mm²) provides, especially, an interesting balance between Gaussian and non-Gaussian diffusion effects.

Directions in Space: Diffusion Tensor Imaging (DTI)

An important consequence of the diffusion MRI encoding process (compared with other MRI approaches) is that diffusion, although a 3D process, is only measured along one direction at a time determined by the orientation in space of the gradient pulses. Most often, diffusion is isotropic (the same in all directions), so this spatial orientation does not matter. In some tissues, however, such as brain white matter or muscle fibers, diffusion is anisotropic, and diffusion effects strongly depend on the direction of the gradient pulse. It is often thought by those in clinical practice and by MRI manufacturers that one obtains a mean diffusivity effect by averaging out images sequentially acquired with gradients oriented along three perpendicular directions. It can easily be shown that this is only an approximation,[30] which may lead to a large overestimation of the true mean ADC in tissues experiencing anisotropic diffusion, especially when diffusion pulses are oriented along multiple axes at the same time (to minimize TE and increase SNR). For instance, even if the diffusion-encoding gradient pulses are oriented only along the X-axis, any gradient pulse present on the Y- or Z-axis will combine with the diffusion encoding pulses on the X-axis and also contribute to the diffusion signal if diffusion coupling terms (e.g., D_{xy}, D_{xz}) exist, which is the case when the tissue feature axes do not perfectly coincide with the gradient directions used for measurements. This "mean" ADC is then *not* rotationally invariant (i.e., values vary according to the measurement direction).

Anisotropic diffusion cannot be correctly described by three diffusion coefficients along three directions but requires the acquisition of diffusion-weighted images along at least six different directions (diffusion tensor imaging [DTI]).[30,31] DTI is the framework that replaces DWI in the presence of anisotropic diffusion. Anisotropic diffusion is observed in the presence of aligned tissue structures, mainly in the heart, muscle, and brain white matter, but other tissues may unexpectedly also show signs of anisotropy, such as the breast.[32] With DTI one can get the "trace" of the diffusion tensor, which represents the true rotation invariant, mean diffusivity (MD), indices of the degree of anisotropy (e.g., fractional anisotropy); and so-called "eigenvectors," which point to the directions along which diffusion is the fastest or the slowest, corresponding in general to the directions parallel or perpendicular to the tissue fibers, respectively.[30,31] DTI has served as the basis for brain white matter tractography, but more advanced techniques are currently used to take into account voxels with multiple fiber orientations.[30]

It has been suggested that diffusion anisotropy in the breast might originate from the presence of ducts that are oriented toward the nipple, and that lesions may partially alter this anisotropy, which could aid in detection (see more details in Section 3). However, the presence or not of diffusion anisotropy in the breast has been a subject of some controversy,[33,34] as DTI parameters (except MD) are very sensitive to noise due to the strongly nonlinear nature of the DTI processing algorithm: noise in DTI data may easily create anisotropy where there is none.[16]

Pitfalls, Challenges, and Common Issues Found in Clinical Practice

IMAGE QUALITY

The single-shot echo-planar imaging (EPI) technique is the method of choice for in vivo diffusion imaging, as it allows efficient, ultrafast acquisition of multiple diffusion-weighted images (different *b* values) without in-plane motion artifacts to which diffusion MRI is notoriously sensitive. Nonetheless, EPI has several limitations related to spatial resolution, artifacts, and signal to noise.

First, as EPI requires switching gradient pulses for the signal readout at a high frequency, there is a limit to the spatial resolution that can be reached depending on the gradient hardware system. This means that small lesions (<2 mm) might be undetectable, whereas they are readily visible on the high-resolution T1w images used with Dynamic Contrast Enhanced (DCE) MRI. Segmented EPI acquisitions[35] (e.g., RESOLVE, MUSE, IRIS; please see the Vendor section of this book) may overcome this limitation at the expense of longer diffusion times and sensitivity to motion between acquired segments that must be corrected using ad hoc approaches during image reconstruction. Recently developed "parallel" acquisition techniques, which allow signals to be collected simultaneously using an array of several radiofrequency coils, appear promising to correct for these limitations.[36]

Second, EPI requires a homogeneous magnetic field. Magnetic interfaces between bone (e.g., ribs) or air-filled cavities (e.g., lungs, sinuses) and water-containing tissues result in local image distortion or signal dropout. For breast imaging, this can be most pronounced at the air/tissue interface at the anterior breast. Another source of geometrical distortion comes from the interaction between the gradient pulses used for diffusion encoding and for imaging. Especially, the strong diffusion-encoding gradient pulses often generate eddy currents in the MRI scanner, which results in gradients that interfere with those used for image encoding. As a consequence, the degree of geometrical distortion increases with the *b* value, a source of artifact in the ADC images, and ADC measurements (Fig. 1.9).

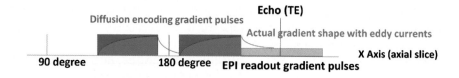

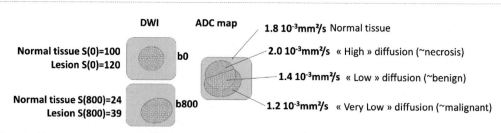

Fig. 1.9 Effect of eddy currents and geometrical distortions. Geometrical distortions may be the source of detrimental artifacts, qualitatively and quantitatively (apparent diffusion coefficient [ADC] and other metrics), especially in small lesions. Eddy currents generated by the gradient coils are the main but not sole source of geometrical distortions (gradient nonlinearities and presence of interfaces with bone or air also contribute). In plane, eddy currents alter the theoretical rectangular shape of the gradient pulses, which "leak" during signal readout *(top)*. The effect increases with the gradient strength, hence the amount of distortion increases with *b* value. When the ADC image is calculated on a pixel-by-pixel value without correction for the distortion, lesions may appear with three parts. Only the central part displays the correct ADC value (here corresponding to a benign lesion), whereas the other parts overestimate (mimicking necrosis) or underestimate (mimicking malignancy) ADC values. The distortion effect along the slice encoding direction is more insidious, as not readily visible. The leakage of the diffusion-encoding gradient pulses on the slice-selection gradient pulses decreases the slice thickness when the *b* value increases (which decreases with *b* value). The overall ADC then becomes larger than it should be but uniformly across the lesion.

Incorrect fat suppression may also lead to erroneous interpretation of diffusion MRI, as residual fat present in breast tissue leads to low diffusion values, mimicking malignancy both visually and quantitively (ADC values). The spectrally adiabatic inversion recovery (SPAIR) method has been recommended for breast imaging.[15] For all of those reasons, it is highly advisable to have MRI system performance checked on a regular basis by vendor technicians. This is especially important if quantitative data are used for multicenter studies, which require rigorous standardization practices. The use of dedicated phantoms made of various materials (e.g., alkanes, ice water) can further help calibrate the overall gradient performances (e.g., gradient pulses intensity, *b* value accuracy, eddy currents, direction, stability).

DWI, CALCULATED DWI, AND SYNTHESIZED DWI

Some vendors provide with their console software "calculated," "extrapolated," or "synthesized" DWI features. Basically, the idea is to simulate images that would be acquired at a given *b* value from images acquired with lower *b* values.[37] For instance, one would wish to see virtual images corresponding to $b = 1500 \, \text{s/mm}^2$ from images acquired at, let us say, $b = 800 \, \text{s/mm}^2$. The motivation is twofold: saving on acquisition time (because only a smaller number of *b* values would be acquired; for instance, $b = 0$ and $800 \, \text{s/mm}^2$) and increasing contrast to detect lesions while avoiding the SNR penalty that appears when acquiring high *b* value images. Indeed, malignant lesions typically exhibit slower diffusion than benign lesions, which in turn exhibit slower diffusion than normal background tissues. Hence by going to high *b* values, the signal attenuation is less in malignant lesions versus benign lesions and background tissue. With sufficiently high *b* values the background signal drops to noise level and lesions become much easier to identify. This is true both for images directly acquired at $b = 1500 \, \text{s/mm}^2$ and for simulated images at this

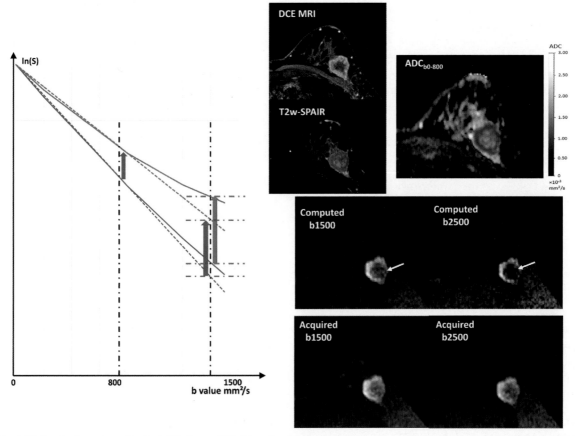

Fig. 1.10 Acquired versus synthesized diffusion-weighted imaging (DWI). *Left:* Synthesized b = 1500 s/mm² images are obtained from images acquired at lower *b* values (e.g., b = 800 s/mm²), assuming free or Gaussian diffusion, that is, by extrapolating the DWI signal decay as a straight line beyond b = 800 s/mm² with the ADC_{0-800} slope. Plot depicts acquired *(solid lines)* and synthesized *(dotted lines)* DWI signal, for both malignant and benign tissues *(red and blue, respectively)*. By doing so, the signal difference (contrast) between low apparent diffusion coefficient (ADC) lesions and higher ADC tissues (e.g., background tissue) increases *(blue arrows)*. However, this contrast would be even larger when using directly acquired b = 1500 s/mm² images, which are more sensitive to diffusion hindrance effects reflected in the curvature of the signal decay *(red arrow)*. Malignant lesions that have both lower ADC values at b = 800 s/mm² and larger hindrance effects at b = 1500 s/mm² will thus appear with increased contrast than in synthesized b = 1500 s/mm² images, providing signal-to-noise ratio (SNR) remains high enough. *Right:* Example in a breast tumor with a nonenhancing central area exhibiting a high ADC_{0-800} value. As a result, the signal drops out on the computed DWI images at b = 1500 and 2500 s/mm² *(arrow)*, suggesting necrosis (free diffusion). However, the corresponding acquired images exhibit a plateau, suggesting instead somewhat hindered diffusion (possible fibrosis), which would also match the not so high T2 in the tumor core. Furthermore, the contrast-to-noise ratio for the calculated images is 3.0 and 2.2 (b = 1500 and 2500 s/mm², respectively) and 3.9 and 3.4 for the acquired b = 1500 and 2500 s/mm² images (e.g., a 22.1% difference at b = 1500 s/mm² and a 37% difference at b = 2500 s/mm²). (Reprinted with permission from lima M, Partridge SC, Le Bihan D Six DWI questions you always wanted to know but were afraid to ask: clinical relevance for breast diffusion MRI. *Eur Radiol*. 2020;30:2561–2570.)

high *b* value, with the advantage that the amount of noise in the simulated images is less, corresponding to that found in the acquired b = 800 s/mm² images, a good example of avoiding noise effects.

By using such calculated high *b* value images, however, one should realize that we completely miss out on the potential diagnostic advantage offered by high *b* values as described above: the sensitivity to tissue microstructure, which appears in the curvature of the DWI signal attenuation when *b* increases (Fig. 1.10). Indeed, the underlying hypothesis behind the calculated or extrapolated DWI concept is Gaussian (or free) diffusion: the signal is extrapolated, assuming that the DWI attenuation curve is linear; in other words, the ADC does not depend on the *b* value but remains constant, which is true only for Gaussian diffusion, as we have seen. Using signals acquired at $b = 0$ (S_0) and $b = 800$ s/mm^2 (S_{800}), one has

$$\text{ADC} = \ln(S_0/S_{800})/800$$

This ADC is assumed to be the same when obtained with $b = 1500$ s/mm^2:

$$\text{ADC} = \ln(S_0/S^*_{1500})/1500 \qquad [3]$$

where S^*_{1500} is the *synthesized* signal for $b = 1500$ s/mm^2.

Rearranging those two equations, one obtains

$$
\begin{aligned}
S^*_{1500} &= S_0 \exp(-1500 * \text{ADC}) \\
&= S_0 \exp(-1500 * \ln(S_0/S_{800})/800) \\
&= S_{800}{}^{\wedge(1500/800)} = S_{800}{}^{\wedge 1.875} \qquad [4]
\end{aligned}
$$

Hence the extrapolated signal has nothing to do with $b = 1500$ s/mm^2; it is no more and no less than the signal acquired by $b = 800$ s/mm^2 elevated to the power of a particular value (here 1.875). However, this value is arbitrary, so why not take 2 or 2.5 to boost contrast even further? Clearly, the simulated image holds no additional information whatsoever that is not already present in the $b = 800$ s/mm^2 image. The power elevation is just a mathematical trick that boosts contrast, spreading the signal intensity range between lesions and normal tissue background and even burying background tissue to the noise, which might be advantageous for lesion detection but does not add value for lesion characterization.

Indeed, those synthesized $b = 1500$ s/mm^2 images lack part of the content present in acquired $b = 1500$ s/mm^2 images, which in addition carry valuable hindrance effects related to tissue microstructural characteristics not clearly present in the $b = 800$ s/mm^2 images. Not only will acquired high b value images further increase contrast compared with calculated images (as hindrance effects are usually greater in malignant lesions than benign lesions and even more than background tissue), but they will also add some specificity in lesion classification. In particular, some tissues that remain in the acquired $b = 1500$ s/mm^2 images may disappear in the synthesized images, resulting in possible interpretation errors (see Fig. 1.10).

This does not mean at all that calculated or extrapolated DWI are not useful and should not be utilized. It is a useful trick to highlight lesions to increase sensitivity for screening (detection); we should just be aware of the limitations and the occurrence of possible errors in interpretation. Whenever possible, directly acquiring images at $b = 1500$ s/mm^2 (or higher) should be preferred over synthesizing, as the acquired images may further increase contrast and specificity to recognize malignant lesions.

NOISE

Finally, diffusion-weighted images are often noisy, especially at high b values, as by principle the signal is heavily attenuated from the diffusion effect. Noise is a vicious enemy, as it is not always visible yet has a profound influence on the parameter values estimated with the various models available (e.g., DTI parameters as shown above), including the ADC. Noise is still another cause of curvature of the signal attenuation than non-Gaussian diffusion at high b values (see Figs. 1.4 and 1.11).

At high b values, because of the nature of the MRI signal (a "magnitude" signal that cannot be negative) there is always some background noise signal left and the diffusion signal remains above a threshold (the "noise floor") instead of asymptotically approaching 0, thus mimicking a curvature effect[38] and no longer reflecting the real amount of diffusion-driven attenuation, which results in underestimated ADC values. If one classifies lesions (e.g., benign versus malignant) based on the ADC threshold values, it is easy to see that this pitfall of underestimated ADC could lead to a severe bias toward a "malignant" nature of the lesions. As an example, let us consider a tissue with a theoretical ADC value (in the absence of noise) of 1.5×10^{-3} mm^2/s (see Fig. 1.11). Assuming the ADC threshold for malignancy is 1.3×10^{-3} mm^2/s, this tissue should be considered benign. In the presence of a noise floor, the signal at $b = 800$ s/mm^2 is higher than it is in the absence of noise. As a result, the ADC value is lower, here 1.0×10^{-3} mm^2/s, and the tissue will be wrongly classified as malignant. This underestimated ADC value will not only reflect the amount of noise in the lesion (instead of genuine diffusion) but also the amount of T1 and mainly T2 weighting in the tissue, as the ADC underestimation will depend on the

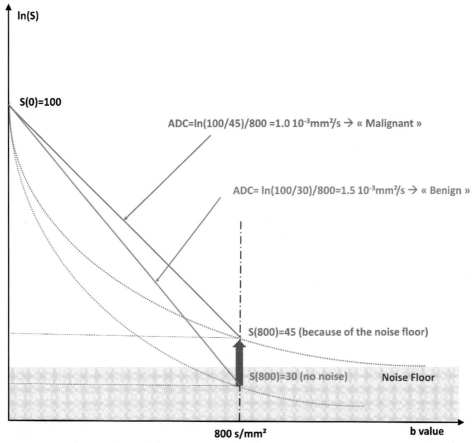

Fig. 1.11 Effect of the noise floor on the apparent diffusion coefficient (ADC). Because of the nature of the noise associated to magnetic resonance imaging (MRI) images, even in the presence of pure noise, the average signal cannot reach 0 but remains at a positive level (so-called noise floor) depending on the amount of noise. Hence although at high *b* values the signal should come close toward 0 *(green curve)*, it reaches a plateau *(red curve)*. As a consequence, the signal used to calculate the ADC is overestimated, which in turn results in an underestimation of the ADC, potentially leading to a misclassification of the tissue nature based on an ADC threshold (here malignant instead of benign).

overall DWI signal level (hence tissues with long T1s and/or short T2s will have lower signal and therefore lower ADC values).

Hence, adequate signal to noise must be obtained to avoid over- or underestimation of the model outputs (e.g., ADC, kurtosis, IVIM fraction), which is not a trivial matter. One may, for instance, increase the voxel size (at the expense of spatial resolution) or repeat image acquisitions at higher *b* values for signal averaging (which unfortunately increases the acquisition time). Several approaches have been proposed to correct the noise at high *b* values, either by retrieving signal values from noise-corrupted data[39,40] or by

using a simple procedure where a noise correction factor is estimated through a phantom calibration process,[38] but these approaches are not easy to implement clinically. Noise effects may partly explain discrepancies in the literature on the various diffusion MRI and IVIM parameter reported values.

Conclusion

Since the mid-1980s diffusion MRI has established itself as a reliable and very powerful imaging modality that has been used for a great number of clinical and research applications, qualitatively and quantitatively, as will be reviewed in Chapters 3 to 7 and 13. The original diffusion metric, ADC, has shown a remarkable resilience and remains by far the most used diffusion MRI quantitative marker. Still, technical advancements in MRI scanners, notably for gradient hardware and fast imaging, are facilitating exploration of new features beyond ADC by allowing perfusion-driven IVIM to become more reliable, providing access to non-Gaussian diffusion through high b values and investigation of diffusion time effects (see Chapter 8). This increasing flexibility for diffusion MRI acquisitions supports expansion of more complex models, leading to a better understanding of the relationship between diffusion MRI parameters and underlying tissue microscopic features (see Chapters 9 and 10). This is especially true in breast imaging, where a wide variety of diffusion MRI techniques demonstrate great potential for clinical applications in the breast (see Chapters 11 and 12). Given this large palette, standardization efforts are necessary (see Chapter 14). A special section of the book dedicated to vendors will highlight what is currently or will soon be available (see Chapters 15–18).

REFERENCES

1. Le Bihan D, Breton E. Imagerie de diffusion in-vivo par résonance magnétique nucléaire. *Comptes-Rendus de l'Académie des Sciences*. 1985;93(5):27–34.
2. Le Bihan D, Breton E, Lallemand D, Grenier P, Cabanis E, Laval-Jeantet M. MR imaging of intravoxel incoherent motions: application to diffusion and perfusion in neurological disorders. *Radiology*. 1986;161(2):401–407.
3. Taouli B, Beer AJ, Chenevert T, et al. Diffusion-weighted imaging outside the brain: consensus statement from an ISMRM-sponsored workshop. *J Magn Reson Imaging*. 2016;44:521–540.
4. Padhani AR, Liu G, Koh DM, et al. Diffusion-weighted magnetic resonance imaging as a cancer biomarker: consensus and recommendations. *Neoplasia*. 2009;11:102–125.
5. Iima M, Le Bihan D. Clinical intravoxel incoherent motion and diffusion MRI imaging: past, present, and future. *Radiology*. 2016;278:13–32.
6. Einstein A. *Investigations on the Theory of the Brownian Movement*. Courier Dover Publications; 1956.
7. Le Bihan D, Breton E, Lallemand D, Aubin ML, Vignaud J, Laval-Jeantet M. Separation of diffusion and perfusion in intravoxel incoherent motion MR imaging. *Radiology*. 1988;168(2):497–505.
8. Le Bihan D. Apparent diffusion coefficient and beyond: what diffusion MR imaging can tell us about tissue structure. *Radiology*. 2013;268(2):318–322.
9. Le Bihan D, Iima M, Federeau C, Sigmund ES. *Intravoxel Incoherent Motion (IVIM) MRI: Principles and Applications*. Pan Stanford Publishing; 2019.
10. Dixon WT. Separation of diffusion and perfusion in intravoxel incoherent motion MR imaging: a modest proposal with tremendous potential. *Radiology*. 1988;168(2):566–567.
11. Le Bihan D. Intravoxel incoherent motion perfusion MR imaging: a wake-up call. *Radiology*. 2008;249(3):748–752.
12. High WA, Ayers RA, Cowper SE. Gadolinium is quantifiable within the tissue of patients with nephrogenic systemic fibrosis. *J Am Acad Dermatol*. 2007;56(4):710–712.
13. ACR Manual on Contrast Media. https://www.acr.org/-/media/ACR/files/clinical-resources/contrast_media.pdf. 2013.
14. Kanda T, Ishii K, Kawaguchi H, Kitajima K, Takenaka D. High-signal intensity in the dentate nucleus and globus pallidus on unenhanced T1-weighted MR images: relationship with increasing cumulative dose of a gadolinium-based contrast material. *Radiology*. 2014;270(3):834–841.
15. Baltzer P, et al. Diffusion-weighted imaging of the breast: a consensus and mission statement from the EUSOBI International Breast Diffusion-Weighted Imaging working group. *Eur Radiol*. 2020;30(3):1436–1450.
16. Iima M, Partridge SC, Le Bihan D. Six DWI questions you always wanted to know but were afraid to ask: clinical relevance for breast diffusion MRI. *Eur Radiol*. 2020;30:2561–2570.
17. Chabert S, Meca C, Le Bihan D. *Relevance of the information about the diffusion distribution in vivo given by kurtosis in q-space imaging*. Kyoto, Japan: Proceedings of the 12th Annual Meeting of ISMRM; May 15-21, 2004:1238.
18. Jensen JH, Helpern JA, Ramani A, Lu H, Kaczynski K. Diffusional kurtosis iwwmaging: the quantification of non-Gaussian water diffusion by means of magnetic resonance imaging. *Magn Reson Med*. 2005;53(6):1432–1440.
19. Mulkern RV, Haker SJ, Maier SE. On high b diffusion imaging in the human brain: ruminations and experimental insights. *Magn Reson Imaging*. 2009;27(8):1151–1162.
20. Yablonskiy DA, Bretthorst GL, Ackerman JJ. Statistical model for diffusion attenuated MR signal. *Magn Reson Med*. 2003;50(4):664–669.
21. Bennett KM, Schmainda KM, Bennett RT, Rowe DB, Lu H, Hyde JS. Characterization of continuously distributed cortical water diffusion rates with a stretched-exponential model. *Magn Reson Med*. 2003;50(4):727–734.

22. Hall MG, Barrick TR. From diffusion-weighted MRI to anomalous diffusion imaging. *Magn Reson Med.* 2008;59(3):447–455.

23. Zhou XJ, Gao Q, Abdullah O, Magin RL. Studies of anomalous diffusion in the human brain using fractional order calculus. *Magn Reson Med.* 2010;63(3):562–569.

24. Wu D, Li G, Zhang J, Chang S, Hu J, Dai Y. Characterization of breast tumors using diffusion kurtosis imaging (DKI). *PLoS One.* 2014;9(11):e113240.

25. Grinberg F, Farrher E, Ciobanu L, Geffroy F, Le Bihan D, Shah NJ. Non-Gaussian diffusion imaging for enhanced contrast of brain tissue affected by ischemic stroke. *PLoS One.* 2014;9(2):e89225.

26. Anderson SW, Barry B, Soto J, Ozonoff A, O'Brien M, Jara H. Characterizing non-gaussian, high b-value diffusion in liver fibrosis: Stretched exponential and diffusional kurtosis modeling. *J Magn Reson Imaging.* 2014;39(4):827–834.

27. Yuan J, Yeung DKW, Mok GS, et al. Non-Gaussian analysis of diffusion weighted imaging in head and neck at 3T: a pilot study in patients with nasopharyngeal carcinoma. *PLoS One.* 2014;9(1):e87024.

28. Filli L, Wurnig M, Nanz D, Luechinger R, Kenkel D, Boss A. Whole-body diffusion kurtosis imaging: initial experience on non-Gaussian diffusion in various organs. *Invest Radiol.* 2014;49(12):773–778.

29. Zhang H, Schneider T, Wheeler-Kingshott CA, Alexander DC. NODDI: practical in vivo neurite orientation dispersion and density imaging of the human brain. *Neuroimage.* 2012; 61(4):1000–1016.

30. Le Bihan D, Mangin JF, Poupon C, et al. Diffusion tensor imaging: concepts and applications. *J Magn Reson Imaging.* 2001;13(4):534–546.

31. Basser PJ, Mattiello J, LeBihan D. MR diffusion tensor spectroscopy and imaging. *Biophys J.* 1994;66(1):259–267.

32. Eyal E, Shapiro-Feinberg M, Furman-Haran E, et al. Parametric diffusion tensor imaging of the breast. *Invest Radiol.* 2012; 47(5):284–291.

33. Iima M, Honda M, Sigmund EE, Ohno Kishimoto A, Kataoka M, Togashi K. Diffusion MR of the breast: current status and future directions. *J Magn Reson Imaging.* 2019; https://doi.org/10.1002/jmri.26908.

34. Baxter GC, Graves MJ, Gilbert FJ, Patterson AJ. A meta-analysis of the diagnostic performance of diffusion MRI for breast lesion characterization. *Radiology.* 2019;291:632–641.

35. Porter DA, Heidemann RM. High resolution diffusion-weighted imaging using readout-segmented echo-planar imaging, parallel imaging and a two-dimensional navigator-based reacquisition. *Magn Reson Med.* 2009;62:468–475.

36. Heidemann RM, Özsarlak Ö, Parizel PM, et al. A brief review of parallel magnetic resonance imaging. *Eur Radiol.* 2003;13:2323–2337.

37. Blackledge MD, Leach MO, Collins DJ, Koh D-M. Computed diffusion-weighted MR imaging may improve tumor detection. *Radiology.* 2011;261:573–581.

38. Iima M, Yano K, Kataoka M, et al. Quantitative non-Gaussian diffusion and intravoxel incoherent motion magnetic resonance imaging: differentiation of malignant and benign breast lesions. *Invest Radiol.* 2015;50(4):205–211.

39. Brion V, Poupon C, Riff O, et al. Parallel MRI noise correction: an extension of the LMMSE to non central χ distributions. In: Brion V, Poupon C, Riff O, et al, eds. *Medical Image Computing and Computer-Assisted Intervention–MICCAI 2011.* Springer; 2011:226–233.

40. Koay CG, Basser PJ. Analytically exact correction scheme for signal extraction from noisy magnitude MR signals. *J Magn Reson.* 2006;179(2):317–322.

41. Partridge SC, Nissan N, Rahbar H, Kitsch AE, Sigmund EE. Diffusion-weighted breast MRI: clinical applications and emerging techniques. *J Magn Reson Imaging.* 2016;45:337–355.

Chapter 2

Conventional Breast Imaging

Ritse Mann MD, PhD

Before the development of mammography, the detection of abnormalities in the breast was largely based on visual inspection and palpation. This has dramatically changed in the last half of the 20th century. The successive development of mammography, ultrasound, and breast magnetic resonance imaging (MRI) has made imaging of the breast indispensable. Moreover, the development of image-guided needle biopsy has virtually obviated the need for surgery of benign breast lesions.

Imaging Techniques and Image-Guided Biopsy

MAMMOGRAPHY

Mammography is an x-ray-based technique that makes use of the different absorption rates of fatty and fibroglandular tissue (FGT) in the breast. Because the breast consists only of soft tissues, a low-energy spectrum is used. Typical settings for mammography are between 25 and 35 kV.[1] Whereas original mammography consisted of little more than an x-ray tube placed against the breast with a film on the opposite side, currently mammography is performed with dedicated mammography machines.

In addition to the x-ray tube and detector, these machines also include a compression mechanism that is used to flatten the breast on the detector plate. This leads to a better spread of the FGT and thus better interpretability of the resulting image. Furthermore, it also lowers the dose needed for high-quality images, as that is mainly dependent on the breast thickness. Besides, it prevents motion artifacts that would otherwise obscure the fine details in the image.[2]

A standard mammogram consists of two views per breast. The standard views are mediolateral oblique (MLO) and craniocaudal (CC). As the glandular structures in the breast have a teardrop-like configuration with the tail in the direction of the axilla, the MLO view is usually perpendicular to this and therefore shows most of the breast parenchyma as well as part of the pectoral muscle. The CC view depicts part of the medial breast that is inaccessible in the MLO view and also enables a somewhat higher compression, as it does not include muscles, which is beneficial to discriminate small masses from FGT. Strict quality control is usually employed for these acquisitions.[3] Images are considered adequate when the whole fibroglandular disc is depicted, the nipple shows in profile, and no folds are present. In MLO acquisitions, the pectoral muscle should be visible from the level of the nipple; in CC acquisitions, the pectoral muscle should just be visible on the dorsal side of the breast, although particularly the latter often shows infeasible.

In case the standard views do not sufficiently show the breast tissue, several additional views are commonly performed. These include nipple views to show the retroareolar area, the axillary view (Cleopatra view) that better depicts the axillary tail, and the cleavage view that shows the medial part of both breasts. In women with breast implants, an Eklund view is sometimes performed, in which the prosthesis is pushed to the back and only the FGT of the breast is compressed.

Mammography requires a very high spatial resolution to accurately depict the structures in the breast. Typical voxel sizes are below 100×100 microns. Although tumors detected with mammography are on average about 15 to 20 mm in size,[4] the high resolution enables accurate assessment of the lesion margins. Moreover, the high resolution enables the depiction of calcifications in the breast that may be associated with breast cancer. These calcifications commonly have a size of less than 200 microns and are therefore only visible when such high spatial resolutions are achieved.[5]

In the second decade of the 21st century, digital breast tomosynthesis (DBT) emerged as the better mammogram. In DBT, the same machinery is used but the x-ray tube is moved over the breast in a limited angular range (15–50 degrees, depending on the machine used).[6] During this movement, multiple acquisitions are obtained, which are subsequently reconstructed to provide a pseudo-3D stack of images that provides some depth information of the imaged breast. This sometimes enables visualization of lesions that would otherwise be hidden in the normal FGT, and conversely may enable discarding potential lesions that are caused by the projection of overlapping fibroglandular structures. Consequently, it was reported that sensitivity for cancer increases; specificity also increases, albeit especially the latter is strongly dependent on the threshold used for mammographic recall. It is possible to create a synthetic mammogram from the tomographic projections that, when used in conjunction with the tomosynthesis stack, obviates the creation of a regular mammography, which limits the radiation dose applied.[7]

When evaluating a mammogram or DBT, the first objective is to assess whether the obtained views meet the quality criteria for each view. Subsequently, the normal breast configuration is assessed. This includes an assessment of the relative amount of FGT in the breast, which is commonly referred to as density. Density is typically described according to the Breast Imaging Reporting and Data System (BI-RADS) that

discerns these four categories: (1) almost entirely fatty tissue, (2) scattered FGT, (3) heterogeneous FGT, and (4) extremely dense FGT (Fig. 2.1).[8] However, there are currently several commercial applications available that automatically determine density from a mammogram and have been shown to be more stable than human assessment.[9] With increasing density, the sensitivity of mammography for breast cancer decreases, as tumors may be masked by overprojecting FGT, and this effect is still present when using DBT. In addition, the risk of developing breast cancer increases with increasing density.[10]

Lesions depicted on mammography and DBT are also reported according to the BI-RADS lexicon.[8] Lesions are being classified as either a mass, calcifications, architectural distortion, or asymmetry. Masses typically have convex margins and are visible in two directions. Assessment is based on their shape, margin, and density. A typical malignant mass is irregular in shape, has a spiculated margin, and is hyperdense compared with the FGT (Fig. 2.2). Typical benign masses are oval, well circumscribed, and hypo- to isodense to the normal breast parenchyma. Calcifications can roughly be divided between calcifications that are certainly benign and those that may be associated with malignant breast lesions. Calcifications that are associated with malignant breast disease in general develop within the ductal structures, either due to impaction of locally trapped fluids or to local necrosis and subsequent calcification. Consequently, these calcifications

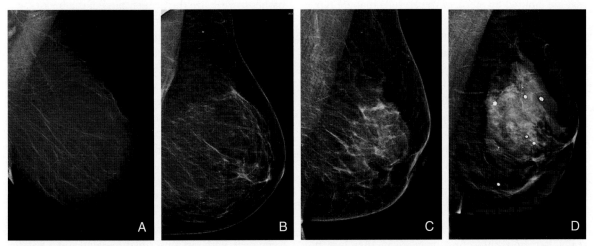

Fig. 2.1 Normal left mediolateral oblique mammography views showing the different density categories. (A) Almost entirely fatty tissue, (B) scattered FGT, (C) heterogeneously dense FGT, and (D) extremely dense FGT. *FGT*, Fibroglandular tissue.

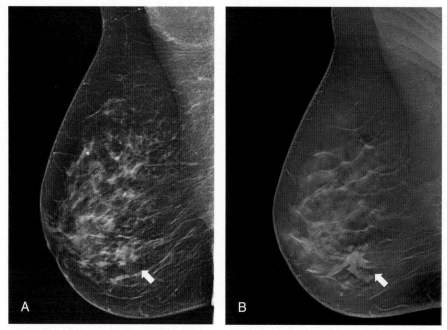

Fig. 2.2 Synthetic mediolateral oblique mammographic view of the right breast of a 47-year-old woman and corresponding tomosynthesis slice showing an irregular spiculated mass in the lower inner quadrant. There is heterogeneously dense fibroglandular tissue that largely obscures the present lesion *(arrows)*.

are tiny and grouped. Single calcifications are hardly ever a cause for worry. Coarse calcifications are likewise virtually always related to benign abnormalities.

ULTRASOUND

Ultrasound imaging makes apt use of ultrasonic waves that are emitted by piezoelectric crystals that are typically embedded in handheld transducers. Common frequencies for clinical ultrasound range between 4 and 20 MHz.[11] The emitted sound waves reflect on tissue transition boundaries and are received by the emitting transducer. Assuming a fixed speed of sound of ultrasound waves in soft tissues (roughly 1500 m/s), the time between emission and reception of the reflection can be used to calculate the depth of the tissue boundary that is causing the reflection, which is subsequently translated into an image.

The first ultrasound studies of the breast were reported in 1952. Since then, the quality of ultrasound images has dramatically improved. The current conversion of reflected sound waves into an image is really fast, and ultrasound images can therefore be viewed in real time.[12] For breast imaging, typically,

linear, high-frequency transducers (14 MHz or more) are used that create high-resolution images of all the tissue that is directly under the probe.[13] The downside of the use of high-frequency probes is that the penetration depth is limited, and in women with very large breasts, it may be required to use lower frequency probes to visualize the deeper parts of the breast.

Breast ultrasound is mainly a targeted technique, which means that it is used to evaluate focal abnormalities primarily detected by other means.[14] This includes both clinical symptoms (palpable lesions) and findings from other imaging tests. Assessment of ultrasound images is performed using the BI-RADS lexicon for breast ultrasound. Most lesions in ultrasound can be characterized as a mass, for which typically shape, margin, orientation, internal echo pattern, and posterior acoustic features are reported (Fig. 2.3). Associated features include architectural distortion, duct changes, and skin abnormalities. Typical malignant lesions present as irregular hypoechoic masses with posterior acoustic shadowing. Benign lesions tend to be oval, with circumscribed margins and a parallel orientation. Posterior acoustic features are commonly

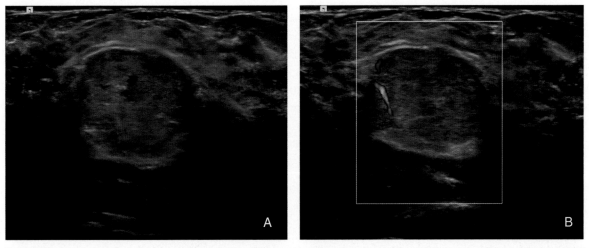

Fig. 2.3 Ultrasound evaluation of a new palpable mass in a 23-year-old woman. There is an oval mass with a partly noncircumscribed, somewhat irregular margin. There is an heterogeneous internal echo pattern, increased vascularization, and posterior acoustic enhancement. The lesion does not conform to the typical appearance of a fibroadenoma and was hence classified as BI-RADS 4. Histological evaluation showed a benign phyllodes tumor that was surgically removed.

absent. Fluid-rich lesions will show posterior acoustic enhancement.

To improve the classification of lesions on ultrasound, the use of Doppler and elastography can be considered. Malignant lesions have a stronger vascularization than benign lesions and a different orientation of feeding vessels (more perpendicular to the lesion), which can be used to strengthen the suspicion.[15] However, the flow in peritumoral vessels is often too slow to be picked up by even state-of-the-art high-resolution Doppler techniques, which implies that absence of Doppler signals is not very informative. Elastography may be used to probe the stiffness of a lesion, as malignant lesions are commonly stiffer than benign lesions; this may be used to avoid biopsy in very soft lesions that are not very suspicious on morphological evaluation but would warrant further evaluation.

MRI

Breast MRI was first employed in the early 1980s. Initial studies used T1 and T2 weighting and showed a similar sensitivity for the detection of breast cancer as could be obtained with mammography. Breast MRI only became viable in clinical practice after the introduction of gadolinium-based contrast media for MRI.[16,17] These proved to be a real game changer.

Contrast-enhanced breast MRI was soon shown to have a much higher comparative sensitivity for breast cancer than either mammography or ultrasound, which is still true despite significant improvements in the other techniques.

Gadolinium-based contrast agents are paramagnetic and therefore enhance T1-weighted relaxation, thus leading to a signal increase in T1-weighted images.

Despite the limited flow signals seen in Doppler ultrasound, virtually all breast cancers are highly vascularized. It is this feature that is exploited by contrast-enhanced imaging. Vessels in malignant breast lesions are different from those observed in healthy tissue.[18] They are the result of angiogenic stimulation by the tumor, and these vessels typically are not properly developed; moreover, they are commonly incapable of dealing with the increased pressure that occurs due to the arteriovenous shunting that occurs in a tumor. Neovascularization is therefore characterized by tortuous vessels with improper endothelial lining, widened interendothelial gaps, and even absence of the basal membrane. In these vessels the applied gadolinium chelates (usually at a dose of 0.1 mmol/kg) can easily extravasate and thus induce a signal change in the extravascular extracellular space.[19]

Current breast MRI thus heavily relies on contrast-enhanced T1-weighted imaging. Adequate enhancement is reached in most lesions approximately 1 to 2 minutes after contrast administration, which is commonly referred to as peak enhancement. This is because in many malignant lesions, maximum enhancement occurs around this moment and contrast starts washing out of the tissue after this time[20]; however, benign lesions and normal FGT generally reach their peak enhancement only later.

In a standard T1-weighted image, fat also has a high signal, and it can therefore be difficult to observe small enhancing lesions on a postcontrast T1-weighted image only. In practice, this is tackled by two approaches: fat suppression and image subtraction.[21]

Fat suppression, either using fat saturation, water selective excitation, or a Dixon-based approach, enables direct evaluation of the postcontrast acquisitions and is commonly used to observe lesions in the context of the surrounding breast parenchyma. However, it should be realized that some other structures in the breast may also have a high T1 signal that is not affected by fat saturation and may thus resemble enhancing lesions (e.g., commonly a high intensity is observed in the larger ducts due to protein-containing fluid). Subtraction (postcontrast minus precontrast) only shows enhancing structures but is susceptible to motion artifacts. However, when registration of pre- and postcontrast acquisitions is good, subtracted images can be used to generate a maximum intensity projection that enables a direct visualization of most enhancing structures in the breast, which is a good start for the evaluation of breast MRI acquisitions.

Evaluation of breast MRI according to the BI-RADS lexicon starts with the assessment of the amount of FGT and the amount of background parenchymal enhancement (BPE). BPE is assessed in series obtained approximately 90 to 120 seconds after contrast administration and classified as minimal, mild, moderate, or marked. The stronger BPE, the more likely that enhancing lesions are missed, albeit this effect is not as well documented as the effect of density in mammography (marked BPE is relatively rare).[22] BPE is dependent on the menstrual cycle and roughly lowest between day 3 and 14, albeit variation is large. To optimize the value of breast MRI, it is commonly recommended to plan the examination accordingly. It should, however, be noted that in women taking oral contraceptives, the normal menstrual cycle is often absent, and also in women with hormone-releasing intrauterine devices (IUDs) the cycle is not normal (the use of such IUDs tends to lead to quite strong BPE).

Enhancing lesions in the breast are classified as focus, mass, or nonmass enhancement. For masses, further morphological description includes shape, margin, and internal enhancement pattern; for nonmass enhancement, distribution and internal enhancement pattern are reported. Foci are generally smaller than 5 mm, but more importantly, they are not further classifiable as either mass or nonmass enhancement. Like in mammography and ultrasound, most cancers present as an irregular mass with an irregular or spiculated margin. Nonmass enhancement corresponding to malignancy is typically segmental in distribution and shows clumped internal enhancement.

In addition, the physiological enhancement behavior of a lesion is evaluated. As described earlier, the fact that cancers commonly have very leaky vessels leads to rapid early enhancement and wash-out after approximately 2 minutes. This is commonly referred to as a type 3 curve, and is clearly associated with malignancy (Fig. 2.4). A type 2 curve shows a plateau in the late phase (i.e., there is a balance between inflow and outflow of contrast), and a type 1 curve describes continuously increasing enhancement during the period of imaging (typically about 7 minutes). A type 1 curve is rare in malignant lesions but may occur in lesions without extensive neovascularization (e.g., low-grade ductal carcinoma in situ [DCIS] or very diffusely growing invasive lobular carcinoma [ILC]).[20] As the enhancement curves provide a proxy for the leakiness of the vessels in a lesion, similar information can be obtained using ultrafast MRI acquisitions from the inflow phase of contrast (i.e., before peak enhancement is reached). When vessels are large and leaky and shunting occurs, enhancement in a lesion is both early (typically within 10 seconds from the descending aorta) and fast (>13.5%/s), which is typical for malignant lesions. Vice versa, when vessels are not so leaky and shunting is absent, enhancement is later (>15 seconds) and slower (<6.4%/s).[23]

Other contrasts in breast MRI currently provide mainly supplemental value. Besides diffusion-weighted imaging (DWI), which is the topic of this book and therefore not discussed in detail in this chapter, T2-weighted acquisitions are commonly

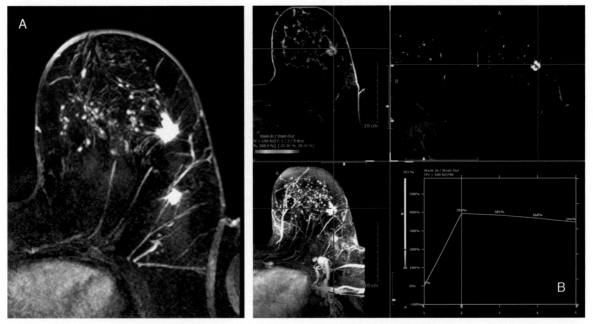

Fig. 2.4 Breast magnetic resonance imaging (MRI) scan of the left breast of a 54-year-old woman with a bifocal tumor in the lateral upper quadrant. (A) Shows a 1-cm multi-planar reconstruction (MPR) of the subtracted T1 series, which enables visualization of two masses and their respective positioning within the breast. In (B), a dynamic analysis is shown. The larger irregular and spiculated mass clearly shows rim enhancement and has a type 3 curve with rapid initial enhancement and washout in the late phase.

obtained. Fat-saturated T2-weighted acquisitions are particularly good for the documentation of cysts. Non-fat-saturated T2-weighted images often better allow the visualization of the architectural distortion that is caused by the tumor in the breast and the presence or absence of edema surrounding a lesion.[21] Most malignant lesions are relatively hypointense at T2-weighted acquisitions due to a low water content. However, especially high-grade lesions may have a more intermediate T2 signal.[24] Central necrosis may be visualized as high signal within an otherwise low signal intensity lesion. Rapidly enhancing oval masses with a sharp margin and a high T2 signal in young women are usually myxoid fibroadenomas, albeit especially in women at increased risk, care must be taken not to misclassify rapidly growing cancers.

IMAGE-GUIDED BIOPSY

Despite the many classifying features that can be collected from multimodal and multiparametric imaging many breast lesions cannot be fully classified by imaging alone. In lesions that have a likelihood of more than 2% to be malignant (BI-RADS 4; see later), tissue sampling is generally recommended. Besides, in case the imaging features are clearly malignant tissue, sampling is still required to determine optimal treatment, as that is also dependent on receptor status and tumor grade. Hence biopsy is indispensable in breast radiology, and an essential part of the toolbox of each breast radiologist.[25,26]

Tissue sampling should be an image-guided procedure, and due to the real-time feedback that can be obtained by using ultrasound, this is in general the first choice. Under ultrasound guidance, many different needles can be used. For cytological procedures, a standard 21 G injection needle is usually employed. However, the reported accuracy of cytology is highly variable and largely dependent on the experience of the pathologists involved. Moreover, in malignant lesions, cytology is not able to differentiate between in situ and invasive disease. Consequently, for the assessment of breast lesions, cytology should be used selectively and should be followed by histological tumor sampling when findings are not conclusively benign.

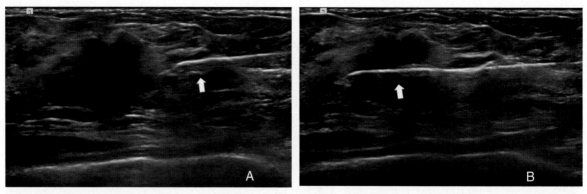

Fig. 2.5 **Ultrasound-guided large-core biopsy in a 52-year-old woman presenting with a palpable lump in the right breast.** The palpable abnormality corresponds to a hypoechoic irregular mass. In (A), the needle *(arrow)* is positioned in the prefire position with the tip just before the abnormality. (B) Shows the postfire image *(arrow)*, which proves that the obtained sample comes from the lesion.

For histological sampling under ultrasound guidance, typically 14 G large-core needles are used that obtain samples with a diameter of about 1 mm (usually about 2 cm in length). The fact that it is possible to document the position of the needle within the lesion enables relatively straightforward radiological-pathological correlation (Fig. 2.5). Typically, two to three cores are sufficient to obtain a reliable diagnosis. Most care should be taken in very small lesions (<5 mm) and solid components in predominantly cystic lesions. Very small lesions may move when firing the needle when they are stiffer than the surrounding parenchyma. Images could, in this case, deceptively show the needle in the lesion when in fact it moved just on its side, and therefore only regular breast tissue is sampled. In predominantly cystic lesions, biopsy might break the wall of the cyst and therefore render small solid components suddenly invisible.

To overcome these issues, it might be feasible to use larger (11–7 G) vacuum-assisted needles.[27] These should be positioned underneath the lesion to be biopsied, with the biopsy chamber pointing toward the transducer. This enables verification of the representativeness of the biopsy sample and therefore may prevent sampling errors.

The same technique can be used to sample more tissue, when an initial large core biopsy reveals lesions of uncertain malignant potential, such as atypical ductal hyperplasia or complex sclerosing lesions. Using this approach, it is also possible to remove lesions completely, which is mainly practiced for the removal of symptomatic fibroadenomas.[28]

Not all lesions are visible with ultrasound, and therefore guidance of the other imaging modalities employed should always be possible. Typical lesions that are only visible on mammography and DBT are grouped calcifications that only rarely have a clear ultrasound correlate. Such calcifications are typically associated with the presence of DCIS but are not very specific, thus these should be biopsied under mammographic or DBT guidance. Classic mammographic guidance makes use of stereotactic views obtained under slight angulation of the x-ray tube to obtain depth information, DBT inherently obtains these views and therefore provides the required depth information automatically.[29] Different from ultrasound guidance, direct imaging feedback of the needle position in the lesion is not possible; rather, correlation is obtained by controlling the needle position before biopsy and the location of the hematoma and marker after the procedure. Furthermore, the lesions are typically more diffuse and therefore harder to classify for pathologists. To obtain a reliable diagnosis, more tissue should be removed than is typically done under ultrasound guidance. Vacuum-assisted biopsy is most common, and six 9 G cores seems to be the minimum.[30] To guarantee that the targeted lesion is indeed biopsied, specimen x-rays are acquired that should show that at least some of the targeted calcifications are removed.

The relatively high sensitivity of MRI for breast cancer implies also that MRI leads to the detection of lesions that have no correlate on other imaging tests and hence should be biopsied under MRI guidance. These include in general small masses and areas of nonmass

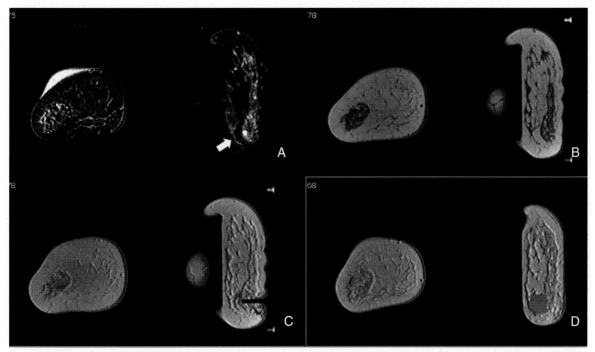

Fig. 2.6 Magnetic resonance imaging (MRI)-guided biopsy of a small, round, enhancing lesion in a 32-year-old woman with a known BRCA2 mutation. (A) Shows the subtracted images before and after contrast administration. The lesion is located at 6 o'clock in the compressed left breast *(arrow)*. (B) Shows the native prebiopsy T1-weighted image. In (C), a coaxial needle is placed at the biopsy site. The needle position for biopsy can be observed in (C) by the signal void that is caused by the plastic placeholder that is inserted for this control scan. (D) Shows the postbiopsy T1-weighted image; note that the hematoma includes the lesion area. Pathology showed a small fibroadenoma.

enhancement. The biopsy procedure is in essence similar to that for stereotactic biopsy.[31] The true 3D nature of MRI makes it relatively easier to check the position of the needle relative to the lesion; however, there is still no real-time imaging feedback. The fact that usually small or diffuse lesions are targeted makes the use of vacuum-assisted needles indispensable. Different from mammographically detected lesions, there is no possibility to check whether the obtained specimen truly includes the targeted lesion. Accuracy of the procedure is therefore checked by assessing whether the location of the hematoma after biopsy corresponds to the location of the original lesion (Fig. 2.6).

Using Conventional Breast Imaging in Clinical Practice

The type and amount of breast imaging used is highly dependent on the clinical scenario and the questions to be answered. In general, four categories can be discerned: (1) screening of asymptomatic women, (2) assessment of patients with breast findings, (3) staging and monitoring of patients with proven breast cancer, and (4) follow-up of treated patients. The latter basically returns to the first situation (i.e., surveillance is a form of screening). In each setting the demands of imaging differ, and consequently the respective roles of the different imaging modalities vary.

BI-RADS SCORES

Assessment of images should lead to a clear evaluation that can easily be understood by others, and that heralds the next steps in the evaluation program. There are several systems around that try to summarize the findings in a number that is simple to interpret. By far, the most commonly used approach is the BI-RADS score, which runs from 0 to 6.[8] BI-RADS scores and their meaning are given in Table 2.1.

BI-RADS 4 is further subdivided in 4A (2%–9%), 4B (10%–49%), and 4C (50%–94%). In essence, BI-RADS scores 4 and 5 imply that a lesion should be biopsied.

TABLE 2.1	BI-RADS Scores	
BI-RADS 0	Incomplete	Additional imaging necessary
BI-RADS 1	Negative	No abnormalities
BI-RADS 2	Benign	0% likelihood of malignancy
BI-RADS 3	Probably benign	<2% likelihood of malignancy
BI-RADS 4	Suspicious for malignancy	2%–94% likelihood of malignancy
BI-RADS 5	Highly suggestive of malignancy	>95% likelihood of malignancy
BI-RADS 6	Known biopsy-proven malignancy	

For lesions interpreted as BI-RADS 3, short-term follow-up may be recommended. However, to downgrade a lesion from BI-RADS 3 to BI-RADS 2 requires 2 years of negative follow-up, and many women prefer biopsy over this extensive surveillance.

SCREENING OF ASYMPTOMATIC WOMEN

In 1968 the World Health Organization listed criteria that should be applicable when offering screening for a disease.[32] These criteria are listed in Table 2.2 and are still applicable generally.

There is no doubt that breast cancer is an important health problem, considering the fact that in 2018 almost 700,000 women died from this disease, despite the presence of a treatment.[33] Screening for breast cancer is built on the paradigm that breast cancer–specific survival increases because earlier treatment is more effective. It should be realized that this is not necessarily true. When breast cancer is in general already metastasized from its onset, then earlier treatment of the disease locally will not make a difference. Moreover, when tumor stage at detection neither affects survival nor the selection/aggressiveness of therapy, the screening paradigm will be broken. However, currently, this is far from reality.

Randomized controlled trials performed with mammography in the second half of the 20th century proved that the screening paradigm was valid. Average tumor size in most studies decreased, and with it the breast cancer–specific mortality decreased. In meta-analysis of these studies, the invitation to screen leads to a mortality reduction of approximately 20%.[34] This says little about the actual effect of screening, but it also takes the acceptability of the screening test for the population into account. Case-control studies in which women actually screened are compared with those who are not screened report a much higher reduction

TABLE 2.2	Criteria for Screening According to Wilson and Junger (World Health Organization)
•	The condition should be an important health problem.
•	There should be a treatment for the condition.
•	Facilities for diagnosis and treatment should be available.
•	There should be a latent stage of the disease.
•	There should be a test or examination for the condition.
•	The test should be acceptable to the population.
•	The natural history of the disease should be adequately understood.
•	There should be an agreed policy on whom to treat.
•	The total cost of finding a case should be economically balanced in relation to medical expenditure as a whole.
•	Case-finding should be a continuous process, not just a "once and for all" project.

of mortality due to mammographic screening on the order of 40%.[35] Current international recommendations uniformly recommend screening in women between the ages of 50 and 70. Variations occur due to differences in the age groups invited (range roughly 40–75) and the frequency at which the screening test is offered (annually or once every 2–3 years). These variations are based on the expected efficiency of the screening test in the population and the value attributed to early cancer detection relative to the negative values attributed to the downsides of screening.[36]

Apart from having to undergo the screening test, screening comes with two typical disadvantages. The first is overdiagnosis, which refers to the detection of cancers that would never become symptomatic in the woman's lifetime. This defines the upper age limit to which screening is useful, because after that age earlier detection of breast cancer is unlikely to contribute to better survival (i.e., the fraction of overdiagnosis goes up with increasing age).[37]

The second disadvantage is the detection of false positives. This refers to a situation in which the screening test points to a possible abnormality that might or might not be breast cancer but that turns out to be benign after further workup. In essence, "false positive" is a misnomer, as screening is aimed to separate women who are most likely cancer-free from those who may or may not have breast cancer. For the latter group, the investigation is simply not finished but requires additional imaging tests or even image-guided biopsy before a final verdict can be given (see Fig. 2.6). Nonetheless, such supplemental studies have been shown to temporarily increase the stress women experience and should thus be limited as much as possible.[38] False-positive findings occur more frequently when the screening test is repeated more frequently, and thus they are affected by the screening frequency. However, by comparing the new screening examination to prior studies, the number of false positives can be strongly reduced (depending on the country and the recall policy, between 2% and 10%).

The biggest shortcoming of mammographic screening is not in its findings, however; rather, it is the underdiagnosis of relevant cancers (i.e., the lack of findings in women who actually do have significant breast cancer).[39] This is evident in the fact that even in women screened, a significant fraction of cancers

presents with symptoms in between two screening rounds (i.e., interval cancers), and also from the fact that a significant fraction of cancers detected through screening are over 2 cm in size and/or already have lymph node metastasis at the time of detection. Consequently, there is a strong need to improve breast cancer screening.

In the last decade, much effort has been put into evaluation of tomosynthesis as an alternative screening test. Several large case-control studies showed increased cancer detection with tomosynthesis over mammography, usually on the order of 1 to 2 in 1000 screens.[40] In the United States, where recall rates are traditionally high, the use of tomosynthesis leads to an increase in specificity. However, in Europe, where recall rates are traditionally much lower, the effect is reversed, and the increased detection of cancer with DBT also slightly reduces the specificity. Overall, the cancers detected with DBT are similar to those observed on mammography, both in size and nodal status. However, follow-up on several of these studies now seems to show an overall reduction of interval cancers, with reported values ranging from 0% to 40%.[41] Thus DBT seems to be somewhat better than mammography for screening purposes. However, this comes at a price that is mainly problematic in population-based screening programs. Reading tomosynthesis takes on average about twice the time that is required for assessing a mammogram and therefore would require a strong increase in the number of evaluating radiologists in such programs.[42] This is not so much an issue in the United States, where screening is mainly hospital based; therefore DBT has been largely embraced as the new screening modality in the United States, whereas it is not commonly used within Europe for screening.

Ultrasound is not commonly used as a first-line screening technique but rather as a supplement to mammographic screening. Although the sensitivity of ultrasound for breast cancer is likely higher than that of mammography, it is much harder to document the entire breast with ultrasound. A structured assessment of both breasts is reported to take approximately 21 minutes and requires a skilled operator.[43] Because only abnormalities are structurally documented, it is also much harder to compare new ultrasound acquisitions to prior images, which adds to the already high false positive rates. Still, in women with dense breasts, ultrasound is commonly used as a supplemental screening technique. Reported supplemental cancer detection rates after negative mammography range between 1 and 7 in 1000 screens.[44] In direct comparison to tomosynthesis, the yield is approximately double.[45] The use of ultrasound as a supplemental screening technique was reported to reduce the interval cancer rate by 50%.[46] However, reported false-positive rates are up to 25%, which seriously hampers the implementation. In practice, the recall rate is usually lowered by only including clearly solid suspicious lesions and leaving out all probably benign lesions. Consequently, the increase in cancer detection is much lower than in the prospective studies. For example, Lee and colleagues reported no increase in cancer detection in women screened with mammography and ultrasound over mammography alone (5.4/1000 vs. 5.5/1000) but did report a strong increase in false-positive findings leading to biopsy (52/1000 vs. 22/1000).[47] This implies that the use of ultrasound for screening is somewhat questionable even when it is undoubtedly true that ultrasound can show cancers that are not visible on mammography.

Breast MRI has been tested as a supplemental screening modality since the start of this century, and its role has been ever expanding.[48] MRI is primarily used in populations with a high likelihood of developing breast cancer, in which conventional screening with mammography and DBT is particularly poor. Based on a number of large comparative multicenter studies, which showed that breast MRI roughly doubles the sensitivity of mammography, in 2007 the American Cancer Society issued guidelines to define who to screen with breast MRI.[49] They concluded that combined mammography and MRI screening was indicated in women with hereditary breast cancer, including those with BRCA1, BRCA2, PTEN, and STK11 mutations that all lead to a lifetime risk of more than 50% to develop breast cancer. Moreover, screening in these women should start at the age of 25, as they are prone to breast cancer development much earlier than the general population. This list was later supplemented with other genetic mutations that also lead to increased risk for the development of breast cancer, such as CDH1, PALB2, and ATM. Apart from these groups of women with hereditary gene

mutations, also women with a personal history of chest irradiation during puberty (usually for lymphoma/leukemia) were deemed eligible for MRI screening, as their risk is more or less similar. Reported positive predictive values of breast MRI in a screening setting range between 20% and 40%; these are generally comparable to those from mammography and much better than those reported for ultrasound. Still, it should be realized that this leads to somewhat higher absolute numbers of false-positive findings, as the number of cancers detected is higher.

Although the American Cancer Society also recommended to screen women with a lifetime risk of between 20% and 50% based on family history with supplemental MRI screening, this recommendation was followed less often due to concerns about cost-effectiveness. However, this was recently shown to be both effective and cost-effective[50] (Fig. 2.7). In the last decade, research on the value of breast MRI for screening focused mostly on women in such intermediate risk groups and even in women at average risk. It was shown that breast MRI has far higher sensitivity than mammography in women with a personal history of breast cancer,[51] women with lobular carcinoma in situ, atypical ductal hyperplasia, and other epithelial atypias on biopsy.[52] Also, MRI outperforms mammography in women with extremely or heterogeneously dense breasts on mammography, and even in women at average risk in general.[53] In a landmark randomized controlled trial in women with extremely dense breasts (Dense Tissue and Early Breast Neoplasm Screening [DENSE]), supplemental cancer detection after a negative mammogram was 16.5 in 1000.[54] It was shown that breast MRI reduces the rate of interval cancers by approximately 85% and causes a major stage shift that leads to all cancers detected in follow-up screening rounds to be stage 0 or 1 and all node negative.[55]

It should be noted that in women screened with MRI, the complementary value of other screening tests is relatively limited. In women under 50, more than 1000 mammograms need to be obtained to find a single additional cancer, and most of those are DCIS.[56] The addition of ultrasound in women screened with MRI was repeatedly shown to be useless and only lead to more false positives; and thus it should be avoided.[57,58] It should therefore be no surprise that in the cost-effectiveness analysis of the DENSE trial,

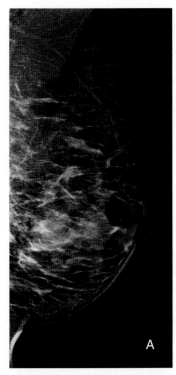
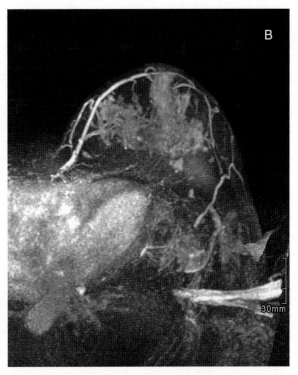

Fig. 2.7 Screening mammogram and magnetic resonance imaging (MRI) of the left breast of a 40-year-old woman with increased familial risk. There is a somewhat obscured mass present retroareolar. The MRI shows almost diffuse nonmass enhancement throughout the left breast, which corresponded with a large, diffuse, growing HER2-positive cancer.

all dominating screening strategies consist of breast MRI only, with only the frequency of the screening test being dependent on the willingness to pay.

In terms of cost-effectiveness, the price of MRI itself always appears to be the major driver. Since 2014 efforts have been made to reduce the price of breast MRI, predominantly by shortening the protocols, known as abbreviated MRI.[59] In practice, many different protocols for abbreviated MRI have been proposed. They all have in common that they focus predominantly on T1-weighted acquisitions during the inflow and peak phase of contrast administration, abandoning late-phase images and most other contrasts. This allows to obtain a breast MRI scan within approximately 5 minutes and thus to increase the throughput per MRI scanner to four or five patients per hour instead of the typical one to two (patients still need to be positioned on the table, which becomes the limiting factor). These abbreviated protocols were repeatedly shown to be as sensitive as

conventional multiparametric breast MRI, with only a very limited reduction of specificity. Therefore in the screening setting, abbreviated MRI is rapidly becoming standard.[60]

However, abbreviated MRI is still a contrast-enhanced technique that requires the use of an intravenous cannula and administration of a contrast agent that can potentially lead to allergic reactions. Noncontrast approaches are currently not good enough to replace contrast-enhanced breast MRI, but they are potentially as good as the combination of DBT and ultrasound.

ASSESSMENT OF PATIENTS WITH BREAST FINDINGS

There are two routes that may lead to a breast finding: recall from screening and the presence of symptoms. Breast symptoms are frequent, and many women do visit a breast clinic during their lives.[61,62] In fact, this group of women is about twice the size of the group that is recalled from screening, albeit in general the likelihood that the symptoms are caused by breast cancer is lower than for screen-detected findings. For the first group, an imaging evaluation is already present (typically mammography), whereas for the latter group no images are available yet. Out of habit, most women presenting with breast complaints therefore undergo a mammography or DBT examination as their baseline examination. This examination may or may not show the abnormality and its effects on the surrounding breast parenchyma, and in addition it provides an overview of the breast that enables the detection of lesions apart from the complaint. Regardless of the outcome of the mammographic assessment, however, targeted ultrasound is usually employed to assess the nature of the breast complaint. In younger women (the upper age limit varies around the world but is roughly between ages 30 and 40), mammography is not recommended, as the relative high amount of FGT, in combination with the low risk of breast cancer, has rendered the examination obsolete.[63]

In women with breast complaints, both the type of symptoms and the underlying pathology are highly dependent on age.[64] Palpable lumps in women aged 20 to 35 are usually fibroadenomas. These are characterized as oval, circumscribed masses with a horizontal orientation that may have a few lobulations.

Fibroadenomas that meet these criteria in women without specific risk factors may be classified as such by imaging alone. Fibroadenomas may still grow in a developing breast, hence growth is not by definition indicative of malignancy. Although rare in this age group, in atypical lesions and in women at increased risk, the presence of cancer always needs to be excluded, either by short-term follow-up or biopsy. Palpable lumps in women aged 40 to 55 tend to be caused by simple cysts that develop in regressing FGT. Cysts are easy to recognize on ultrasound, as their fluid content does not reflect sound waves, hence they are oval, well circumscribed, and anechoic (Fig. 2.8). Puncture and aspiration are only indicated when in doubt or when the cyst gives physical complaints. In this age group, cancer is, however, no longer rare and is a major differential. In women over 60, new, palpable lumps are commonly caused by cancer. A typical malignant lesion appears as a hypoechoic mass with hyperechoic halo, a noncircumscribed and commonly spiculated margin, an antiparallel orientation, and posterior shadowing. However, it should be noted that more aggressive cancers tend to be more oval and wetter, which leads to mixed posterior acoustic effects or even posterior enhancement.

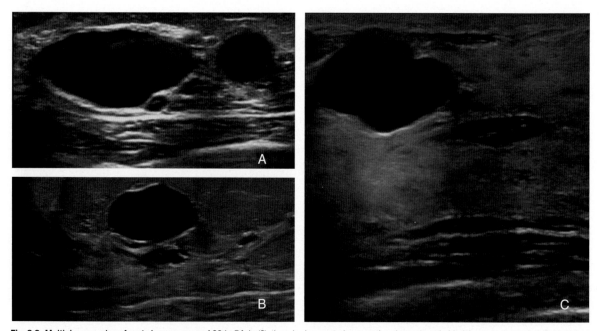

Fig. 2.8 Multiple examples of cysts in women aged 38 to 54. In (C), there is clear posterior acoustic enhancement behind the cysts due to their fluid content.

Many women also visit the breast clinic for focal or diffuse breast pain. This is sometimes caused by focal inflammation of the breast tissue or inflamed cysts but usually goes without any imaging correlate. Cancer is only rarely associated with focal pain and is relatively unlikely in this setting; however, obviously suspicious imaging findings should be further explored. In the absence of underlying imaging findings, adequate patient information is essential.[14]

Another typical complaint that leads to a visit to the breast clinic is nipple discharge. Physiological nipple discharge is usually bilateral and clear, white, yellow, or greenish. Suspicious nipple discharge is usually spontaneous, unilateral, and brown to bloody. Common causes for this are intraductal papillomas, duct ectasias, and DCIS. Papillomas usually show on ultrasound as small, clearly intraductal, round to oval homogeneous masses. However, they are considered lesions of uncertain malignant potential, because up to 10% of these are associated with atypia, and some may even contain DCIS. DCIS may present as an intra-ductal proliferation on ultrasound and may also be evident from grouped calcifications on the mammogram, but it is commonly occult. In this setting, breast MRI is often used as a problem solver in order to exclude underlying pathology. However, in cases of persistent bloody nipple discharge without an imaging correlate (even on MRI), microdochectomy may be considered to assess the underlying cause.[65]

Women may also present with spontaneous nipple retraction. This is usually due to loose skin that drops over the nipple, because it is more firmly attached to the pectoral wall by Cooper ligaments. In these cases, it should be possible to push the nipple outward, and there should not be any palpable mass behind the nipple. However, it is also possible that a tumor pulls on the Cooper ligaments and thus forces the nipple inward. Consequently, adequate evaluation of the area behind the nipple is mandatory in such circumstances. Mammographic nipple views and ultrasound may show the presence of a mass in this setting. It should be noted that in the case of symptoms, many lesions in fact classify as BI-RADS 4 and will therefore undergo biopsy.

Many studies have explored the value of different techniques to reduce the need for biopsy. In ultrasound (power) Doppler, elastography and contrast-enhanced ultrasound have been shown to allow a reduction in the need for biopsy.[66] Likewise, optoacoustic imaging has successfully been tested.[67]

The role of breast MRI in this setting is relatively limited. Although in meta-analysis the absence of enhancement in solid masses virtually rules out the presence of malignancy,[68] performing a biopsy is usually easier, more rapidly available, and gives a more indisputable answer than another imaging test and is therefore commonly the first choice of action. However, MRI may prove valuable in women in whom the imaging and clinical findings are discrepant (Fig. 2.9).

Women recalled from screening are likewise evaluated by ultrasound. In general, a mammogram is already available for these women, and the ultrasound examination is targeted to the findings there. Additional views may sometimes enable to differentiate true masses from overprojecting FGT, rendering the need for ultrasound obsolete. In the remainder, ultrasound may either show the lesion or not. In case the lesion is visible, evaluation is similar as in women presenting with symptomatic abnormalities. Especially small cysts and intramammary lymph nodes may be classified based on the imaging appearance alone.[14] In case there is no ultrasound correlate to a screen-detected finding, the lesion should not be ignored. Grouped calcifications are hardly ever visible under ultrasound. MRI can also not reliably rule out malignancy in these women, and calcifications are therefore usually biopsied under stereotactic guidance.[26]

For MRI detected lesions the same holds true: only about 58% have an ultrasound correlate (masses more often than nonmass enhancement), and therefore MRI-guided biopsy should be available for women presenting with MRI-detected suspicious lesions.[69]

STAGING AND MONITORING OF PATIENTS WITH PROVEN BREAST CANCER

In women diagnosed with breast cancer, imaging aims at staging of the known cancer and searching for occult second cancers. The latter is a form of screening and generally not thought of as part of the staging procedure. Mammography detects an asymptomatic contralateral cancer in roughly 5% of patients with unilateral cancer. In women with a negative contralateral mammogram, 3% to 5% will still prove to have bilateral cancer after MRI.[70,71] Hence particularly in

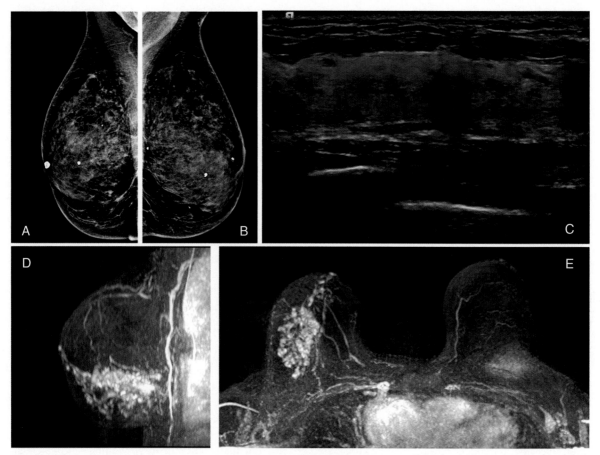

Fig. 2.9 A 56-year-old woman presenting with a palpable mass in the right breast. Mammography (A and B) was rated to be normal. Also ultrasound (C) did not show any abnormality. A breast MRI was made to exclude malignancy; however, it shows a large segmental nonmass enhancement in the lower outer quadrant of the right breast (D and E). This was subsequently biopsied under magnetic resonance imaging (MRI) guidance and corresponded to a large grade 3 ductal carcinoma in situ (DCIS).

young women in whom the detection of these second cancers is unquestionably clinical relevant, MRI should be performed.

Staging of breast cancer is done according to the TNM (tumor, node, metastasis) classification as shown in Table 2.3.[72] From imaging, the clinical TNM stage is obtained (i.e., cTNM), which is usually replaced later by the pathological TNM stage (pTNM) in patients who undergo surgery as the first therapeutic procedure. In women who undergo primary systemic therapy, the pathological TNM is denoted as ypTNM, to indicate that it is not the original tumor stage.

It is thus evident that for prognostic purposes, it is essential to measure the size of the tumor and to evaluate the presence of axillary metastasis.

Of note is that the size of the tumor is described as the maximum size of the largest continuous tumor area. For example, a mass of 5.5 cm in diameter is a T3 carcinoma, but a region within the breast of 5.5 cm with several small masses up to 1 cm is a T1b cancer; the fact that there are multiple masses is indicated with a bracketed "m" for multiple (i.e., T1b[m]). Although the size of the multifocal cancer is thus much smaller, the extent of both cancers is the same. For surgical planning the extent is more important than the size, but for prognosis the latter is more relevant.

To assess the size of cancer within the breast, many studies have shown that MRI is the technique of choice.[21] Mammography tends to strongly underestimate the size of breast cancer, whereas ultrasound may

TABLE 2.3 Tumor (pT) and Lymph Node (pN) Classes and the Overall Disease Stage According to the TNM Classification					
Pathological Tumor Class (pT)		**Pathological Lymph Node Class (pN)**		**Breast Cancer Stage**	
Tis	DCIS, LCIS, Paget disease	pN0	No lymph node metastases	0	DCIS
T1mic	<1 mm	pN1mic	Micro >0.2 –2 mm	Ia	T1N0
T1a	<5 mm	pN1a	1–3 axillary lymph nodes	Ib	T0–1 N mic
T1b	5–10 mm	pN1b	Sentinel lymph node procedure shows ipsilateral intramammary lymph node metastasis	IIa	T0–1N1 T2N0
T1c	>10–20 mm	pN1c	a + b	IIb	T2N1 T3N0
T2	>20–50 mm	pN2a	4–9 axillary lymph nodes	IIIa	T0–2N2 T3N1–2
T3	>50 mm	pN2b	Enlarged intramammary lymph nodes based on metastases	IIIb	T4N0–2
T4a	Extension to chest wall	pN3a	10 or more axillary nodes, or infraclavicular nodes	IIIc	Any T, N3
T4b	Extension to skin	pN3b	Axillary and enlarged intramammary nodes	IV	Systemic metastasis
T4c	a + b	pN3c	Supraclavicular lymph node metastasis		
T4d	Inflammatory breast cancer				

DCIS, Ductal carcinoma in situ; *LCIS,* lobular carcinoma in situ.

also not show intraductal extensions and small satellites. Despite being the best imaging test for breast cancer size estimation, MRI is not free from error. Roughly 75% is accurately measured, whereas compared with pathology, about 10% to 15% are respectively under- and overestimated by at least 5 mm.[73,74] Considering the underlying physiology, this should not be a surprise, as bulky tumors will have significant enhancement, but more indolent or diffuse growing parts may remain partly occult. On the other hand, the release of angiogenic stimulants is not restricted to the actual tumor area but may also cause vasogenic alterations in the tissue surrounding the tumor that will therefore also enhance. This implies that additional findings on MRI that will change the therapeutic approach should

be histologically verified, which also means that access to MRI-guided breast biopsy is mandatory.

Still, it remains questionable whether MRI is always needed or should be used for selective subsets of patients only. In many women, a mammogram is already present that can be used as a first-line staging examination, and when the breast is relatively fatty and the tumor is well visible, this could be enough. One should not forget that surgeons are relatively coarse in their approach and remove much more tissue than what is obviously affected on imaging. Moreover, already in the 1980s it was shown that after breast-conserving therapy, in up to 40% of women residual cancer is left in the breast that is effectively treated by adjuvant therapies, particularly radiotherapy.[75]

Due to the simple fact that more cancer is visible with MRI, it became harder for surgeons to leave cancer behind in the treated breast, which subsequently translates to a somewhat increased mastectomy rate (about 10%), which should be weighed against a reduction in reexcision rates of about 3.5%.[76] However, one should keep in mind that in practice, MRI is reserved for the patients in whom a therapeutic plan is hardest to make. In centers with extensive experience, for example, MRI images are often also used to attempt breast-conserving and oncoplastic procedures that would not have been possible without accurate 3D information.

Although initially preoperative staging was, as its name indicates, predominantly an investigation to assess the size of the tumor and tell the surgeon what to remove, its current prime goal is to select the optimal therapy, which may include primary surgery; very often it also consists of neoadjuvant therapy. For that, it is essential to be aware of the fact that breast cancer is not a single disease but rather includes many different types of cancer.

In practice, different histological types and different molecular subtypes are recognized. The most common histological type is invasive ductal carcinoma of no special type (IDC-NST), commonly referred to as IDC (80%–85%). ILC, a subtype characterized by the absence of the adhesion molecule e-cadherin, which is characterized by a much more diffuse growth pattern, comes second (10%–15%). For this specific subtype, MRI is always strongly advised because mammography is very unreliable.[77,78] Further, there are other specific breast cancer subtypes characterized by specific growth patterns or cells of origin. Based on the amount of mitosis, the nuclear polymorphism, and the tubule formation, histological grades (1–3) are defined. Moreover, breast cancers are subdivided by their molecular profile.[79] Because this is from origin a genetic signature, cancers are generally placed in one or the other category based upon the receptor status on the cell membrane. For accurate classification, the estrogen receptor (ER), progesterone receptor (PR), and human epidermal growth factor receptor 2 (HER2) are essential. ER-positive cancers are collectively called luminal, and within this group three subtypes are recognized. Luminal A cancers are slow-growing,

low-proliferative cancers. Luminal B cancers are more proliferative and may in fact be quite aggressive. These can either be HER2-positive or HER2-negative. Then there are the so-called HER2+ cancers, which are ER- and PR-negative, and finally the triple negative (TN) cancers that do not present with any of the aforementioned receptors on their cell membranes. In general, the TN cancers are highly aggressive and rapidly growing, although the group is quite heterogeneous and not all cancers have the same poor prognosis.

To choose an appropriate therapy for a cancer, its stage, grade, and molecular subtype should be known. For example, HER2-positive cancers are virtually always treated with neoadjuvant systemic therapy (e.g., pertuzumab, trastuzumab) because they respond very well to targeted therapy that blocks the HER2 receptor. Conversely, luminal A cancers may be quite resistant to chemotherapy but respond well to neo-endocrine therapy. However, to cure such cancers, direct surgery is often the better choice. Imaging features correlate to the overall cancer type.[80] TN cancers are often round and show central necrosis and rim enhancement (Fig. 2.10). HER2-positive cancers are commonly multifocal and are more often associated with microcalcifications. Luminal cancers are usually spiculated masses. Moreover, the molecular subtype of a cancer influences the accuracy of MRI assessment.[81] Imaging features should thus be correlated to pathological findings in order to confirm and understand the type of cancer present.

Spatial heterogeneity should also be taken into account, however. Currently, we have no good ways to document the presence and extent of heterogeneity within a tumor.[82] Still, this is the most likely explanation for the partial response that is commonly observed. Because nonresponding clones may eventually cause mortality,[83] this is a serious issue that should be tackled. Potentially, the use of radiomics (i.e., the structured and automated assessment of quantified imaging characteristics) may provide relevant information about this that can eventually be used to adapt treatment, although there is currently no clinically applicable model available for this.[84]

It should be realized that when cancers are treated neoadjuvantly, no adequate surgical specimen is present, and it may be very hard to retrieve the original

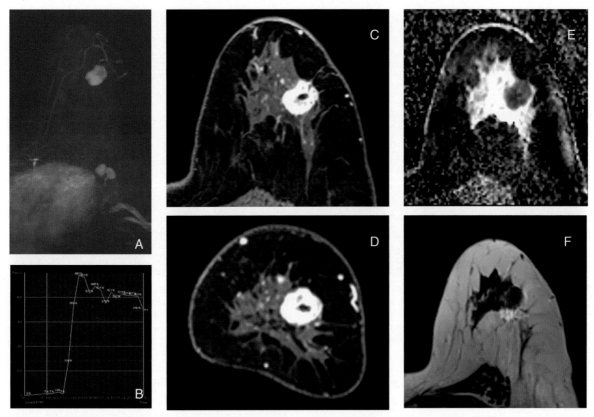

Fig. 2.10 Multiparametric breast magnetic resonance imaging (MRI) shows an oval mass that enhances rapidly. (A) Shows the maximum intensity projection 8 seconds after aortic enhancement, and (B) shows the corresponding curve. In (C) and (D), morphology can be best appreciated, showing an oval mass with a sharp margin, rim enhancement, and central necrosis. A marker is dropped in the necrotic core. The lesion has a very low ADC level (E), measured as 0.78, and clear perifocal edema (F). The lesion was proven to be a triple negative grade 3 carcinoma. *ADC,* Apparent diffusion coefficient.

tumor bed. Consequently, adequate marking of the original tumor is necessary. In smaller and bulky cancers, a single marker in the center of the lesion may be adequate. In larger lesions, bracketing the cancer area or marking the dominant tumor areas is a must.[85]

In follow-up of patients treated with neoadjuvant surgery, imaging and particularly MRI may guide the subsequent surgery, by indicating the level of response of the tumor and the extent of residual disease. For this, it is important to look at late-phase images, as the vasculature also lessens due to neoadjuvant therapy, and hence enhancement slows.[86] Moreover, when showing a radiological complete response, it is essential to realize that MRI is more trustworthy in HER2+ and TN cancers than in luminal tumors[87,88] (Fig. 2.11). In general, MRI

alone is not sufficient to obviate surgery.[89] However, studies are continuing to explore biopsy methods to detect residual disease and obviate surgery.[90]

Assessment of the axillary lymph nodes is an integral part of cancer staging. Often this is already done at the time of biopsy. The method of choice for the evaluation of the axilla is ultrasound, as lymph nodes are quite recognizable, and the very high resolution can be used to evaluate the cortex in which metastasis is located. A normal lymph node has a fatty hilum and a thin cortex. In clearly pathological lymph nodes, the hilum is compressed or obliterated, but most often the cortex is only slightly thickened. Biopsy of lymph nodes with a cortex thickness of more than 2.3 to 3 mm is done to also detect small lymph node metastasis.[91] This cannot exclude the presence

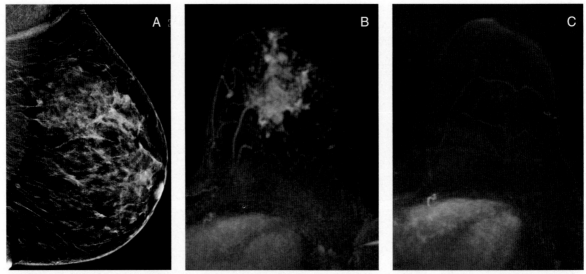

Fig. 2.11 55-year-old woman presenting with left nipple retraction. (A) In the MLO mammogram of the left breast, there is an architectural distortion at 12 o'clock. Biopsy under ultrasound guidance revealed an invasive lobular cancer. Magnetic resonance imaging (MRI) was performed for staging (B), showing that there is a very large diffuse tumor behind the nipple in the left breast. The woman was treated with neoadjuvant chemotherapy, and the follow-up MRI was rated as a radiological complete response (C). However, there was an almost 5-cm residual tumor remaining at final histopathology, which is quite typical for treatment of ILC with neoadjuvant chemotherapy. *ILC,* Invasive lobular carcinoma; *MLO,* mediolateral oblique.

of lymph node metastasis but is quite useful when cancer is detected. Because neoadjuvant therapy is also capable of downstaging the axilla, the presence of axillary metastasis is an additional justification to select a neoadjuvant versus adjuvant treatment strategy. It can eventually prevent axillary nodal clearance (lymph node dissection) and the associated morbidity. Accordingly, marking of axillary lymph nodes that are proven affected is essential, as these can be removed after neoadjuvant therapy to prove the complete response of the tumor in the lymph nodes.[92] Considering the fact that studies like AMAROS and Z011 showed that axillary clearance is not necessary when sentinel lymph node biopsy shows at most two positive lymph nodes,[93,94] it is very likely that in women without pathological lymph nodes on ultrasound, all axillary surgery (including sentinel lymph node biopsy) may be spared, which would eventually lead to even less morbid therapy. However, studies confirming whether this approach is safe are still ongoing, and results should be awaited.[95] Neither mammography nor MRI has a large role in the assessment of the axilla. However, MRI does show the whole thoracic area, and in case of clearly abnormal nodes

either in the axilla or along the intramammary lymph node chain, these should be investigated. A negative MRI has similar to a negative ultrasound a quite high negative predictive power for pN2 disease.[96]

DWI of the Breast

It is against the aforementioned backdrop that the role of DWI in the breast should be appreciated. Its potential applications will be discussed within the context of this book. For the moment, it is strongly advocated for improving lesion discrimination in MRI. In this context it has been shown to lead to a reduction in the need for biopsy, as it enables to classify a proportion of suspicious lesions on contrast-enhanced MRI as certainly benign. Still, most women with abnormalities in the breast do not undergo breast MRI for lesion classification when biopsy can be performed, and this is unlikely to change unless biopsy can be avoided in the large majority of women, which is currently not yet the case.

Clearly DWI would be valuable in MRI screening, where it may reduce recall rates. However, there is some tension in the fact that for cost-effectiveness, current screening breast MRI protocols are limited to minimal acquisition time. When image quality can be substantially improved and standardized, however, DWI may offer a very interesting approach for non-contrast-enhanced screening. In women with proven breast cancer, DWI may be used to evaluate additional findings on staging MRI and prevent needless biopsies for supplemental findings. Moreover, it can provide more certainty about the actual spread of the cancer and provide valuable quantitative data for cancer classification and therapeutic assessment. To what extent that can be used to better tailor therapy remains to be seen. The current status and future perspectives will be discussed to a much further extent in the remainder of this book.

REFERENCES

1. Gennaro G, Bernardi D, Houssami N. Radiation dose with digital breast tomosynthesis compared to digital mammography: per-view analysis. *Eur Radiol.* 2018;28(2):573–581.
2. Zuley ML. The basics and implementation of digital mammography. *Radiol Clin N Am.* 2010;48(5):893–901.
3. Perry N, Broeders M, de Wolf C, Törnberg S, Holland R, von Karsa L. European guidelines for quality assurance in breast cancer screening and diagnosis. Fourth edition—summary document. *Ann Oncol.* 2008;19(4):614–622.
4. Burke JP, Power C, Gorey TF, Flanagan F, Kerin MJ, Kell MR. A comparative study of risk factors and prognostic features between symptomatic and screen detected breast cancer. *Eur J Surg Oncol.* 2008;34(2):149–153.
5. Tot T, Gere M, Hofmeyer S, Bauer A, Pellas U. The clinical value of detecting microcalcifications on a mammogram. *Semin Cancer Biol.* 2021;72:165–174.
6. Sechopoulos I. A review of breast tomosynthesis. Part I. The image acquisition process. *Med Phys.* 2013;40(1):014301.
7. Skaane P, Bandos AI, Eben EB, et al. Two-view digital breast tomosynthesis screening with synthetically reconstructed projection images: comparison with digital breast tomosynthesis with full-field digital mammographic images. *Radiology.* 2014;271(3):655–663.
8. D'Orsi CJ, Sickles EA, Mendelson EB, et al. ACR BI-RADS® Atlas, Breast Imaging Reporting and Data System. American College of Radiology; 2013.
9. Holland K, van Zelst J, den Heeten GJ, et al. Consistency of breast density categories in serial screening mammograms: a comparison between automated and human assessment. *Breast.* 2016;29:49–54.
10. Boyd NF, Guo H, Martin LJ, et al. Mammographic density and the risk and detection of breast cancer. *N Engl J Med.* 2007;356(3):227–236.
11. Aldrich JE. Basic physics of ultrasound imaging. *Crit Care Med.* 2007;35(5 suppl):S131–S137.
12. Dempsey PJ. The history of breast ultrasound. *J Ultrasound Med.* 2004;23(7):887–894.
13. Candelaria RP, Hwang L, Bouchard RR, Whitman GJ. Breast ultrasound: current concepts. *Semin Ultrasound CT MR.* 2013;34(3):213–225.
14. Evans A, Trimboli RM, Athanasiou A, et al. Breast ultrasound: recommendations for information to women and referring physicians by the European Society of Breast Imaging. *Insights Imaging.* 2018;9(4):449–461.
15. Mehta TS, Raza S, Baum JK. Use of Doppler ultrasound in the evaluation of breast carcinoma. *Semin Ultrasound CT MR.* 2000;21(4):297–307.
16. Heywang SH, Hahn D, Schmidt H, et al. MR imaging of the breast using gadolinium-DTPA. *J Comput Assist Tomogr.* 1986;10(2):199–204.
17. Kaiser W. MRI of the female breast. First clinical results. *Arch Int Physiol Biochim.* 1985;93(5):67–76.
18. Carmeliet P, Jain RK. Angiogenesis in cancer and other diseases. *Nature.* 2000;407(6801):249–257.
19. Knopp MV, Weiss E, Sinn HP, et al. Pathophysiologic basis of contrast enhancement in breast tumors. *J Magn Reson Imaging.* 1999;10(3):260–266.
20. Kuhl CK, Mielcareck P, Klaschik S, et al. Dynamic breast MR imaging: are signal intensity time course data useful for differential diagnosis of enhancing lesions? *Radiology.* 1999;211(1):101–110.
21. Mann RM, Cho N, Moy L. Breast MRI: state of the art. *Radiology.* 2019;292(3):520–536.
22. Liao GJ, Henze Bancroft LC, Strigel RM, et al. Background parenchymal enhancement on breast MRI: A comprehensive review. *J Magn Reson Imaging.* 2020;51(1):43–61.
23. Mann RM, Mus RD, van Zelst J, Geppert C, Karssemeijer N, Platel B. A novel approach to contrast-enhanced breast magnetic resonance imaging for screening: high-resolution ultrafast dynamic imaging. *Invest Radiol.* 2014;49(9):579–585.
24. Santamaría G, Velasco M, Bargalló X, Caparrós X, Farrús B, Luis Fernández P. Radiologic and pathologic findings in breast tumors with high signal intensity on T2-weighted MR images. *Radiographics.* 2010;30(2):533–548.
25. Sanderink WBG, Mann RM. Advances in breast intervention: where are we now and where should we be? *Clin Radiol.* 2018;73(8):724–734.
26. Bick U, Trimboli RM, Athanasiou A, et al. Image-guided breast biopsy and localisation: recommendations for information to women and referring physicians by the European Society of Breast Imaging. *Insights Imaging.* 2020;11(1):12.
27. Heywang-Köbrunner SH, Heinig A, Hellerhoff K, Holzhausen HJ, Nährig J. Use of ultrasound-guided percutaneous vacuum-assisted breast biopsy for selected difficult indications. *Breast J.* 2009;15(4):348–356.
28. Mathew J, Crawford DJ, Lwin M, Barwick C, Gash A. Ultrasound-guided, vacuum-assisted excision in the diagnosis and treatment of clinically benign breast lesions. *Ann R Coll Surg Engl.* 2007;89(5):494–496.
29. Rochat CJ, Baird GL, Lourenco AP. Digital mammography stereotactic biopsy versus digital breast tomosynthesis-guided biopsy: differences in biopsy targets, pathologic results, and discordance rates. *Radiology.* 2020;294(3):518–527.
30. den Dekker BM, van Diest PJ, de Waard SN, Verkooijen HM, Pijnappel RM. Stereotactic 9-gauge vacuum-assisted breast biopsy, how many specimens are needed? *Eur J Radiol.* 2019;120:108665.
31. Santiago L, Candelaria RP, Huang ML. MR imaging-guided breast interventions: indications, key principles, and imaging-pathology correlation. *Magn Reson Imaging Clin N Am.* 2018;26(2):235–246.
32. Wilson JMG, Junger G. Principles and Practice of Screening for Disease. *World Health Organisation.* 1968.

33. Bray F, Ferlay J, Soerjomataram I, Siegel RL, Torre LA, Jemal A. Global cancer statistics 2018: GLOBOCAN estimates of incidence and mortality worldwide for 36 cancers in 185 countries. *CA Cancer J Clin.* 2018;68(6):394–424.

34. Marmot MG, Altman DG, Cameron DA, Dewar JA, Thompson SG, Wilcox M. The benefits and harms of breast cancer screening: an independent review. *Lancet.* 2012;380(9855):1778–1786.

35. Broeders M, Moss S, Nyström L, et al. The impact of mammographic screening on breast cancer mortality in Europe: a review of observational studies. *J Med Screen.* 2012;19(suppl 1): 14–25.

36. Nelson HD, Pappas M, Cantor A, Griffin J, Daeges M, Humphrey L. Harms of breast cancer screening: systematic review to update the 2009 U.S. Preventive Services Task Force recommendation. *Ann Intern Med.* 2016;164(4):256–267.

37. Wallis MG. How do we manage overdiagnosis/overtreatment in breast screening? *Clin Radiol.* 2018;73(4):372–380.

38. Brewer NT, Salz T, Lillie SE. Systematic review: the long-term effects of false-positive mammograms. *Ann Intern Med.* 2007;146(7):502–510.

39. Kuhl CK. Underdiagnosis is the main challenge in breast cancer screening. *Lancet Oncol.* 2019;20(8):1044–1046.

40. Alabousi M, Wadera A, Kashif Al-Ghita M, et al. Performance of digital breast tomosynthesis, synthetic mammography and digital mammography in breast cancer screening: a systematic review and meta-analysis. *J Natl Cancer Inst.* 2021;113(6):680–690.

41. Johnson K, Lång K, Ikeda DM, Åkesson A, Andersson I, Zackrisson S. Interval breast cancer rates and tumor characteristics in the prospective population-based Malmö Breast Tomosynthesis Screening Trial. *Radiology.* 2021;299(3):559–567.

42. Tagliafico AS, Calabrese M, Bignotti B, et al. Accuracy and reading time for six strategies using digital breast tomosynthesis in women with mammographically negative dense breasts. *Eur Radiol.* 2017;27(12):5179–5184.

43. Berg WA, Blume JD, Cormack JB, et al. Combined screening with ultrasound and mammography vs mammography alone in women at elevated risk of breast cancer. *JAMA.* 2008;299(18):2151–2163.

44. Vourtsis A, Berg WA. Breast density implications and supplemental screening. *Eur Radiol.* 2019;29(4):1762–1777.

45. Tagliafico AS, Mariscotti G, Valdora F, et al. A prospective comparative trial of adjunct screening with tomosynthesis or ultrasound in women with mammography-negative dense breasts (ASTOUND-2). *Eur J Cancer.* 2018;104:39–46.

46. Ohuchi N, Suzuki A, Sobue T, et al. Sensitivity and specificity of mammography and adjunctive ultrasonography to screen for breast cancer in the Japan Strategic Anti-cancer Randomized Trial (J-START): a randomised controlled trial. *Lancet.* 2016;387(10016):341–348.

47. Lee JM, Arao RF, Sprague BL, et al. Performance of screening ultrasonography as an adjunct to screening mammography in women across the spectrum of breast cancer risk. *JAMA Intern Med.* 2019;179(5):658–667.

48. Mann RM, Kuhl CK, Moy L, Contrast-enhanced MRI. for breast cancer screening. *J Magn Reson Imaging.* 2019;50(2):377–390.

49. Saslow D, Boetes C, Burke W, et al. American Cancer Society guidelines for breast screening with MRI as an adjunct to mammography. *CA Cancer J Clin.* 2007;57(2):75–89.

50. Geuzinge HA, Obdeijn IM, Rutgers EJT, et al. Cost-effectiveness of breast cancer screening with magnetic resonance imaging for women at familial risk. *JAMA Oncol.* 2020;6(9):1381–1389.

51. Cho N, Han W, Han BK, et al. Breast cancer screening with mammography plus ultrasonography or magnetic resonance imaging in women 50 years or younger at diagnosis and treated with breast conservation therapy. *JAMA Oncol.* 2017;3(11):1495–1502.

52. Schwartz T, Cyr A, Margenthaler J. Screening breast magnetic resonance imaging in women with atypia or lobular carcinoma in situ. *J Surg Res.* 2015;193(2):519–522.

53. Kuhl CK, Strobel K, Bieling H, Leutner C, Schild HH, Schrading S. Supplemental breast MR imaging screening of women with average risk of breast cancer. *Radiology.* 2017;283(2):361–370.

54. Bakker MF, de Lange SV, Pijnappel RM, et al. Supplemental MRI screening for women with extremely dense breast tissue. *N Engl J Med.* 2019;381(22):2091–2102.

55. Veenhuizen SGA, de Lange SV, Bakker MF, et al. Supplemental breast MRI for women with extremely dense breasts—results of the second screening round of the DENSE trial. *Radiology.* 2021;299(2):278–286.

56. Vreemann S, van Zelst JCM, Schlooz-Vries M, et al. The added value of mammography in different age-groups of women with and without BRCA mutation screened with breast MRI. *Breast Cancer Res.* 2018;20(1):84.

57. Sardanelli F, Podo F, Santoro F, et al. Multicenter surveillance of women at high genetic breast cancer risk using mammography, ultrasonography, and contrast-enhanced magnetic resonance imaging (the high breast cancer risk Italian 1 study): final results. *Invest Radiol.* 2011;46(2):94–105.

58. Riedl CC, Luft N, Bernhart C, et al. Triple-modality screening trial for familial breast cancer underlines the importance of magnetic resonance imaging and questions the role of mammography and ultrasound regardless of patient mutation status, age, and breast density. *J Clin Oncol.* 2015;33(10):1128–1135.

59. Leithner D, Moy L, Morris EA, Marino MA, Helbich TH, Pinker K. Abbreviated MRI of the breast: does it provide value? *J Magn Reson Imaging.* 2019;49(7):e85–e100.

60. Comstock CE, Gatsonis C, Newstead GM, et al. Comparison of abbreviated breast MRI vs digital breast tomosynthesis for breast cancer detection among women with dense breasts undergoing screening. *JAMA.* 2020;323(8):746–756.

61. Appelman L, Appelman PTM, Siebers CCN, et al. The value of mammography in women with focal breast complaints in addition to initial targeted ultrasound. *Breast Cancer Res Treat.* 2021;185(2):381–389.

62. Lehman CD, Lee CI, Loving VA, Portillo MS, Peacock S, DeMartini WB. Accuracy and value of breast ultrasound for primary imaging evaluation of symptomatic women 30-39 years of age. *AJR Am J Roentgenol.* 2012;199(5):1169–1177.

63. Houssami N, Ciatto S, Irwig L, Simpson JM, Macaskill P. The comparative sensitivity of mammography and ultrasound in women with breast symptoms: an age-specific analysis. *Breast.* 2002;11(2):125–130.

64. Feig SA. Breast masses. Mammographic and sonographic evaluation. *Radiol Clin N Am.* 1992;30(1):67–92.

65. Gupta D, Mendelson EB, Karst I. Nipple discharge: current clinical and imaging evaluation. *AJR Am J Roentgenol.* 2021;216(2):330–339.

66. Kapetas P, Clauser P, Woitek R, et al. Quantitative multiparametric breast ultrasound: application of contrast-enhanced ultrasound and elastography leads to an improved differentiation of benign and malignant lesions. *Invest Radiol.* 2019;54(5):257–264.

67. Neuschler EI, Butler R, Young CA, et al. A Pivotal study of optoacoustic imaging to diagnose benign and malignant breast masses: a new evaluation tool for radiologists. *Radiology*. 2018;287(2):398–412.

68. Bennani-Baiti B, Bennani-Baiti N, Baltzer PA. Diagnostic performance of breast magnetic resonance imaging in non-calcified equivocal breast findings: results from a systematic review and meta-analysis. *PLoS One*. 2016;11(8):e0160346.

69. Spick C, Baltzer PA. Diagnostic utility of second-look US for breast lesions identified at MR imaging: systematic review and meta-analysis. *Radiology*. 2014;273(2):401–409.

70. Brennan ME, Houssami N, Lord S, et al. Magnetic resonance imaging screening of the contralateral breast in women with newly diagnosed breast cancer: systematic review and meta-analysis of incremental cancer detection and impact on surgical management. *J Clin Oncol*. 2009;27(33):5640–5649.

71. Lehman CD, Gatsonis C, Kuhl CK, et al. MRI evaluation of the contralateral breast in women with recently diagnosed breast cancer. *N Engl J Med*. 2007;356(13):1295–1303.

72. Giuliano AE, Connolly JL, Edge SB, et al. Breast cancer—major changes in the American Joint Committee on Cancer eighth edition cancer staging manual. *CA: Cancer J Clin*. 2017;67(4):290–303.

73. Luparia A, Mariscotti G, Durando M, et al. Accuracy of tumour size assessment in the preoperative staging of breast cancer: comparison of digital mammography, tomosynthesis, ultrasound and MRI. *Radiol Med*. 2013;118(7):1119–1136.

74. Ramirez SI, Scholle M, Buckmaster J, Paley RH, Kowdley GC. Breast cancer tumor size assessment with mammography, ultrasonography, and magnetic resonance imaging at a community based multidisciplinary breast center. *Am Surg*. 2012;78(4):440–446.

75. Holland R, Veling SH, Mravunac M, Hendriks JH. Histologic multifocality of Tis, T1-2 breast carcinomas. Implications for clinical trials of breast-conserving surgery. *Cancer*. 1985;56(1):979–990.

76. Sardanelli F Preoperative staging with MRI: did the MIPA trial solve all issues? Insights into Imaging - ECR 2018 - BOOK OF ABSTRACTS. 92018:106..

77. Mann RM, Veltman J, Barentsz JO, Wobbes T, Blickman JG, Boetes C. The value of MRI compared to mammography in the assessment of tumour extent in invasive lobular carcinoma of the breast. *Eur J Surg Oncol*. 2008;34(2):135–142.

78. Wong SM, Prakash I, Trabulsi N, et al. Evaluating the impact of breast density on preoperative MRI in invasive lobular carcinoma. *J Am Coll Surg*. 2018;226(5):925–932.

79. Curigliano G, Burstein HJ, P Winer E, et al. De-escalating and escalating treatments for early-stage breast cancer: the St. Gallen International Expert Consensus Conference on the Primary Therapy of Early Breast Cancer 2017. *Ann Oncol*. 2019;30(7):1181.

80. Wu J, Sun X, Wang J, et al. Identifying relations between imaging phenotypes and molecular subtypes of breast cancer: model discovery and external validation. *J Magn Reson Imaging*. 2017;46(4):1017–1027.

81. Yoo EY, Nam SY, Choi HY, Hong MJ. Agreement between MRI and pathologic analyses for determination of tumor size and correlation with immunohistochemical factors of invasive breast carcinoma. *Acta Radiol*. 2018;59(1):50–57.

82. Gillies RJ, Balagurunathan Y. Perfusion MR imaging of breast cancer: insights using "habitat imaging." *Radiology*. 2018;288(1):36–37.

83. Chaudhury B, Zhou M, Goldgof DB, et al. Heterogeneity in intratumoral regions with rapid gadolinium washout correlates with estrogen receptor status and nodal metastasis. *J Magn Reson Imaging*. 2015;42(5):1421–1430.

84. Pinker K, Chin J, Melsaether AN, Morris EA, Moy L. Precision medicine and radiogenomics in breast cancer: new approaches toward diagnosis and treatment. *Radiology*. 2018;287(3):732–747.

85. Dash N, Chafin SH, Johnson RR, Contractor FM. Usefulness of tissue marker clips in patients undergoing neoadjuvant chemotherapy for breast cancer. *AJR Am J Roentgenol*. 1999; 173(4):911–917.

86. Kim SY, Cho N, Park IA, et al. Dynamic contrast-enhanced breast MRI for evaluating residual tumor size after neoadjuvant chemotherapy. *Radiology*. 2018;289(2):327–334.

87. Loo CE, Straver ME, Rodenhuis S, et al. Magnetic resonance imaging response monitoring of breast cancer during neoadjuvant chemotherapy: relevance of breast cancer subtype. *J Clin Oncol*. 2011;29(6):660–666.

88. van Ramshorst MS, Loo CE, Groen EJ, et al. MRI predicts pathologic complete response in HER2-positive breast cancer after neoadjuvant chemotherapy. *Breast Cancer Res Treat*. 2017;164(1):99–106.

89. Yu N, Leung VWY, Meterissian S. MRI performance in detecting pCR after neoadjuvant chemotherapy by molecular subtype of breast cancer. *World J Surg*. 2019;43(9):2254–2261.

90. Heil J, Kuerer HM, Pfob A, et al. Eliminating the breast cancer surgery paradigm after neoadjuvant systemic therapy: current evidence and future challenges. *Ann Oncol*. 2020;31(1):61–71.

91. Schipper RJ, van Roozendaal LM, de Vries B, et al. Axillary ultrasound for preoperative nodal staging in breast cancer patients: is it of added value? *Breast*. 2013;22(6):1108–1113.

92. Donker M, Straver ME, Wesseling J, et al. Marking axillary lymph nodes with radioactive iodine seeds for axillary staging after neoadjuvant systemic treatment in breast cancer patients: the MARI procedure. *Ann Surg*. 2015;261(2):378–382.

93. Giuliano AE, Ballman KV, McCall L, et al. Effect of axillary dissection vs no axillary dissection on 10-year overall survival among women with invasive breast cancer and sentinel node metastasis: the ACOSOG Z0011 (Alliance) Randomized Clinical Trial. *JAMA*. 2017;318(10):918–926.

94. Boughey JC. How do the AMAROS trial results change practice? *Lancet Oncol*. 2014;15(12):1280–1281.

95. Reimer T, Engel J, Schmidt M, Offersen BV, Smidt ML, Gentilini OD. Is axillary sentinel lymph node biopsy required in patients who undergo primary breast surgery? *Breast Care (Basel)*. 2018;13(5):324–330.

96. van Nijnatten TJA, Ploumen EH, Schipper RJ, et al. Routine use of standard breast MRI compared to axillary ultrasound for differentiating between no, limited and advanced axillary nodal disease in newly diagnosed breast cancer patients. *Eur J Radiol*. 2016;85(12):2288–2294.

Overview of Breast DWI: Diagnosis of Suspicious Lesions Using DWI in Combination With Standard MRI

Pascal A. T. Baltzer, MD

The Need for Reducing Unnecessary Biopsies in Breast MRI

Dynamic contrast-enhanced (DCE) magnetic resonance imaging (MRI) of the breast—referred to as standard breast MRI throughout this chapter—is considered the most sensitive test for diagnosis of malignant breast lesions.[1-3] Standard breast MRI relies on highlighting tumor vasculature by means of intravenously applied gadolinium (Gd)-based contrast media. Because (biologically active) cancers require nutrients, a complex cascade of cytokines induces the growth of new vessels, a process known as neoangiogenesis.[4] This ensures that practically all breast cancers show contrast uptake on DCE MRI images. A lack of enhancement in a technically adequate breast MRI examination excludes biologically significant breast cancer with high certainty. Nonenhancing breast cancers are uncommon,[5] and the negative predictive value of a negative MRI scan for invasive breast cancer has been reported as 99% in two meta-analyses.[6,7] The high sensitivity is the reason why—besides classical indications, such as high-risk screening and staging and therapy monitoring of breast cancer—breast MRI is gaining increasing acceptance for applications of problem-solving and intermediate risk screening.[1,8-10] On the other hand, enhancement itself is not specific: benign ductal proliferation and ductal carcinoma in situ (DCIS) can show similar patterns of angiogenesis as invasive breast cancer.[11-13] Breast MRI reporting according to the Breast Imaging Reporting and Data System (BI-RADS) lexicon is standardized, but BI-RADS does not include a clinical decision rule such as PI-RADS for the prostate.[14,15] The lack of formal guidance makes breast MRI interpretation a subjective, experience-dependent task.[16] In addition, BI-RADS semantic features contain redundant information[17] and show significant overlap between benign and malignant lesions.[18,19] Insecurity of the reporting physician will lead to biopsy and follow-up recommendations that are ultimately unnecessary. False-positive findings pose a challenge to the broad implementation of breast MRI, as the availability of MRI-guided biopsy facilities is limited, and cost-effectiveness of supplemental breast MRI screening in women with dense breasts critically depends on MRI specificity.[8,20]

Diffusion-weighted imaging (DWI) can help with this clinical problem: it provides additional quantitative information that is fast to acquire. Malignant neoplastic tissue changes cause a characteristic decrease in water diffusivity as measured by the apparent diffusion coefficient (ADC) in standard DWI. This can be put to clinical use, as the probability of cancer decreases with increasing ADC values, so that breast cancer can be excluded practically beyond a certain ADC threshold.

DWI and the ADC in Clinical Practice

CHOICE OF *b* VALUES

The general physical principle of DWI is covered in Chapter 1 in this book. From a clinical perspective, DWI is a technique sensitive to the molecular (Brownian) motion of water and, in some circumstances, the "pseudoincoherent motion" caused by flowing blood in small vessels (perfusion).[21] To assess water diffusion in a quantitative manner, at least two sets of images must be acquired. The first set of images is a non- (or very low) diffusion-weighted image with recommended b values of 0 (or at least lower than 50) s/mm^2. As the clinical relevance of using nonzero low b values for suppressing signal from larger vessels in the breast is less evident than in the liver, for example, there is no clear benefit of using b50 s/mm^2 instead of b0 s/mm^2 images. The second set of images is diffusion weighted, and a b value of 800 s/mm^2 is currently recommended. This b value is determinant for the DWI contrast level and the calculated ADC value. The simple diffusion model used for DWI assumes a monoexponential signal loss, independent of the choice of b value, assuming free (not hindered) water diffusion. However, in tissues, water diffusion is highly hindered, which results in a decrease of the amount of signal loss when the b value increases. This hindrance is what makes DWI so sensitive to changes in tissue microstructure, as seen in tumors, but it also implies that choice of b values is a major issue for DWI acquisition standardization. Other less important issues for standardization are the pulse gradient setup and timing, which might also affect the ADC to some degree. It is recommended to perform the acquisition of DWI before contrast medium injection, as the local background magnetic gradient created by Gd-filled vessels might result in small ADC underestimation.[22,23] However, this effect has not been shown to be clinically significant in measuring breast lesion ADC, so that the acquisition of DWI after DCE MRI might be acceptable when clinically necessary. Calculation of the ADC is usually automatically performed by scanner software; the main adjustment that can be performed is a low b value filter that ignores voxels with a base signal below the chosen arbitrary value. This reduces noisy voxels, including those covering suppressed fat signal, but it may make anatomical orientation and correlation with anatomical images difficult. The ADC map itself is a parametric map, the signal intensity of each voxel corresponds to an ADC value that can be considered a spatially resolved quantitative imaging biomarker.

INTEGRATING DWI IN THE OVERALL MULTIPARAMETRIC BREAST MRI PROTOCOL

A standard breast MRI protocol comprises T2- and T1-weighted MRI sequences, the latter being repeated

as a part of the DCE protocol. DWI usually comes as an added MRI sequence that should ideally be performed before DCE.[23,24] DWI should be performed in axial orientation using an echo-planar imaging (EPI) sequence. Recommended acquisition parameters are a repetition time (TR) of ≥3000 ms, a minimal echo time (TE), an in-plane resolution ≤2 × 2 mm^2, a slice thickness ≤4 mm, and application of parallel imaging to reduce image distortion. Fat suppression is commonly incorporated in breast MRI sequences and is mandatory for DWI. There are different fat suppression techniques available, which vary in their robustness and signal-to-noise ratio (SNR). The spectrally adiabatic inversion recovery (SPAIR) technique has been recommended for breast DWI as the best compromise between signal and robustness.[25] T2-weighted acquisitions can be acquired with an acquisition time of 2 to 4 minutes. Although some authors suggested that $b = 0$ images with submillimeter resolution (using 7T MRI) might be used as a replacement of T2w images—providing the T2-weighted contrast while saving on acquisition times—currently, low b value images acquired at 1.5T and 3T cannot replace T2-weighted TSE images.[25] The total DWI sequence can be acquired within 2 to 4 minutes only if the relevant two b values are acquired. The central part of the breast MRI protocol is a DCE T1-weighted sequence acquired before and several times after contrast (see Chapter 2). This sequence is used to identify lesions, and in addition to the enhancement curve type, most other BI-RADS features are obtained from these images. The higher the temporal resolution, the higher the degree of information available from signal intensity curve type analysis, and the higher the spatial resolution, the higher the amount of diagnostic data available from contrast enhancement morphology. The necessary trade-off in clinical practice usually does favor spatial over temporal resolution, though there are multiple acceleration techniques able to alleviate this loss of temporal resolution. There are only loose recommendations regarding how the technique should be acquired, but usually 5 minutes postcontrast scanning suffices to identify wash-out curves and enhancement heterogeneity[24] (see Chapter 2). Further techniques, such as MR spectroscopy and T1 or T2 mapping, are currently not recommended in standard protocols due

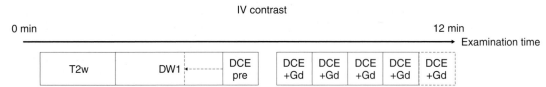

Fig. 3.1 Typical multiparametric breast magnetic resonance imaging (MRI) protocol combining T2w, DWI, and DCE acquisitions. After a localizer of less than 1 minute, an anatomical axial T2w sequence is acquired. Using a long echo time of >170 ms and no fat suppression, an acquisition time of around 2 minutes is feasible. The DWI sequence is assumed here with an acquisition time of 4 minutes, which can be shortened if the need arises *(dashed line and arrow)*. It is immediately followed by a standard clinical T1w sequence for dynamic imaging with an assumed temporal resolution of 1 minute. After the precontrast scan, IV contrast is given, and after an injection delay of 30 seconds, postcontrast scanning continues over 5 minutes; again, that may possibly be shortened by 1 minute *(dashed line)*. The total protocol should thus not take more than around 12 minutes magnet time, and it has been successfully used in the last decade. *DCE*, Dynamic contrast enhancing; *DWI*, diffusion-weighted imaging; *IV*, intravenous. (As described in Dietzel M, Baltzer PAT. How to use the Kaiser score as a clinical decision rule for diagnosis in multiparametric breast MRI: a pictorial essay. *Insights Imaging.* 2018;9:325–335. https://doi.org/10.1007/s13244-018-0611-8.)

to the lack of consensus regarding their integration in multiparametric protocols, while their incremental diagnostic value is not entirely clear.[9,24,26–28] A full multiparametric breast MRI therefore can take less than 15 minutes in total acquisition time,[24] as shown in Fig. 3.1.

Analysis of DWI Images

QUALITATIVE ASSESSMENT

What diagnostic information does the DWI sequence provide? As malignant lesions show a typical diffusion hindrance, they appear of intermediate to high signal on high b value ($b \geq 800\,s/mm^2$) images. Though the appearance of malignant lesions on DWI is highly variable regarding shape, margins, and mass-like features and thus not very specific, these images could be used to potentially detect cancer lesions (see Chapter 6). This use of DWI is hampered by the fact that not only malignant lesions show high signal on high b value DWI images: complicated cysts with bloody, putrid, or proteinaceous content all show high to very high signal and may thus impair the ability of the reading physician to identify breast cancer, and some cancers are not visible on DWI images. Therefore cancer detection currently relies on the contrast-enhanced T1w images. DWI can further provide fluid-sensitive T2w contrast on low b value (e.g., $b = 0\,s/mm^2$) images, similar to that of the T2w sequence though usually at lower image quality and spatial resolution, which may be helpful to identify cysts, edema, and masses with very high signal intensity that often represent benign fibroadenoma. Finally, DWI provides the ADC map in

which diffusivity may be assessed quantitatively. For this purpose, the DWI images are carefully compared with the contrast-enhanced and T2w images in order to localize the lesion.

QUANTITATIVE ASSESSMENT: DOWNGRADING SUSPICIOUS CONTRAST-ENHANCING LESIONS BY MEANS OF THE ADC

Quantitative assessment of ADC maps requires drawing a region of interest (ROI) around the lesion either directly on the ADC map or copied from DWI images.[24,29,30] The positioning of the ROI may greatly influence ADC measurements, so ROIs must be placed with great care to avoid cystic or necrotic areas and rather target the biologically most active parts of the lesions. Malignant lesions show a typical diffusion hindrance reflected by low ADC values, whereas a substantial number of benign lesions present with high ADC values.[31] But how can the ADC be put to use in clinical practice? The dilemma is the same as with other diagnostic features: does the absence of diffusion hindrance overrule a suspicious wash-out curve type? Should a lesion presenting with a low ADC value be biopsied despite benign morphological features and curve type? The ultimate aim in breast imaging to detect as many cancers as possible while keeping the costs as low as possible in terms of false-positive biopsy and follow-up recommendations.[32] As the sensitivity of contrast-enhanced MRI is without question, reducing false-positive findings without compromising sensitivity is what best describes the clinical need. A number of authors have addressed the topic. The most straightforward approach is applying a high ADC cutoff value above which a lesion is automatically downgraded, thereby omitting biopsy. More complicated algorithms adapting the ADC threshold to the specific lesion type and contrast-enhanced MRI BI-RADS category assignment were also successfully developed and tested[33,34] (Fig. 3.2).

The feasibility of such thresholds has been proven multiple times in small single-center studies, but the suggested ADC cutoffs varied, and the community

discussed whether extensive standardization procedures are required before a general ADC threshold can be recommended. One issue is the choice of b value, as explained earlier. Other factors, such as the diffusion gradient timing, the amount of image noise and the applied noise filters, insufficient fat suppression, and so forth can potentially confound the ADC.[23] A study investigating the influence of different software calculating the ADC of the same DWI acquisitions found

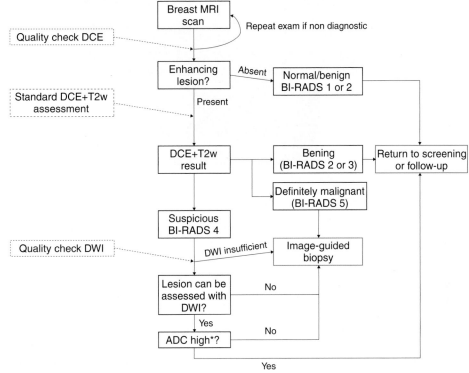

Fig. 3.2 Flowchart demonstrating the current place of DWI in the reading process of a breast magnetic resonance imaging (MRI) examination in clinical practice. Before the breast MRI is read, a basic quality check ensures that the DCE sequence is of diagnostic quality. Nondiagnostic examinations due to a misinjection of IV contrast or incomplete image acquisition due to premature termination of the examination or severe motion artifacts may require a repeat examination. The first step is to screen for enhancing lesions. For the sake of brevity, assessment of fibroglandular tissue, cysts, and background parenchymal enhancement is omitted here. If absent, the examination is considered negative in terms of possible breast cancer, and the patient is returned to screening or subjected to follow-up as clinically appropriate. If an enhancing lesion is present, regular assessment of the lesion by interpretation of morphological and kinetic features is performed, and a BI-RADS category is assigned. Benign lesions again are returned to screening or subjected to follow-up as clinically appropriate. Definitely malignant lesions (e.g., spiculated masses with wash-out enhancement curve) require immediate biopsy. In all these lesions, DWI is not really helpful to meaningfully influence the logical decision process and change clinical management. However, if an enhancing BI-RADS 4 lesion is identified, DWI can be used for further assessment of this lesion. First, DWI quality must be checked. If DWI quality is globally insufficient, the lesion must undergo biopsy. The same applies if DWI is of sufficient quality but cannot be located on DWI (i.e., DWI images and ADC map), for example, due to a very small finding or geometrical distortions, as the wrong area could be interrogated on the ADC map. If DWI is of sufficient quality and the lesion can be confidently located on DWI, the ADC is measured using an ROI.[23] If the ADC does exceed a threshold currently suggested around 1.3–1.5×10^{-3} mm^2/s,[23,35–37] the lesion could be downgraded and biopsy avoided. Whether a simplified categorization of ADC values[23] could be used for the same purpose has not been tested clinically yet. The patient is then subjected to follow-up imaging as clinically indicated. If the ADC is not high, biopsy is indicated, as malignancy cannot be excluded reliably. *ADC*, Apparent diffusion coefficient; *BI-RADS*, Breast Imaging Reporting and Data System; *DCE*, dynamic contrast enhancing; *DWI*, diffusion-weighted imaging; *IV*, intravenous; *ROI*, region of interest.

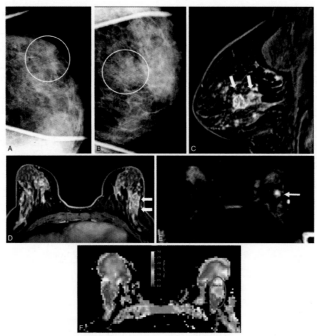

Fig. 3.3 Two clinical cases acquired in different institutions using different magnetic resonance imaging (MRI) equipment evident from differences in SNR, contrast, and spatial resolution. (A)–(C) A postmenopausal woman who underwent problem-solving MRI at 1.5T that revealed an early enhancing mass with heterogeneous internal enhancement and a feeding vessel (*arrow* in A; subtracted early T1w). On the ADC map (B, calculated from $b = 0\,s/mm^2$ and $b = 800\,s/mm^2$ with a high noise filter setting), the lesion is barely distinguishable from the breast parenchyma, whereas the $b = 800\,s/mm^2$ image shows the lesion as hyperintense (*arrow* in C). The ADC value was $1.73 \times 10^{-3}\,mm^2/s$. Because of an elevated risk for breast cancer, the patient received a biopsy that revealed a benign fibroadenoma. (D)–(F) A perimenopausal patient who underwent assessment of findings in the right contralateral breast. The 3T scan revealed a heterogeneous regional nonmass enhancement (*dashed circle* in A; early contrast-enhanced T1w subtraction). The corresponding ADC map showed the enhancing parts of the nonmass lesion as hypointense compared with the breast parenchyma (B, ADC map calculated from $b = 50\,s/mm^2$ and $b = 800\,s/mm^2$ with a low noise filter setting), whereas the calculated $b = 1600\,s/mm^2$ image (C) reveals a modest hyperintensity. The corresponding ADC values were measured as $1.55 \times 10^{-3}\,mm^2/s$ and higher, pointing out benign changes. The patient requested an MRI-guided biopsy that revealed benign epithelial hyperplasia without atypia. *ADC*, Apparent diffusion coefficient; *SNR*, signal-to-noise ratio.

that interreader variation—meaning the manual placement of ROIs—was more important than variations in the reconstructed ADC.[38] Overall, reproducibility and repeatability of DWI measurements including quantitative ADC maps is high, as shown in an intraindividual comparison study.[39] The specific ADC cutoff is still debated: a value of $1.3 \times 10^{-3}\,mm^2/s$ has been suggested[25] to classify malignant versus benign lesions and decrease false positives in cancer detection. A recent prospective multicentric study identified a safe ADC cutoff value of $1.5 \times 10^{-3}\,mm^2/s$ to downgrade suspicious enhancing MRI lesions in which biopsy was recommended without missing any cancers.[36] This cutoff was confirmed in a large multicentric data set in which the DWI acquisition technique varied, thus

proving the immediate clinical applicability of a high ADC cutoff to downgrade BI-RADS 4 lesions even without in-depth standardization[37] (Fig. 3.3).

This does not mean that standardization in DWI acquisition is not an issue but rather that ADC values can be applied in clinical decision-making immediately. It goes without saying that improving DWI standardization will reduce variable rates of avoidable biopsies between centers and thus help use the full potential of DWI.[23,37] One step toward this goal might be a BI-RADS–analogous categorization of the ADC value[23] (Table 3.1). These categories could be helpful to simplify ADC interpretation similar to the categorization of enhancement time curves in DCE MRI of the breast.

TABLE 3.1 Categorization Proposal	
ADC Category[a]	**ADC Range (in 10^{-3} mm^2/s)**
Very low	≤ 0.9
Low	$>0.9-\leq1.3$
Intermediate	$>1.3-\leq1.7$
High (normal)	$>1.7-\leq2.1$
Very high	>2.1

[a]The categories comprise ADC ranges typically associated with cancer (very low), possibly malignant lesions (low), likely benign lesions (intermediate), normal breast tissue (high), and cysts (very high).
ADC, Apparent diffusion coefficient.
As suggested in Baltzer P, Mann RM, Iima M, et al; EUSOBI International Breast Diffusion-Weighted Imaging Working Group. Diffusion-weighted imaging of the breast—a consensus and mission statement from the EUSOBI International Breast Diffusion-Weighted Imaging Working Group. *Eur Radiol.* 2020;30:1436–1450. https://doi.org/10.1007/s00330-019-06510-3

Considerations for Implementing ADC Measurements in Clinical Practice

Though the ADC is a powerful quantitative imaging biomarker and its clinical value proven at a high level of evidence, its broad implementation faces certain challenges. The first is optimization and standardization of the image acquisition. EPI-based DWI requires fat suppression to minimize chemical shift and ghosting artifacts due to phase mismatch that may render the image or part of the image nondiagnostic.[40] Robustness and SNR of fat suppression techniques show a trade-off: spectral fat suppression shows high SNR and low robustness, whereas the short tau inversion recovery (STIR) technique provides high stability while providing limited SNR. Therefore the European Society of Breast Imaging (EUSOBI) International DWI Working Group recommends to use the SPAIR technique, which combines the advantages of both mentioned methods while avoiding most of the disadvantages.[23] The diffusion weighting is defined as the *b* value that is influenced by diffusion sensitizing gradient strength (G), duration (δ), and temporal spacing between these gradients (Δ). Most vendors, however, do not provide the opportunity to adjust these single parameters and,

subsequently, diffusion time. Though the resulting diffusion times for most clinical DWI sequences will be in the range of 50 to 100 ms, they will nevertheless vary, and thereby the resulting ADC will be influenced by varying degrees of diffusion hindrance and restriction.[41] More pronounced are potential differences if the *b* value itself is altered. Dorrius and colleagues investigated the effect of *b* values on the resulting ADC in a meta-analysis of 26 studies and demonstrated a decrease of ADC values with increasing *b* values.[22] They attributed this effect mainly to suppression of microperfusion effects,[22] though the increasing relevance of non-Gaussian diffusion has to be considered as well.[41] They further identified the largest difference between mean ADC values of benign and malignant lesions at 1000 s/mm^2, though diagnostic test performance did not differ from studies using, for example, $b = 800$ s/mm^2 (a value afterward recommended by the EUSOBI International Working Group[23]). Finally, Dorrius and colleagues investigated the effect of intravenous (IV) Gd-based contrast media on ADC values and did not find significant differences between DWI acquired before or after IV contrast.[22] Based on these findings, basic standardization would require a recommendation of *b* values as has been recognized by the EUSOBI International Working Group, who suggested to use two *b* values of 0 or 50 s/mm^2 and 800 s/mm^2 for ADC calculation.[23]

Second, variability of postprocessing and ADC quantitation methods is a challenge affecting overall diagnostic performance. An ADC map based on the same DWI source images may show minor variations if calculated by different software with different low *b* value noise filtering.[38,42] This bias, however, is negligible considering the larger intra- and interreader variation of ADC measurements from ADC maps even under controlled conditions.[38,39] One of the primary factors influencing ADC measurements is the choice of the ROI and the ADC metric (e.g., mean, minimum maximum): most combinations of ROI type and ADC metric show similar diagnostic performance, whereas quantitative ADC values and their reproducibility differ.[29] Although a recent systematic review and meta-analysis further investigated the topic and could not identify a preferred ROI method due to a lack of empirical evidence of one above the other,[30]

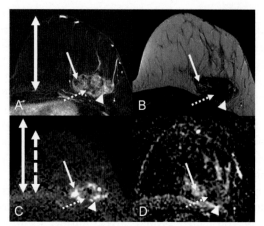

Fig. 3.4 Images of a 47-year-old woman with an invasive ductal cancer G3 in the left breast. (A) Contrast-enhanced subtraction, (B) T2w-TSE, (C) calculated $b = 1400\,s/mm^2$, (D) ADC map (in $10^{-6}\,mm^2/s$). A heterogeneous enhancing mass with multiple feeding vessels is shown (A). The less or nonenhancing parts correspond to T2w hyperintense necrotic *(small arrow)* and T2w hypointense fibrotic *(small dashed arrow)* areas within the lesion. Here, the corresponding ADC is either too high *(small arrow* in D) or too low *(small dashed arrow* in D) if the ROI is placed only in these areas and will be elevated or decreased if a larger ROI encompasses them. To correctly determine the ADC of vital lesion parts, the ROI *(arrowhead* on A–D) must be placed in the contrast-enhancing part that does not show artifacts or signs of necrosis/fibrosis on T2w (B) and DWI images (C). The position must be carefully compared between anatomical and DWI images as geometrical compression is present in the DWI images *(large dashed arrow* in C and D) in phase-encoding direction (anterior-posterior) and leads to a distortion of the breast in this direction compared with the anatomical images *(large arrow)*. *ADC,* Apparent diffusion coefficient; *DWI,* diffusion-weighted imaging; *ROI,* region of interest.

ADC thresholds will differ according to the measurement used. The EUSOBI International Working Group has issued a recommendation to measure the mean ADC value in a small ROI that should be placed in a vital, contrast-enhancing part of the interrogated lesion, avoiding fibrosis and necrosis[23] (see example in Fig. 3.4).

Finally, the examined tissue itself may not be well suited for DWI with quantitative ADC mapping: in the case of a low underlying T2-signal, such as in low water conditions like fibrotic and scar tissue, applying diffusion sensitizing gradients will fail to detect a significant signal decrease due to the noise floor. The ADC fitting procedure will result in very low ADC values that are not based on water diffusion but noise, also referred to as T2-signal blackout,[23] and such areas

of ADC maps must be considered nondiagnostic (also depicted in Fig. 3.4).

Future Considerations

For the radiologist working in clinical breast imaging, DWI is an exciting technique: it provides remarkable potential while not requiring IV contrast and using only limited acquisition time. Although this chapter focuses on the assessment of contrast-enhancing lesions by DWI, an optimized DWI technique could potentially be used as a stand-alone diagnostic test[43,44] (see Chapter 6). The quantitative ADC already can be used to downgrade MRI-suspicious lesions to avoid unnecessary invasive procedures.[36,37] Still, standardization issues in image acquisition and a lack of robustness of fat suppression and image quality remain and require vendor collaboration.[23] Specifically, image quality limits the clinical use of DWI: radiologists not used to this technique see noisy, low-resolution images that are prone to geometrical distortions in phase encoding direction. Consequently, small lesions can be difficult to spot, and geometrical distortions do not allow for direct copying of ROIs from contrast-enhanced images to the ADC map. Software providing coregistration and distortion correction would be highly desirable and could be combined with color-coded overlays suggesting nondiagnostic areas in the DWI/ADC image due to artifacts, low water signal, or fluid collections. These issues require to be solved before newer, likely more specific DWI techniques including advanced DWI modeling can be used clinically outside research centers. Finally, though the potential of using a high ADC threshold to avoid unnecessary biopsies has been proven on a high level of evidence, no interventional study has actually applied this knowledge to actually do so and report on outcomes and long-term oncological safety.

REFERENCES

1. Bakker MF, de Lange SV, Pijnappel RM et al, DENSE Trial Study Group. Supplemental MRI screening for women with extremely dense breast tissue. *N Engl J Med.* 2019;381:2091–2102. https://doi.org/10.1056/NEJMoa1903986
2. Warner E, Messersmith H, Causer P, Eisen A, Shumak R, Plewes D. Systematic review: using magnetic resonance imaging to screen women at high risk for breast cancer. *Ann Intern Med.* 2008;148:671–679.

3. Houssami N, Ciatto S, Macaskill P, et al. Accuracy and surgical impact of magnetic resonance imaging in breast cancer staging: systematic review and meta-analysis in detection of multifocal and multicentric cancer. *J Clin Oncol.* 2008;26:3248–3258. https://doi.org/10.1200/JCO.2007.15.2108.

4. Folkman J. Role of angiogenesis in tumor growth and metastasis. *Semin Oncol.* 2002;29:15–18. https://doi.org/10.1053/sonc.2002.37263.

5. Baltzer PAT, Benndorf M, Gajda M, Kaiser WA. An exception to tumour neoangiogenesis in a malignant breast-lesion. *Breast J.* 2010;16:197–198. https://doi.org/10.1111/j.1524-4741.2009.00875.x.

6. Bennani-Baiti B, Bennani-Baiti N, Baltzer PA. Diagnostic performance of breast magnetic resonance imaging in non-calcified equivocal breast findings: results from a systematic review and meta-analysis. *PLoS One.* 2016;11:e0160346. https://doi.org/10.1371/journal.pone.0160346.

7. Bennani-Baiti B, Baltzer PA. MR imaging for diagnosis of malignancy in mammographic microcalcifications: a systematic review and meta-analysis. *Radiology.* 2017;283:692–701. https://doi.org/10.1148/radiol.2016161106.

8. Clauser P, Mann R, Athanasiou A, et al. A survey by the European Society of Breast Imaging on the utilisation of breast MRI in clinical practice. *Eur Radiol.* 2018;28:1909–1918. https://doi.org/10.1007/s00330-017-5121-4.

9. Mann RM, Balleyguier C, Baltzer PA, et al. European Society of Breast Imaging (EUSOBI), with language review by Europa Donna—the European Breast Cancer Coalition, Breast MRI: EUSOBI recommendations for women's information. *Eur Radiol.* 2015;25:3669–3678. https://doi.org/10.1007/s00330-015-3807-z.

10. Kuhl CK. Abbreviated magnetic resonance imaging (MRI) for breast cancer screening: rationale, concept, and transfer to clinical practice. *Ann Rev Med.* 2019;70:501–519. https://doi.org/10.1146/annurev-med-121417-100403.

11. Bluff JE, Menakuru SR, Cross SS, et al. Angiogenesis is associated with the onset of hyperplasia in human ductal breast disease. *Br J Cancer.* 2009;101:666–672. https://doi.org/10.1038/sj.bjc.6605196.

12. Carpenter PM, Chen W-P, Mendez A, McLaren CE, Su M-Y. Angiogenesis in the progression of breast ductal proliferations. *Int J Surg Pathol.* 2011;19:335–341. https://doi.org/10.1177/1066896909333511.

13. Engels K, Fox SB, Whitehouse RM, Gatter KC, Harris AL. Distinct angiogenic patterns are associated with high-grade in situ ductal carcinomas of the breast. *J Pathol.* 1997;181:207–212. https://doi.org/10.1002/(SICI)1096-9896(199702)181:2<207::AID-PATH758>3.0.CO;2-4.

14. Edwards SD, Lipson JA, Ikeda DM, Lee JM. Updates and revisions to the BI-RADS magnetic resonance imaging lexicon. *Magn Reson Imaging Clin N Am.* 2013;21:483–493. https://doi.org/10.1016/j.mric.2013.02.005.

15. Weinreb JC, Barentsz JO, Choyke PL, et al. PI-RADS Prostate Imaging—Reporting and Data System: 2015, Version 2. *Eur Urol.* 2016;69:16–40. https://doi.org/10.1016/j.eururo.2015.08.052.

16. Baltzer PAT, Kaiser WA, Dietzel M. Lesion type and reader experience affect the diagnostic accuracy of breast MRI: a multiple reader ROC study. *Eur J Radiol.* 2015;84:86–91. https://doi.org/10.1016/j.ejrad.2014.10.023.

17. Benndorf M, Baltzer PAT, Kaiser WA. Assessing the degree of collinearity among the lesion features of the MRI BI-RADS lexicon. *Eur J Radiol.* 2011;80:e322–e324. https://doi.org/10.1016/j.ejrad.2010.11.030.

18. Gutierrez RL, DeMartini WB, Eby PR, Kurland BF, Peacock S, Lehman CD. BI-RADS lesion characteristics predict likelihood of malignancy in breast MRI for masses but not for nonmass-like enhancement. *AJR Am J Roentgenol.* 2009;193:994–1000. https://doi.org/10.2214/AJR.08.1983.

19. Baltzer PAT, Benndorf M, Dietzel M, Gajda M, Runnebaum IB, Kaiser WA. False-positive findings at contrast-enhanced breast MRI: a BI-RADS descriptor study. *AJR Am J Roentgenol.* 2010;194:1658–1663. https://doi.org/10.2214/AJR.09.3486.

20. Kaiser CG, Dietzel M, Vag T, Froelich MF. Cost-effectiveness of MR-mammography vs. conventional mammography in screening patients at intermediate risk of breast cancer—a model-based economic evaluation. *Eur J Radiol.* 2020;136:109355. https://doi.org/10.1016/j.ejrad.2020.109355.

21. Le Bihan D, Breton E, Lallemand D, Aubin ML, Vignaud J, Laval-Jeantet M. Separation of diffusion and perfusion in intravoxel incoherent motion MR imaging. *Radiology.* 1988;168:497–505.

22. Dorrius MD, Dijkstra H, Oudkerk M, Sijens PE. Effect of b value and pre-admission of contrast on diagnostic accuracy of 1.5-T breast DWI: a systematic review and meta-analysis. *Eur Radiol.* 2014;24:2835–2847. https://doi.org/10.1007/s00330-014-3338-z.

23. Baltzer P, Mann RM, Iima M, et al.; EUSOBI International Breast Diffusion-Weighted Imaging Working Group. Diffusion-weighted imaging of the breast—a consensus and mission statement from the EUSOBI International Breast Diffusion-Weighted Imaging Working Group. *Eur Radiol.* 2020;30:1436–1450. https://doi.org/10.1007/s00330-019-06510-3.

24. Dietzel M, Baltzer PAT. How to use the Kaiser score as a clinical decision rule for diagnosis in multiparametric breast MRI: a pictorial essay. *Insights Imaging.* 2018;9:325–335. https://doi.org/10.1007/s13244-018-0611-8.

25. Bogner W, Pinker K, Zaric O, et al. Bilateral diffusion-weighted MR imaging of breast tumors with submillimeter resolution using readout-segmented echo-planar imaging at 7 T. *Radiology.* 2015;274:74–84. https://doi.org/10.1148/radiol.14132340.

26. Mann RM, Cho N, Moy L. Breast MRI: state of the art. *Radiology.* 2019;292:520–536. https://doi.org/10.1148/radiol.2019182947.

27. Marino MA, Helbich T, Baltzer P, Pinker-Domenig K. Multiparametric MRI of the breast: a review. *J Magn Reson Imaging.* 2018;47:301–315. https://doi.org/10.1002/jmri.25790.

28. Sardanelli F, Boetes C, Borisch B, et al. Magnetic resonance imaging of the breast: recommendations from the EUSOMA Working Group. *Eur J Cancer.* 2010;46:1296–1316. https://doi.org/10.1016/j.ejca.2010.02.015.

29. Bickel H, Pinker K, Polanec S, et al. Diffusion-weighted imaging of breast lesions: region-of-interest placement and different ADC parameters influence apparent diffusion coefficient values. *Eur Radiol.* 2017;27:1883–1892. https://doi.org/10.1007/s00330-016-4564-3.

30. Wielema M, Dorrius MD, Pijnappel RM, et al. Diagnostic performance of breast tumor tissue selection in diffusion weighted imaging: a systematic review and meta-analysis. *PLoS One.* 2020;15:e0232856. https://doi.org/10.1371/journal.pone.0232856.

31. Partridge SC, Nissan N, Rahbar H, Kitsch AE, Sigmund EE. Diffusion-weighted breast MRI: clinical applications and emerging techniques. *J Magn Reson Imaging.* 2017;45:337–355. https://doi.org/10.1002/jmri.25479.

32. Baltzer PAT, Kapetas P, Marino MA, Clauser P. New diagnostic tools for breast cancer. *Memo.* 2017;10:175–180. https://doi.org/10.1007/s12254-017-0341-5.

33. Pinker K, Bickel H, Helbich TH, et al. Combined contrast-enhanced magnetic resonance and diffusion-weighted imaging reading adapted to the "Breast Imaging Reporting and Data System" for multiparametric 3-T imaging of breast lesions. *Eur Radiol.* 2013;23:1791–1802. https://doi.org/10.1007/s00330-013-2771-8.

34. Pinker K, Baltzer P, Bogner W, et al. Multiparametric MR imaging with high-resolution dynamic contrast-enhanced and diffusion-weighted imaging at 7 T improves the assessment of breast tumors: a feasibility study. *Radiology.* 2015;276:360–370. https://doi.org/10.1148/radiol.15141905.

35. McDonald ES, Romanoff J, Rahbar H, et al. Mean apparent diffusion coefficient is a sufficient conventional diffusion-weighted MRI metric to improve breast MRI diagnostic performance: results from the ECOG-ACRIN Cancer Research Group A6702 Diffusion Imaging Trial. *Radiology.* 2021;298:60–70. https://doi.org/10.1148/radiol.2020202465.

36. Rahbar H, Zhang Z, Chenevert TL, et al. Utility of diffusion-weighted imaging to decrease unnecessary biopsies prompted by breast MRI: a trial of the ECOG-ACRIN Cancer Research Group (A6702). *Clin Cancer Res.* 2019;25:1756–1765. https://doi.org/10.1158/1078-0432.CCR-18-2967.

37. Clauser P, Krug B, Bickel H, et al. Diffusion-weighted imaging allows for downgrading MR BI-RADS 4 lesions in contrast-enhanced MRI of the breast to avoid unnecessary biopsy. *Clin Cancer Res.* 2021;27(7):1941–1948. https://doi.org/10.1158/1078-0432.CCR-20-3037.

38. Clauser P, Marcon M, Maieron M, Zuiani C, Bazzocchi M, Baltzer PAT. Is there a systematic bias of apparent diffusion coefficient (ADC) measurements of the breast if measured on different workstations? An inter- and intra-reader agreement study. *Eur Radiol.* 2016;26:2291–2296. https://doi.org/10.1007/s00330-015-4051-2.

39. Spick C, Bickel H, Pinker K, et al. Diffusion-weighted MRI of breast lesions: a prospective clinical investigation of the quantitative imaging biomarker characteristics of reproducibility, repeatability, and diagnostic accuracy. *NMR Biomed.* 2016;29:1445–1453. https://doi.org/10.1002/nbm.3596.

40. Partridge SC, McDonald ES. Diffusion weighted magnetic resonance imaging of the breast: protocol optimization, interpretation, and clinical applications. *Magn Reson Imaging Clin N Am.* 2013;21:601–624. https://doi.org/10.1016/j.mric.2013.04.007.

41. White NS, McDonald C, McDonald CR, et al. Diffusion-weighted imaging in cancer: physical foundations and applications of restriction spectrum imaging. *Cancer Res.* 2014;74:4638–4652. https://doi.org/10.1158/0008-5472.CAN-13-3534.

42. Zeilinger MG, Lell M, Baltzer PAT, Dörfler A, Uder M, Dietzel M. Impact of post-processing methods on apparent diffusion coefficient values. *Eur Radiol.* 2017;27:946–955. https://doi.org/10.1007/s00330-016-4403-6.

43. McDonald ES, Hammersley JA, Chou S-HS, et al. Performance of DWI as a rapid unenhanced technique for detecting mammographically occult breast cancer in elevated-risk women with dense breasts. *AJR Am J Roentgenol.* 2016;207:205–216. https://doi.org/10.2214/AJR.15.15873.

44. Baltzer PAT, Bickel H, Spick C, et al. Potential of noncontrast magnetic resonance imaging with diffusion-weighted imaging in characterization of breast lesions: intraindividual comparison with dynamic contrast-enhanced magnetic resonance imaging. *Invest Radiol.* 2018;53:229–235. https://doi.org/10.1097/RLI.0000000000000433.

Chapter 4

Biomarkers, Prognosis, and Prediction Factors

Beatriu Reig, MD, MPH*, Linda Moy, MD, Eric E. Sigmund, PhD and Laura Heacock, MD, MS

Breast cancer is a heterogeneous group of neoplasms originating from the epithelial cells lining the milk ducts. This heterogeneity has been observed in histology for a long time and formed the backbone of the traditional pathology-driven classification of breast cancer. Multiple studies have shown that this heterogeneity in the histopathologic features of breast cancer was associated with clinical outcomes. More recently, the pathology-driven classification has been replaced by molecular classifications based on hormone receptors, human epidermal growth factor receptor 2 (HER2), and Ki-67 status. These molecular classifications reflect genetic tumor heterogeneity and have strong associations with the prognosis of various breast cancers. As a result, there is hope that the development of targeted therapies to these molecular subtypes will lead to improved outcomes of breast cancer. Additionally, a lot of research has been performed to identify imaging features on breast imaging examinations, such as breast magnetic resonance imaging (MRI), that may serve as imaging biomarkers for these molecular subtypes of breast cancer. This chapter reviews the current understanding of the intrinsic molecular subtypes of breast cancer, with emphasis on the imaging features of these molecular subtypes on breast MRI and diffusion-weighted imaging (DWI).

Background

In 2022 an estimated 287,850 new cases of invasive breast cancer are expected to be diagnosed in women in the United States, along with 51,400 new cases of noninvasive (in situ) breast cancer.[1] An estimated 43,250 women are expected to die in 2022 from

breast cancer, making it the second-leading cause of cancer death among women in the United States.[1] Death rates have been steady in women under 50 since 2007 but have continued to drop in women over 50. The overall death rate from breast cancer decreased by 1.3% per year from 2013 to 2017. These decreases are thought to be the result of treatment advances and earlier detection through screening. Although screening mammography accounts for most of this early detection, studies have found that screening with breast MRI leads to earlier detection of biologically relevant cancers among high-risk and average-risk women, which are often occult on mammography.[2–9]

Breast MRI is an indispensable modality, along with mammography and ultrasound (US). Its clinical indications are staging of known cancer, screening for breast cancer in women at increased risk, and evaluation of response to neoadjuvant chemotherapy.[10–13] Unlike conventional mammography and US, MRI is a functional technique. Contrast material-enhanced MRI evaluates the permeability of blood vessels by using an intravenous contrast agent (gadolinium chelate) that shortens the local T1 time, leading to a higher signal on T1-weighted images.[14] The underlying principle is that neoangiogenesis leads to formation of leaky vessels that allow for faster extravasation of contrast agents,[15] thus leading to rapid local enhancement and the detection of breast cancer.

In the specific setting of MRI for high-risk screening in *BRCA1/2* mutation carriers, the reported sensitivities are between 75.2% and 100% and specificities between 83% and 98.4%.[16,17] The cancer detection rate among known *BRCA1/2* carriers was 26.2 per 1000, compared with 5.4 per 1000 in high-risk nonmutation carriers.[2] Compared with the earlier trials, the sensitivities and

*beatriu.reig@nyulangone.org

specificities of breast MRI continue to improve due to two major factors. First, MRI scanners, coils, and scan protocols have evolved, leading to marked improvement in image quality and spatial resolution. Second, radiologists have gained significantly more experience in the interpretation of breast MRI examinations.[10] Despite this progress, false-positive findings remain a limitation of breast MRI examinations.

False-positive MRI lesions have indeterminate morphological and kinetic features that turn out to be benign at biopsy but cannot be classified as certainly benign based upon the imaging examination alone. Because benign breast lesions are frequent, a multiparametric breast MRI examination that includes DWI assists with lesion characterization. DWI can help visualize and quantify random movement of water molecules in tissue, influenced by tissue microstructure and cell density. This is achieved by applying motion-sensitizing gradients (described by the *b* value) to an essentially T2-weighted echo-planar imaging sequence.[18,19] Breast cancers show decreased water diffusion, primarily attributed to increased cell density, leading to higher signal intensity on DWI. The apparent diffusion coefficient (ADC) is a quantitative measure of diffusivity derived from DWI. Values are usually expressed in 10^{-3} mm^2/s. Because of the hindered diffusion in cancers, mean ADCs are generally low (range $0.8–1.3 \times 10^{-3}$ mm^2/s) compared with those in benign lesions (range $1.2–2.0 \times 10^{-3}$ mm^2/s).[20] Consequently, cancers have a low signal intensity on the derived ADC maps, and this feature allows DWI to improve the differentiation between benign and malignant breast lesions.[20,21] Additional roles for DWI include lesion detection on a screening MRI, using DWI as a prognostic indicator, and predicting response to treatment. This chapter will explain how quantitative DWI findings provide information on prognosis and prediction factors of breast cancers and help lesion management. Please see related chapters on breast lesion characterization (see Chapter 3), monitoring response to treatment (see Chapter 5), and multiparametric imaging, radiomics, and artificial intelligence (see Chapter 10).

Classification of Breast Cancer

Breast cancer is a heterogeneous disease comprising several molecular and genetic subtypes, each with characteristic biological behavior and imaging patterns.[22] Traditional classification of breast cancer is based on the clinicopathologic analysis of tumors, with classes of breast cancer defined by histopathologic features, including the pattern of architectural growth (e.g., cribriform, papillary) and the nuclear grade (low, intermediate, or high).[22] Treatment choices are partially determined by the tumor size, local invasion, and lymph node involvement or distant metastases, as defined by the American Joint Committee on Cancer's (AJCC) TNM staging classification (7th edition).[23] However, this traditional classification of breast cancer, based on the histopathologic features, offers limited prognostic value. Although survival rates correlate best with tumor size and the presence of axillary metastasis, breast cancer patients at the same anatomical stage of disease can have markedly different clinical courses and clinical outcomes.[22,24,25] Fortunately, developments in the field of molecular biology have allowed breast cancers to be analyzed by their expression of specific biomarkers. As a result, the eighth edition of the AJCC's TNM staging classification[26] incorporates this genetic information into the traditional classification scheme.

GENOMIC EXPRESSION PATTERN ANALYSIS AND MOLECULAR SUBTYPE OF BREAST CANCER

Technical developments in DNA microarrays, specifically genomic expression pattern analysis using hierarchical clustering, are the basis for the molecular classification of major subtypes of breast cancer. In 2000 Perou and colleagues[27] tested 65 breast tumors against DNA microarrays representing 8102 genes. These investigators noted that the molecular portraits of the tumors, derived from patterns of gene expression, disclosed some groupings. Tumors were clustered in terms of growth rate, activation of specific signaling pathways, and cellular composition.[22,27] For example, the more proliferative tumors overexpressed genes such as Ki-67, a marker of cellular proliferation; this expression correlated with increased mitotic indexes at histopathologic examination. Based on the persistent differences in their gene expression patterns, the authors divided breast cancers into two large categories based on their pattern of gene expression. When tumor cells manifested characteristics similar to the epithelial cells lining the milk ducts, expressing, for example, cytokeratin 8/18 and genes associated with the estrogen receptor (ER), the cancers were labeled luminal cancers. Alternatively, when cancer cells displayed characteristics similar to myoepithelial cells (also known as basal cells) that line the inner surface of the basement membranes, expressing, for example, cytokeratin 5/6 and laminin, the cancers were grouped into the basal category.[22,27]

As a result, two large categories of luminal breast cancers and basal breast cancers were defined and dichotomized on the basis of the presence or absence of ERs. ER biology was identified as a key player in breast carcinogenesis, defining the morphology and the clinical behavior of the final tumor, whereas other parameters, such as tumor grade, were found to be less important.[27–29] Luminal tumors also were generally characterized by an absence of overexpression of the HER2 gene, a proto-oncogene that stimulates cellular growth. Based on genomic profiling at the DNA, microRNA, and protein levels, researchers in The Cancer Genome Atlas (TCGA) Network refined these classifications into four intrinsic molecular subtypes of breast cancer: luminal A, luminal B, HER2-enriched (HER2+), and triple-negative (TN) and/or basal-like tumors (Table 4.1).[30–33] Since then, multiple studies confirmed that each subtype of breast cancer has a unique response to therapy, disease-free survival (DFS), and overall survival (OS). As a result, subtype-based recommendations for systemic therapies have been implemented in clinical practice.[33–35]

DISTRIBUTION AND PROGNOSIS OF MOLECULAR SUBTYPES OF BREAST CANCER

These subtypes are unevenly distributed in breast cancer patients and associated with different tumor phenotypes and distinct variations in response to therapy and survival.[32,36,37] Patients with luminal A tumors have the most favorable prognosis, followed by those with luminal B tumors, who have an intermediate prognosis. On the other end of the spectrum, TN and HER2+ subtypes are associated with an unfavorable prognosis, but with the introduction of targeted drugs, such as trastuzumab or pertuzumab, the natural course of disease of the HER2+ subtype is nowadays more favorable,[38] whereas the triple-negative subtype is associated with an unfavorable prognosis.[33–35]

In the clinical and research settings, molecular subtypes are derived by invasive sampling. Several molecular assays are commercially available, including Oncotype DX (Genomic Health, Redwood City, CA); MammaPrint (Agendia, Irvine, CA); Mammostrat (Clarient Diagnostic Services, Aliso Viejo, CA); PAM50 (Prosigna; NanoString, Seattle, WA); EndoPredict (Sividon/Myriad Genetics, Salt Lake City, UT); and MapQuant Dx Genomic Grade index (Ipsogen/QIAGEN; Venlo, the Netherlands).[33,39–41] Oncotype DX and MammaPrint, both of which are approved by the Food and Drug Administration, have shown predictive and prognostic abilities for evaluating the risk of developing distant metastasis and predicting the benefit of adjuvant chemotherapy.[33,42,43] However, biopsies of small tumor regions may not be representative of the genetic, epigenetic, and/or phenotypic alterations of the entire tumor. A common alternative is to use immunohistochemical (IHC) surrogates for the definition of molecular subtypes (see Table 4.1).[32–34,44] There is variable agreement between classifications via these surrogates and formal genetic testing (41%–100%). Given these limitations and the relatively high cost of assays, there is a strong demand for more accurate, noninvasive means of differentiating molecular subtypes, which presents a unique opportunity for advanced medical imaging, specifically with breast MRI and DWI.[33]

LUMINAL TUMORS

Luminal A tumors are the most common type of breast cancer, accounting for 50% to 55% of all tumors. They are characterized by high genetic expression of the ER and progesterone receptors (PRs), as well as many other genes expressed by the epithelial cells that line the lumen of the terminal duct lobular unit, where most breast cancers arise. These cancers are usually low-grade tumors, without amplification of the HER2/neu proto-oncogene and with a low Ki-67 proliferative index.[36,45,46] Overall, luminal A breast cancer is associated with the most favorable prognosis, with a 5-year OS and relapse-free survival rate of more than 80% in 2001.[28] This excellent prognosis is in part because expression of steroid hormone receptors is predictive of a favorable response to hormonal therapy.[22] Luminal A tumors progress slowly over time, and

TABLE 4.1   Clinical and Immunohistochemical Surrogates for Molecular Subtypes of Breast Cancer

Intrinsic Subtype	Subtype	ER	PR	HER2	Ki-67	Histological Grade	Recurrence Risk Score	Frequency (%)	Comments
Luminal A	Luminal A-like	Positive	Positive>20%	Negative	Low	Generally Grade 1 or 2	Low	50–55	Best prognosis
Luminal B	Luminal B-like (HER2−)	Positive	Negative or low <20%	Negative	High	Generally Grade 3	High	20 (both types of luminal B)	Less favorable than luminal A
	Luminal B-like (HER2+)	Positive	Any	Overexpressed or amplified	Any	Generally Grade 3	High		
ErbB2 overexpression	HER2+ (nonluminal)	Negative	Negative	Overexpressed or amplified	Any	Generally Grade 3	N/A	15	Improved with HER2-targeted therapy
Triple negative	Triple negative	Negative	Negative	Negative	Any	Generally Grade 3	N/A	10–20	May improve with novel agents[a]

[a]Immunotherapy, antibody-drug conjugates (ADCs), and poly (adenosine diphosphate-Q22 a ribose) polymerase inhibitors.
ER, estrogen receptor; *HER2*, human epidermal growth factor receptor 2; *PR*, progesterone receptor.

the chance of DFS survival is higher than with other subtypes.[47]

Luminal B tumors account for 20% of all tumors. These cancers also express ERs and PRs but have greater proliferative activity, as can be assessed through Ki-67 levels; these cancers are usually mid- to high-grade tumors.[22,28] Luminal B breast cancers characteristically do not overexpress HER2/neu, but approximately 30% of them will be HER2-enriched.[22] The prognosis of patients with luminal B breast cancer is often poorer than that for patients with luminal A tumors. Five-year OS and relapse-free survival rates were approximately 40% in 2001.[28] Although ER status and PR status are predictors of response to endocrine therapy, the clinical outcome cannot reliably be predicted solely from the ER and PR status, and analysis of other cellular markers and tumor characteristics is required for optimal assessment of outcome and to determine the need for chemotherapy.[22]

Mammography, Ultrasound, and Magnetic Resonance Imaging Features of Luminal Tumors

Luminal A tumors are most commonly screening-detected masses with spiculated margins and associated architectural distortion.[45,48,49] Luminal B masses exhibit indistinct, microlobulated, or spiculated margins but are less likely to demonstrate distortion.[49,50] Ko and colleagues reported on the appearance of 93 ER-positive (ER+) HER2-negative (HER2-) breast cancers at mammography.[22,50] These cancers appeared most often as irregular masses (45%) or irregular masses with calcifications (28%). Overall, microcalcifications were seen in 41% of these cancers.[50] The typical sonographic appearance of luminal tumors is an irregular mass with angular or microlobulated margins, with posterior acoustic shadowing.[48–50]

On MRI, luminal A and luminal B tumors often present as an enhancing irregular mass with spiculated margins and uncommonly as nonmass enhancement.[45,51,52] Uematsu and colleagues described the appearance of 117 ER+ HER2- breast cancers at MRI.[53] Forty-six percent of these lesions were unifocal, 44% were multifocal, and 9% were multicentric. These investigators reported mass enhancement in the majority of these tumors (67%), with the remainder being areas of nonmass enhancement (33%), most often segmental.[53] The masses were most often

irregular (32%) or oval (38%) in shape, with irregular margins in 86%.[53] Heterogeneous internal enhancement was seen in 97% of the tumors, with plateau or washout kinetics in 79%. Eighty-five percent of the ER+ HER2-tumors were iso- to hypointense on T2-weighted MR images.[22,53]

Diffusion-Weighted Imaging of Luminal Tumors

DWI is a useful tool to differentiate malignant lesions from benign lesions. It also provides information on tumor biology and microstructural features. As a result, studies were conducted to correlate ADC values and breast cancer prognostic factors. We will review the literature on the association of DWI with luminal tumors. Examples of luminal A and luminal B breast cancers evaluated on DWI are illustrated in Figs. 4.1 and 4.2, respectively.

The ability of DWI to serve as an imaging biomarker that is associated with particular molecular subtype and to prognosticate the response to treatment is an area of robust research. Most of these DWI studies are summarized in Table 4.2.[54–73] Some investigators found that the percent of ER or PR expression accounted for differences in ADC values.[56,58–60,62,63,66,69,71–73]

However, the underlying mechanism for the effects of hormone receptor status and its effect on tissue diffusivity remains unknown. It is hypothesized that hormone receptor–positive tumors have lower ADC values than those breast cancers that are hormone receptor–negative secondary to different levels of cell membrane permeability. Springer and colleagues found that ER- or PR-positive tumors have different levels of cell plasma membrane permeability that are attributed to Na^+,K^+-ATPase enzymes. These enzymes play a role in cell membrane permeability and cell density and directly affect the sensitivity of diffusion MRI.[90] Other researchers hypothesize that the hormone receptor status affects a tumor's vascularity and, as a result, the ADC values. Cho and colleagues found a significantly lower ADC value in ER+ tumors, which is speculated to be related to a lower perfusion contribution.[73] Although the results are clearly mixed, smaller ADC related values are found in luminal B, hormone receptor–negative compared with luminal A by some scholars.[70,72,91] Further, some investigations suggest low tissue diffusivity in luminal B, hormone receptor–negative compared with luminal A tumors.

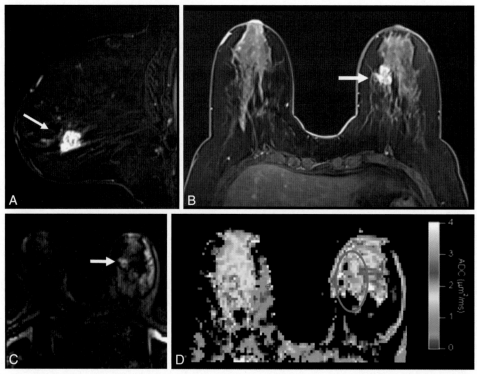

Fig. 4.1 Fifty-five-year-old woman presenting with a newly diagnosed invasive ductal carcinoma, moderately differentiated, luminal A tumor (ER+/PR+, HER2−, Ki-67 10%). (A) Sagittal T1-weighted postcontrast subtraction images and (B) axial T1=weighted postcontrast images shows a 2.2-cm spiculated heterogeneously enhancing mass *(arrow)* in the medial left breast. (C) Diffusion-weighted b_{800} image shows the cancer is hyperintense *(arrow)*. (D) The apparent diffusion coefficient (ADC) map *(red circle)* generated with b_0 and b_{800} values shows low values in the cancer, consistent with restricted diffusion.

Using intravoxel incoherent motion (IVIM) analysis, their study confirmed that the ADC versus ER findings in human breast tumors are indeed vascular, based on the significantly lower Dp kurtosis and skewness in ER+ tumors and the significant negative correlations between fp kurtosis and skewness and Dp kurtosis and skewness with ER expression. Interestingly, mean fp values correlated positively with PR expression.[73] The biological implications of the study seems to confirm that human breast tumors are indeed vascular, based on the significantly lower Dp kurtosis and skewness in ER+ tumors and the significant negative correlations between fp kurtosis and skewness and Dp kurtosis and skewness with ER expression. Interestingly, mean fp values correlated positively with PR expression. Similarities in hormone receptor effects would suggest a negative correlation, as with ER expression; however, PR+ tumors may increase tumor growth by

angiogenesis through the normalization of tumor vasculature, which would allow for proper blood flow. In fact, studies have shown that progesterone may increase angiogenesis through regulation of vascular endothelial growth factor (VEGF) in breast cancer cells.[92]

Finally, given the increased clinical utilization of molecular assays, two groups recently found a correlation between ADC values and Oncotype DX score, a quantitative 21 gene recurrence score test for early ER+ breast cancer patients.[64,85] Additional research is necessary to determine whether DWI may serve as a surrogate genetic biomarker for these expensive molecular assays.

HER2-ENRICHED TUMORS

HER2-enriched tumors are characterized by overexpression of the Erb-B2 oncogene, which encodes a

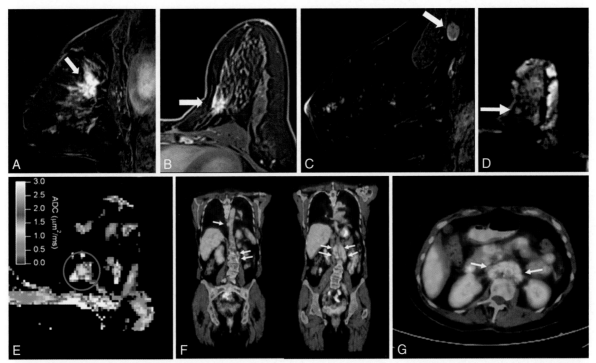

Fig. 4.2 Forty-eight-year-old woman presenting with a palpable mass in the left breast. (A) Sagittal T1-weighted postcontrast subtraction images and (B) axial T1-weighted postcontrast images showed a 3-cm spiculated enhancing mass *(white arrow)* in the left breast. (C) In addition, there is an enlarged lymph node *(arrow)* in the left axilla. (D) Diffusion-weighted b_{800} image shows the cancer is hyperintense *(arrow)*. (E) The apparent diffusion coefficient (ADC) map *(red circle)* (generated with b_0 and b_{800} values) is heterogeneous showing areas with and without restricted diffusion. Subsequent biopsies showed invasive lobular carcinoma, well-differentiated luminal B tumor (ER+/PR+ HER2−, Ki-67 18%) in the left breast and a metastatic lymph node in the left axilla. The patient was treated with lumpectomy followed by chemotherapy and radiation. Nine years later, the patient underwent a positron-emission tomography/computed tomography (PET/CT) for persistent lower back pain after a motor vehicle accident. (E–G) PET/CT showed multiple new hypermetabolic paraesophageal, retrocrural, and retroperitoneum lymph nodes *(arrows)*. Biopsy of a retroperitoneal lymph node confirmed metastatic breast cancer.

transmembrane tyrosine kinase receptor. Binding of this receptor initiates a cascade mediating cell proliferation, differentiation, and ultimately survival. They account for 12% to 20% of all breast cancers and are noted to have both shortened DFS and OS. Luminal cancers, particularly luminal B, can overexpress the Erb-B2 oncogene, whereas tumors that are considered HER2+ show low levels of ER expression. Although HER2+ tumors often lack overexpression of Ki-67 and other proliferation genes, they have a poorer prognosis than luminal cancers. Anti-HER2 therapy for both early and advanced breast cancers has increased time to disease progression, duration of response, and median survival, whereas HER2+ disease continues to have a poor prognosis relative to luminal cancers.[22,45]

Mammography, Ultrasound, and Magnetic Resonance Imaging Features of HER2-Enriched Tumors

Unlike other cancer types, HER2+ tumors are not associated with age, race, or other risk factors.

On mammography, HER2+ tumors classically present as an irregular or spiculated mass with associated pleomorphic or other calcifications. The presence of calcifications may correlate to the high coexistence of DCIS with invasive ductal cancers.[22,45] On sonography, these tumors have irregular margins and are hypoechoic or less commonly isoechoic. Up to one-third of these masses demonstrate an echogenic rim on US; an abrupt interface with the surrounding tissue and posterior acoustic enhancement is more common.[22,45]

TABLE 4.2 Summary of Diffusion-Weighted Imaging Parameters According to Prognostic Factors

Reference	Patients (n)	Field Strength (T)	b-values	Significant Parameters	Significant Outcomes	Nonsignificant Outcomes
Kim et al. 2009[60]	67	1.5	0, 1000	Median ADC	ER (marginal significance)	PR, HER2, p53, Ki-67, EGFR
Jeh et al. 2011[59]	107	1.5, 3	0, 1500 for 1.5 T;0, 750 for 3 T	Mean ADC	ER, HER2	PR, Ki-67, EGFR
Choi et al. 2012[67]	355	1.5	0, 1000	Mean ADC	ER, PR, Ki-67	HER2, LN
Martincich et al. 2012[58]	190	1.5	0, 900	Median ADC	ER, HER2, HER2+ subtype vs. luminal	
Kamitani et al. 2013[66]	81	1.5	0, 500, 1000	Mean ADC	ER, PR, LN	HER2, nuclear grade, vascular invasion
Cipolla et al. 2014[74]	92	3	0, 1000	ADC	Histological grade	
Kim et al. 2015[54]	173	3	0, 750	ADC histogram parameters	HER2, Ki-67, LN, subtypes	HG, ER, PR
Park et al. 2015[65]	110	3	0, 1000	Mean ADC	HER2	HG, LN, ER, PR
Belli et al. 2015[75]	289	1.5	0, 1000	Mean ADC	HG, LN	Tumor size
Molinari et al. 2015[76]	115	1.5	0, 1000	ADC	Ki-67, HG, luminal B vs. other subtypes	
Arponen et al. 2015[77]	112	3	0, 200, 400, 600, 800	ADC	LN, HG, PR, NPI	ER, HER2, Ki-67
Cho et al. 2016[73]	50	3	0, 30, 70, 100, 150, 200, 300, 400, 500, 800	ADC, IVIM parameters (Dt, Dp, fp)	ER, PR, HER2, Ki-67, subtypes	
Kim et al. 2016[72]	275	3	0, 30, 70, 100, 150, 200, 300, 400, 500, 800	ADC, IVIM parameters (Dt, fp)	Ki-67, luminal B vs. other subtypes	
Durando et al. 2016[78]	212	3	0, 1000	ADC	LVI	Tumor size, HG, ER, PR, HER2, LN
Kitajima et al. 2016[79]	214	3	0, 1000	Mean ADC	Ki-67, tumor size, LN, TNM stage, IDC vs. ILC	ER, PR, HER2, subtype

TABLE 4.2 Summary of Diffusion-Weighted Imaging Parameters According to Prognostic Factors—*Continued*

Reference	Patients (*n*)	Field Strength (T)	*b*-values	Significant Parameters	Significant Outcomes	Nonsignificant Outcomes
Shin et al. 2016[80]	138	3	0, 1000	ADC	Tumor cellularity, Ki-67, PLI	TILs, LN, tumor size
Lee et al. 2017[71]	72	3	0, 25, 50, 75, 100, 150, 200, 300, 500, 800	ADC, IVIM parameters (Ds)	ER, HG, subtype, Ki-67	
Kawashima et al. 2017[70]	134	3	0, 20, 40, 80, 120, 200, 400, 600, 800	ADC, IVIM parameters (D)	Luminal A vs. luminal B, Ki-67	
Suo et al. 2017[69]	101	3	0, 10, 30, 50, 100, 150, 200, 500, 800, 1000, 1500, 2000, 2500	ADC, α, Df, Ds, f, DDC, MD	Ki-67, LN, ER	
Fan et al. 2017[81]	82	3	50, 1000	ADC (tumor, peritumoral)	Ki-67	
Vidic et al. 2018[68]	51	3	0, 10, 20, 30, 40, 50, 70, 90, 120, 150, 200, 400, 700	Combined diffusion model	HER2 status of ER+ tumors	
Iima et al. 2018[61]	199	3	5, 10, 20, 30, 50, 70, 100, 200, 400, 600, 800, 1000, 1500, 2000, 2500	$sADC_{200-1500}$	PR, subtypes	
Fan et al. 2018[82]	126	3	50, 1000	Mean ADC	Subtypes	
Liu et al. 2018[56]	151	3	0, 1000	ADC	ER, PR, HER2	
Amornsiripanitch et al. 2018[64]	107	3	0, 800	ADC mean, CNR	HG, Ki-67, Oncotype DX RS	
Shen et al. 2018[55]	71	3	0, 600	ADC	Ki-67, subtypes	
Zhuang et al. 2018[83]	80	3	0, 800	Min ADC, max ADC, ΔADC	Ki-67	
Surov et al. 2018[84]	870	1.5, 3	0, 1000; 0, 900 for 1.5 T; 50, 1000; 0, 0, 800; 0, 1000 for 3 T	Mean ADC	Ki-67	Nuclear grade
Thakur et al. 2018[85]	31	3	0, 600, 1000	Mean ADC	Oncotype DX RS	
Igarashi et al. 2018[86]	140	1.5	0, 1000, 1500	ADC (tumor, peritumoral), ratio	LVI	

(Continued)

TABLE 4.2 **Summary of Diffusion-Weighted Imaging Parameters According to Prognostic Factors—Continued**

Reference	Patients (n)	Field Strength (T)	b-values	Significant Parameters	Significant Outcomes	Nonsignificant Outcomes
Suo et al. 2019[63]	134	3	0, 800, 1500	Mean ADC, entropy of ADC	ER, PR, HER2, Ki-67, luminal vs. HER2+ subtypes	
Horvat et al. 2019[62]	107	3	0, 850	Mean ADC, max ADC	ER, PR, luminal vs. nonluminal subtypes	
Kim et al. 2019[87]	258	3	0, 1000	ΔADC	Distant metastasis-free survival	
Fogante et al. 2019[88]	125	1.5	0, 800	Mean ADC	TILs, IDC vs. ILC	
Tang et al. 2020[89]	114	1.5	50, 800	ADC histogram parameters	TILs, Ki-67	

CNR, Contrast to noise ratio; D, Ds, Dt, true diffusion (or slow) coefficient; DDC, distributed diffusion coefficient; Df, Dp, pseudodiffusion (or fast) coefficient; EGFR, epidermal growth factor receptor; ER, estrogen receptor; f, fp, perfusion fraction; HER2, human epidermal growth factor receptor 2; HG, histological grade; IDC, invasive ductal carcinoma; ILC, invasive lobular carcinoma; LN, axillary lymph nodes status; LVI, lymphovascular invasion; MD, mean diffusivity; NPI, Nottingham Prognostic Index score; PLI, peritumoral lymphocytic infiltrate; PR, progesterone receptor; RS, recurrence score; sADC, synthetic ADC; subtype, molecular subtype; TILs, tumor-infiltrating lymphocyte levels; α, anomalous exponent term of stretched-exponential diffusion model; ΔADC, maximum − minimum apparent diffusion coefficient.

The aggressive tumor growth seen in HER2+ tumors is reflected in its ultrafast washin[93] and type 3 washout kinetics on dynamic contrast-enhanced MRI. Although it most commonly presents as an irregular enhancing mass, it can often be seen as linear nonmass enhancement. Importantly, HER2+ breast cancers are often multifocal and multicentric (up to 50%),[45] and breast MRI can be therefore important in demonstrating extent of disease.

Diffusion-Weighted Imaging of HER2-Enriched Tumors

Examples of HER2+ breast cancers evaluated on DWI are illustrated in Figs. 4.3 and 4.4. Compared with luminal tumors, HER2-enriched tumors have higher ADC values than luminal cancers, suggesting that ADC may hold predictive value for HER2 expression.[59,60,63] Jeh and colleagues investigated 107 women with invasive cancers and found that there was a significant correlation of the ADC_{mean} value with HER2 expression ($P = .018$).[59] Similar results were seen by Kim and colleagues, who determined that for most ADC parameters, the mean values were higher for HER2-enriched cancers than for luminal and triple negative cancers. Their multivariate analysis demonstrated HER2 expression, tumor grade, and Ki-67 were the explanatory prognostic factors for ADC_{median}.[60] More recently, Suo and colleagues evaluated 134 primary breast cancers and found that the HER2-positive subtype tended to display higher mean ADC values and that ADC_{1500} entropy provided superior diagnostic performance over ADC_{800} entropy ($P = .04$). The authors speculated this result likely reflects the high cellularity in HER2-overexpressing breast cancer.[63] Entropy on DWI has been theorized to be associated with higher cellularity and cellular heterogeneity,[94] both of which are

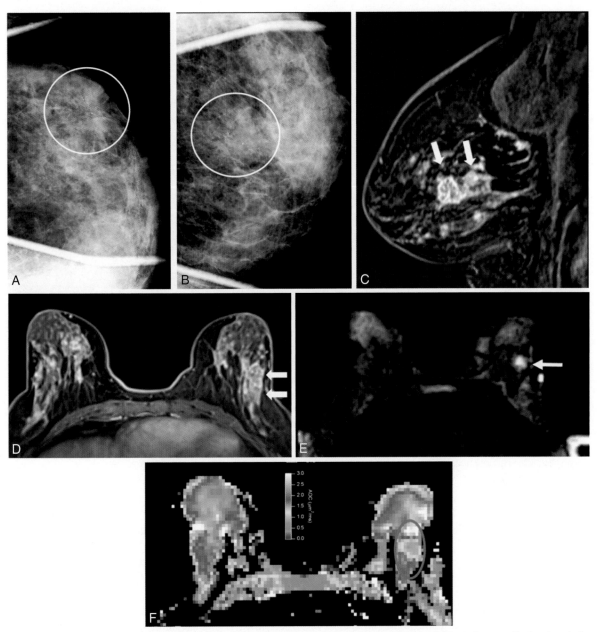

Fig. 4.3 Fifty-year-old asymptomatic woman presenting with indeterminate microcalcifications in the left breast. Spot magnification views in the (A) craniocaudal and (B) lateral view demonstrated grouped heterogeneous calcifications associated with subtle architectural distortion *(circles)*. Stereotactic core biopsy yielded invasive ductal carcinoma, moderately differentiated ER−/PR−, HER2+. (C) Sagittal T1-weighted postcontrast subtraction images and (D) axial T1-weighted postcontrast images showed a 3.5-cm spiculated heterogeneously enhancing mass *(arrow)*. (E) Diffusion-weighted b_{800} image shows the cancer is hyperintense *(arrow)*. (F) Apparent diffusion coefficient (ADC) map, generated with b_0 and b_{800} values, shows lower values in the cancer *(red circle)* than in the adjacent fibroglandular tissue, consistent with restricted diffusion.

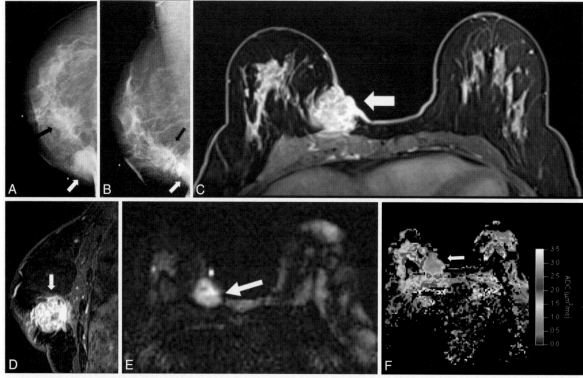

Fig. 4.4 Fifty-two-year-old woman presenting with a palpable mass in the right breast. (A) Craniocaudal and (B) mediolateral oblique mammographic views demonstrate a dense spiculated mass *(white arrow)* in the lower inner quadrant that corresponds with the palpable finding. A second irregular spiculated mass *(black arrow)* was seen in the central region. (C) Axial T1-weighted postcontrast images and (D) sagittal T1-weighted postcontrast subtraction images showed a 4.3-cm irregular, round heterogeneously enhancing mass corresponding to the palpable finding *(arrow)*. (E) Diffusion-weighted b_{800} image shows the mass is hyperintense *(arrow)*. (F) Apparent diffusion coefficient (ADC) map generated with b_0 and b_{800} values shows lower values in the mass *(arrow)* than in the fibroglandular tissue. Pathology yielded an invasive ductal carcinoma, moderately differentiated ER–/PR–, HER2+ for both masses.

noted in HER2-positive breast cancers.[95] Although these results are promising, they have thus far been demonstrated only in small sample sizes.

TRIPLE NEGATIVE BREAST CANCERS

Triple negative breast cancers (TNBCs) account for approximately 15% of all breast cancers. They express many of the same genes found in the basal myoepithelial cells of the terminal ductal lobular unit. They are associated with a failure to express ER and ER-associated genes.[45] As they lack the receptors available for targeted therapy, chemotherapy is the only current option for adjuvant and neoadjuvant therapy. However, due to their high grade and high proliferative index, TNBCs have a higher sensitivity to chemotherapy than any other tumor type. Similar to HER2+

tumors, improved DFS and OS is seen in tumors that demonstrate pathological complete response (pCR) after neoadjuvant therapy. However, overall prognosis remains poor compared with luminal breast cancers.[45]

TNBCs are seen more frequently in premenopausal women and African-American women. Women who are genetic carriers of the BRCA mutations, particularly *BRCA1*, are also more likely to develop basal-like breast cancers.

Mammography, Ultrasound, and Magnetic Resonance Imaging Features of Triple Negative Breast Cancers

Like most cancers, TNBCs most commonly present mammographically as an irregular mass with spiculated margins. However, 8% to 32% of these tumors will appear as round or oval with circumscribed margins, a known pitfall of evaluating these tumors in younger women where they can initially mimic benign lesions. Associated calcifications or architectural distortion are uncommon.[22,45]

Sonographically, TNBCs are most often hypoechoic with irregular or indistinct margins. Similar to their mammographic appearance, up to 20% can have circumscribed margins, and up to 50% can have parallel orientation. The initial similarity to more benign lesions, such as fibroadenomas or complicated cysts, can lead to short-term follow-up and potential delay in diagnosis.[22,45]

On MRI, TNBCs are most commonly round or oval masses with spiculated or irregular margins. Similar to mammography and sonography, approximately 10% are circumscribed. Due to their high grade and proliferative increase, rim enhancement with central tumor necrosis is common. Although they are more likely than HER2+ tumors to be unifocal, MRI can reveal multifocal disease in up to 25% of cases.[22,96]

Diffusion-Weighted Imaging of Triple Negative Breast Cancers

Examples of TNBCs evaluated on DWI are illustrated in Figs. 4.5 and 4.6. Similar to the literature evaluating HER2+ tumors, TNBCs have also been shown to have higher ADC values compared with luminal tumors. Youk and colleagues evaluated 271 breast cancers and found that although tumor subtypes were not readily differentiable or changed in detection by visual assessment of DWI maps, the ADC_{mean} value of TNBC (1.034×10^{-3} mm^2/s) was significantly higher than that of ER+ (0.891×10^{-3} mm^2/s; $P = .002$) and HER2+ tumors (0.839×10^{-3} mm^2/s; $P < .0001$).[96] The authors suggested this may be due to the high rate of intratumoral necrosis seen in TNBC in their study population, as suggested by very high intratumoral signal intensity on T2-weighted imaging.[96] Similar results were found by Choi and colleagues, who found TNBC displayed higher ADC parameters than ER+ subtype breast cancer, with whole-lesion ADC kurtosis significant on multivariate analysis ($P < .001$).[67]

However, these results have not been reproduced in other studies.[58,63] As some studies evaluating TNBC compared with luminal cancers have excluded HER2+ tumors,[67] additional studies with direct comparison between HER2+ to TNBCs are needed.

Diffusion-Weighted Imaging Predicting Markers of Tumor Aggressiveness

The molecular classification of tumors has elucidated some of the heterogeneity inherent to breast cancer. Additional biomarkers such as grade tumor grade and tumor infiltrating lymphocytes also have prognostic and treatment implications,[22] and their association with DWI biomarkers is summarized in Table 4.2.

IN SITU VERSUS INVASIVE

Ductal carcinoma in situ (DCIS) is a noninvasive and nonobligate precursor of invasive breast cancer. DCIS originates in the ductal epithelium and does not infiltrate through the basement membrane. Some DCIS will progress into invasive cancer, whereas some DCIS will remain in situ for many years, possibly for the remainder of the patient's life span. There are ongoing observational studies of DCIS that seek to determine whether some low-risk DCIS may be safely observed rather than treated.[97] As patients in these observational trials will not undergo surgery, it is important to develop imaging biomarkers that could reliably differentiate in situ from invasive lesions. As DCIS is restricted to the intraductal compartment, it may not limit extracellular water diffusion to the same degree an invasive cancer that spreads throughout the breast tissue.

Several studies have shown lower ADC values in invasive carcinomas compared with in situ carcinomas.[67,98–100] Studies have also shown that low-grade DCIS demonstrates significantly different ADC values and other quantitative DWI parameters than high-grade DCIS.[101–103] Note that if imaging is to be used to downstage treatment, then specificity for low-risk DCIS should be very high in order to avoid inclusion of patients with concurrent invasion or microinvasion.[101]

TUMOR GRADE

All invasive breast carcinomas are assigned a histological grade, which is based on the Nottingham classification and is a quantitative assessment of three morphological features (tubule formation, nuclear pleomorphism, and mitotic count).[26] Each component is given a score from 1 (least aggressive) to 3 (most aggressive), and the sum of the three scores

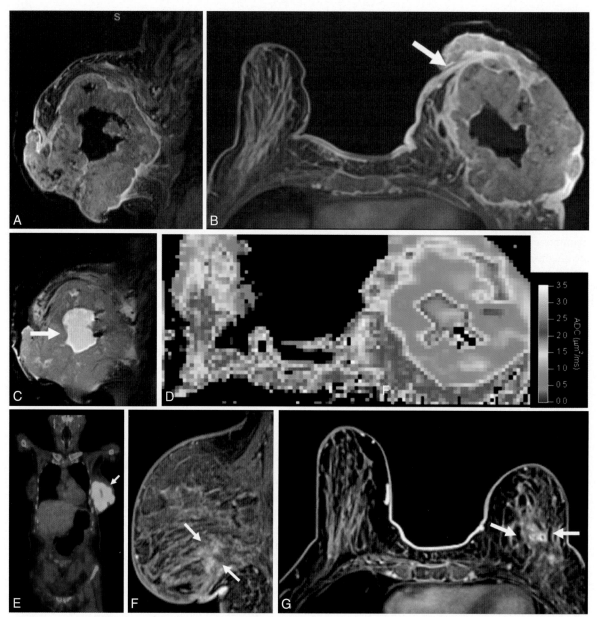

Fig. 4.5 Fifty-five-year-old woman presenting with a large, fungating, ulcerated mass in left breast. (A) Sagittal and (B) axial T1-weighted postcontrast images demonstrates a 13-cm rim-enhancing mass occupying the entire breast. Multiple enlarged blood vessels *(arrow)* are surrounding the mass. (C) Sagittal T2-weighted precontrast image show high signal in the center of the mass consistent with tumor necrosis *(arrow)*. (D) Apparent diffusion coefficient (ADC) map generated with b_0 and b_{800} values shows high signal values in the center of the cancer consistent with tumor necrosis. Low ADC values are seen throughout the rest of the tumor, consistent with restricted diffusion. (E) 2-deoxy-2-[fluorine-18]fluoro-D-glucose positron-emission tomography/computed tomography (PET/CT) showed an avidly enhancing mass *(arrow)* in the left breast. Ultrasound-guided core biopsy yielded a triple negative breast cancer. The patient underwent neoadjuvant therapy with paclitaxel and radiation. Follow-up breast magnetic resonance imaging (MRI) was performed 4 months after the start of therapy. (F) Sagittal and (G) axial T1-weighted postcontrast images demonstrate a 3-cm area of nonmass enhancement *(arrows)*. A modified radical mastectomy identified no residual disease.

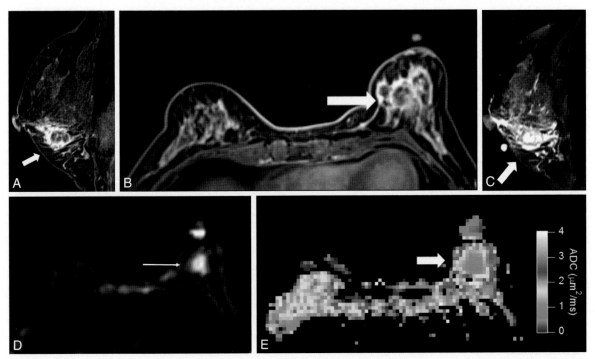

Fig. 4.6 Forty-three-year-old woman presenting with a palpable tender mass in the right breast. (A)-Sagittal T1 weighted postcontrast subtraction images and (B) axial T1-weighted postcontrast images showed a 2.2-cm irregular, round rim enhancing mass corresponding to the palpable finding *(arrow)*. (C) Sagittal T2-weighted precontrast images show the central necrosis *(arrow)*. (D) Diffusion-weighted b_{800} image shows the cancer is hyperintense *(arrow)*. (E) Apparent diffusion coefficient (ADC) map generated with b_0 and b_{800} values shows low signal throughout the tumor, suggestive of diffusion restriction. Ultrasound-guided core biopsy yielded a triple negative breast cancer with a Ki-67 of 70%.

provides the grade. Tumors with scores of 3 to 5 are well-differentiated and low grade, whereas tumors with scores 8 to 9 are poorly differentiated and higher grade. Tumor grade is incorporated into the clinical classification and staging of all breast cancers within AJCC prognostic stage groups. Higher grade is independently predictive of worse disease-specific survival and worse OS.[26]

Given that increased proliferation and mitotic activity are associated with greater cellularity, it is possible that a lower ADC value could predict higher grade. The literature has shown mixed success. Some studies have found a significant relationship between ADC values and tumor grade,[74–76] whereas others did not.[62,67,78,79,84] Among the studies that did not find significance are the two largest studies, analyzing data from 335[67] and 870[84] patients, so the lack of significance was not likely due to underpowering. There is variability in the field strength, DWI sequences, and

b-values used in all of these studies, so lack of standardized technique may account for variable results. In addition, these studies grouped molecular subtypes and histological subtypes in their analyses, possibly confounding the results. Arponen and colleagues[77] found that a significant relationship between ADC and tumor grade was only seen when using a small region of interest (ROI) rather than whole-lesion ROI, which is an area for future study.

Importantly, it should be noted that even if there is a significant association between ADC value and grade, this may not translate into clinical significance. A study compiling data from six centers[84] found that although ADCs were significantly higher in grade 1 lesions compared with grade 2 and 3 lesions, receiver operating characteristic (ROC) analysis showed that using ADC for discrimination of tumor grade had very low sensitivity and specificity (sensitivity 56.2% and specificity 67.9% at the optimal ADC threshold), and the authors concluded that ADC could not be used as a surrogate marker for histological tumor grade.

KI-67

Kim and colleagues evaluated whether the ADC parameters may be associated with prognostic factors and invasive ductal carcinoma subtypes using a histogram analysis. The investigators found that the ADC was most robustly correlated with the Ki-67 labeling index.[54] More recently, Mori and colleagues[104] and Shen and colleagues[55] confirmed these results. Shen and colleagues investigated whether ADC may serve as an imaging biomarker for invasive ductal carcinoma. Among 71 patients who underwent 3.0 Tesla DWI, the authors found that Ki-67 expression and molecular subtype were independently associated with the ADC. The mean ADC was significantly different between Ki-67-positive (low ADC) and Ki-67-negative (high ADC) lesions.[55] On ROC curves, with a diagnostic sensitivity of 1.00 and specificity of 0.432, a cutoff value of 0.97×10^{-3} mm^2/s was identified. Given this negative association between ADC values and Ki-67 labeling index, the authors concluded that ADC may be helpful for predicting Ki-67 expression in invasive ductal carcinoma (IDC) preoperatively.[55]

However, the literature is mixed, and other groups found no correlation between ADC values and Ki-67 labeling index.[56–61] Zhuang and colleagues evaluated 80 IDCs and demonstrated that the ΔADC (ADC$_{max}$ − ADC$_{min}$) showed significant correlations with the Ki-67 labeling index (for all tumors), whereas ADC$_{mean}$ and ADC$_{median}$ did not.[83] Kim and colleagues also explored whether combined minimum ADC and ADC difference value may improve the diagnostic performance of DWI compared with mean ADC.[87] In 25 of the 258 women (9.7%) who developed distant metastasis, the ADC difference value was higher in women with distant metastasis than in those without distant metastasis (mean 0.743×10^{-3} mm^2/s vs. 0.566×10^{-3} mm^2/s, respectively; $P < .001$). Multivariable analysis showed that a higher ADC difference value ($>0.698 \times 10^{-3}$ mm^2/s) (hazard ratio [HR] = 4.5; $P < .001$), presence of axillary node metastasis (HR, 3.3; $P = .02$), and estrogen receptor negativity (HR = 2.6; $P = .02$) were predictive of poorer distant metastasis–free survival.[87] These mixed results were the motivation for a large

multicenter analysis of six sites to explore the relationships between ADC and expression of Ki-67 labeling index and tumor grade in 870 patients.[84] Using a Youden index that identified a threshold ADC value of 0.91 led to a sensitivity of 64%, specificity of 50%, positive predictive value of 67.7%, and negative predictive value of 45.0%. The authors concluded that it was impossible to differentiate high/moderate grade tumors from grade 1 lesions using ADC values.[84] Overall, the mixed results in the literature may be due to the use of different technical approaches for acquisition and analysis, and to not taking into account the molecular subtypes of breast cancers.

LYMPHOVASCULAR INVASION

Lymphovascular invasion (LVI) is defined as cancer within blood or lymph vessels and is an independent risk factor for metastasis, recurrence, and mortality.[78] Multiple studies[78,86,104] have found that ADC values are significantly lower in lesions with LVI. The ratio of peritumor-tumor ADC is also a predictor of LVI[105] and even more significant than tumor ADC value in one study.[104] This ratio is highest in cases with high peritumoral ADC and low tumoral ADC, which are cancers with peritumoral edema due to LVI, and low tumoral ADC values associated with proliferation and tumor aggressiveness.

TUMOR INFILTRATING LYMPHOCYTES

Tumor infiltrating lymphocytes (TILs) are immune cells that when found in the intratumoral stroma correlate with a positive prognosis and improved response to neoadjuvant chemotherapy and immunotherapy.[89] TILs may represent a surrogate for a preexisting favorable host antitumor-activated T cell response. Studies have found that breast cancers with low or absent TILs have a significantly lower mean ADC value than cancers with high TILs.[88,89,106] Tumor molecular subtype should be taken into account in future studies, because there is evidence that different DWI-derived parameters may be better suited to TIL prediction in different subtypes.[80,89]

PERITUMORAL TISSUE

A tumor and its microenvironment have a two-way interaction, as the tumor releases extracellular signals to promote angiogenesis and microvessel density while the microenvironment changes stromal properties to increase rigidity of the tumor-associated stroma.[81] DWI of peritumoral tissue has been shown to be associated with high-risk features. Specifically, high ADC values in the peritumoral tissue are associated with higher grade, lack of ER expression, high Ki-67 levels, and lymph node metastases.[107] In addition, increased ADC heterogeneity in the peritumoral space has also been associated with high-risk features, including Ki-67 levels,[81] lymph node status,[108] and tumor molecular subtype.[82] This suggests that more aggressive tumors have a more heterogeneous tumor microenvironment.

Diffusion-Weighted Imaging for Tumor Staging and Surgical Planning

Current breast cancer staging recommendations[26] incorporate the TNM system and the biomarkers described in the first part of this chapter. Anatomical staging using the TNM system remains relevant, because tumor size (T), lymph node status (N), and presence of metastatic disease (M) partially inform the patient's prognosis and treatment plan. Size of the index tumor is variably predicted on DWI[75,79,80] and better evaluated on dynamic contrast-enhanced MRI (DCE MRI). However, in addition to index tumor size, extent of disease including multifocality is an important factor in surgical planning.

MULTIFOCALITY

Multifocality is the presence of more than one invasive focus in one quadrant, and multicentricity is the presence of invasive foci in different quadrants of the same breast. Rates of multicentricity and multifocality vary among tumor types but are approximately 20% and 25%, respectively.[11] In theory, preoperative MRI to evaluate for multicentricity and multifocality could result in fewer reexcisions for positive margins and decreased local recurrence rates. However, trials have not demonstrated improved outcomes, and preoperative staging MRI remains a common but controversial indication.[10] National and international guidelines vary on recommendations for preoperative MRI, but it may be indicated in women at increased risk of local recurrence, such as those diagnosed at a young age,

women with dense breasts, and women with invasive lobular carcinoma.[10]

In a study of patients found to have additional lesions on preoperative MRI, Song and colleagues[109] found that adding an ADC cutoff value to DCE MRI could dramatically improve specificity (from 18.9% to 82.2%) without significantly decreasing sensitivity (from 98.6% to 90.0%). Park and colleagues[110] similarly studied women with newly diagnosed breast cancer and additional suspicious lesions on preoperative MRI, finding that ADC histogram features could differentiate between benign and invasive lesions.

These studies suggest that adding DWI to preoperative MRI could potentially reduce false-positive additional lesions, leading to decreased biopsies and reducing unnecessarily extensive surgery.

AXILLARY LYMPH NODE METASTASIS

Lymph node status is an important prognostic indicator and may determine the patient's treatment plan. As axillary surgery and radiation may be associated with morbidity such as lymphedema, there is a trend toward de-escalation of treatment in the axilla when appropriate. To minimize morbidity, noninvasive axillary staging with reliable imaging biomarkers would be preferable to surgical staging to help inform treatment decisions.

Several studies have found a significant association between ADC values of the primary tumor and lymph node status,[75,79,111,112] suggesting that lower ADC values correlate with more aggressive cancers with higher metastatic potential. However, this was not confirmed in a large multicenter analysis pooling data for 661 patients, which showed no correlation between primary tumor ADC value and lymph node status.[113]

There is also interest in evaluating the lymph nodes themselves rather than predicting lymph node involvement from the primary tumor, with some mixed results. Some studies show an association between ADC of the axillary lymph nodes and lymph node positivity,[114–118] with metastatic nodes exhibiting lower ADC values versus negative or nonmetastatic nodes.[118] Of note, one study further evaluated only morphologically suspicious lymph nodes and found that the morphologically suspicious benign reactive lymph nodes had similar quantitative DWI features as morphologically suspicious malignant lymph nodes.[118] This suggests that DWI features do not add information beyond what can be determined by qualitative morphological features; this was also supported by a study finding that lymph node diameter is more predictive of lymph node involvement than ADC value.[115]

Future Directions

As discussed in Chapter 10, radiomics and machine learning in breast MRI are rapidly evolving fields that are well suited to the incorporation of imaging biomarkers, such as DWI data. Radiomics is the field in which large numbers of quantitative features are extracted from medical images and pooled in large-scale analysis to create decision support models.[35] The imaging data may be combined with patient-level data such as clinicopathologic features or genetic data (known as radiogenomics) to improve accuracy. Using radiomics-style analysis incorporating DWI data may provide more information than using ADC measurements alone. A few studies using radiomics with DWI have evaluated prediction of axillary lymph node metastases,[119] characterizing benign versus malignant lesions,[120,121] and predicting response to neoadjuvant chemotherapy.[122]

Machine learning is a branch of data science that enables computers to learn from existing "training" data without explicit programming.[35] Machine learning tools have been applied to DWI and multiparametric MRI data to predict response to neoadjuvant therapy[123] and lesion characterization.[68,94]

Conclusions

Breast cancer is a heterogeneous disease comprising different molecular subtypes with distinct genetic profiles. These subtypes have different prognoses and treatment plans. The ability of DWI to serve as an imaging biomarker to predict molecular subtype and to prognosticate the response to treatment is an area of robust research. Additional DWI biomarkers associated with tumor aggressiveness and predictors of invasion and tumor extent are also under investigation. These techniques remain investigational and have not yet reached clinical applicability. In order to achieve clinical relevance, DWI techniques will require standardization, subgroup analysis by patient group and tumor subtype, and independent validation by multiple researchers.

REFERENCES

1. American Cancer Society. Cancer Facts & Figures 2022. Atlanta: American Cancer Society; 2022.
2. Kriege M, Brekelmans CT, Boetes C, et al. Efficacy of MRI and mammography for breast-cancer screening in women with a familial or genetic predisposition. *N Engl J Med.* 2004;351(5):427–437.
3. Kuhl CK, Schrading S, Leutner CC, et al. Mammography, breast ultrasound, and magnetic resonance imaging for surveillance of women at high familial risk for breast cancer. *J Clin Oncol.* 2005;23(33):8469–8476.
4. Leach MO, Boggis CR, Dixon AK, et al. Screening with magnetic resonance imaging and mammography of a UK population at high familial risk of breast cancer: a prospective multicentre cohort study (MARIBS). *Lancet.* 2005;365(9473):1769–1778.
5. Warner E, Plewes DB, Hill KA, et al. Surveillance of BRCA1 and BRCA2 mutation carriers with magnetic resonance imaging, ultrasound, mammography, and clinical breast examination. *JAMA.* 2004;292(11):1317–1325.
6. Bakker MF, de Lange SV, Pijnappel RM, et al. Supplemental MRI screening for women with extremely dense breast tissue. *N Engl J Med.* 2019;381(22):2091–2102.
7. Kuhl CK, Strobel K, Bieling H, Leutner C, Schild HH, Schrading S. Supplemental breast MR imaging screening of women with average risk of breast cancer. *Radiolog.* 2017;283(2):361–370.
8. Riedl CC, Luft N, Bernhart C, et al. Triple-modality screening trial for familial breast cancer underlines the importance of magnetic resonance imaging and questions the role of mammography and ultrasound regardless of patient mutation status, age, and breast density. *J Clin Oncol.* 2015;33(10):1128–1135.
9. Comstock CE, Gatsonis C, Newstead GM, et al. Comparison of abbreviated breast MRI vs digital breast tomosynthesis for breast cancer detection among women with dense breasts undergoing screening. *JAMA.* 2020;323(8):746–756.
10. Mann RM, Cho N, Moy L. Breast MRI: state of the art. *Radiology.* 2019;292(3):520–536.
11. Mann RM, Kuhl CK, Kinkel K, Boetes C. Breast MRI: guidelines from the European Society of Breast Imaging. *Eur Radiol.* 2008;18(7):1307–1318.
12. Sardanelli F, Boetes C, Borisch B, et al. Magnetic resonance imaging of the breast: recommendations from the EUSOMA working group. *Eur J Cancer.* 2010;46(8):1296–1316.
13. American College of Radiology. ACR Practice Parameter for the Performance of Contrast-Enhanced Magnetic Resonance Imaging (MRI) of the Breast. 2014.
14. Knopp MV, Weiss E, Sinn HP, et al. Pathophysiologic basis of contrast enhancement in breast tumors. *J Magn Reson Imaging.* 1999;10(3):260–266.
15. Carmeliet P, Jain RK. Angiogenesis in cancer and other diseases. *Nature.* 2000;407(6801):249–257.
16. Warner E, Messersmith H, Causer P, Eisen A, Shumak R, Plewes D. Systematic review: using magnetic resonance imaging to screen women at high risk for breast cancer. *Ann Intern Med.* 2008;148(9):671–679.

17. Evans DG, Harkness EF, Howell A, et al. Intensive breast screening in BRCA2 mutation carriers is associated with reduced breast cancer specific and all cause mortality. *Hered Cancer Clin Pract*. 2016;14:8.

18. Le Bihan D, Iima M. Diffusion magnetic resonance imaging: what water tells us about biological tissues. *PLoS Biol*. 2015;13(7):e1002203.

19. Partridge SC, McDonald ES. Diffusion weighted magnetic resonance imaging of the breast: protocol optimization, interpretation, and clinical applications. *Magn Reson Imaging Clin N Am*. 2013;21(3):601–624.

20. Shi RY, Yao QY, Wu LM, Xu JR. Breast lesions: diagnosis using diffusion weighted imaging at 1.5 T and 3.0 T: systematic review and meta-analysis. *Clin Breast Cancer*. 2018;18(3):e305–e320.

21. Baltzer P, Mann RM, Iima M, et al. Diffusion-weighted imaging of the breast: a consensus and mission statement from the EUSOBI International Breast Diffusion-Weighted Imaging working group. *Eur Radiol*. 2020;30(3):1436–1450.

22. Trop I, LeBlanc SM, David J, et al. Molecular classification of infiltrating breast cancer: toward personalized therapy. *Radiographics*. 2014;34(5):1178–1195.

23. Edge SB, Compton CC. The American Joint Committee on Cancer: the 7th edition of the AJCC cancer staging manual and the future of TNM. *Ann Surg Oncol*. 2010;17(6):1471–1474.

24. National Cancer Institute. Surveillance, Epidemiology, and End Results (SEER) Program. Accessed November 18, 2021. https://seer.cancer.gov.

25. Van 't Veer LJ, Dai H, van de Vijver MJ, et al. Gene expression profiling predicts clinical outcome of breast cancer. *Nature*. 2002;415(6871):530–536.

26. American Joint Commission on Cancer . AJCC Cancer Staging Manual. 8th ed. Springer International Publishing; 2017.

27. Perou CM, Sorlie T, Eisen MB, et al. Molecular portraits of human breast tumours. *Nature*. 2000;406(6797):747–752.

28. Sorlie T, Perou CM, Tibshirani R, et al. Gene expression patterns of breast carcinomas distinguish tumor subclasses with clinical implications. *Proc Natl Acad Sci U S A*. 2001;98(19):10869–10874.

29. Sotiriou C, Neo SY, McShane LM, et al. Breast cancer classification and prognosis based on gene expression profiles from a population-based study. *Proc Natl Acad Sci U S A*. 2003;100(18):10393–10398.

30. Curtis C. Genomic profiling of breast cancers. *Curr Opin Obstet Gynecol*. 2015;27(1):34–39.

31. Cancer Genome Atlas Network . Comprehensive molecular portraits of human breast tumours. *Nature*. 2012; 490(7418):61–70.

32. Goldhirsch A, Winer EP, Coates AS, et al. Personalizing the treatment of women with early breast cancer: highlights of the St Gallen International Expert Consensus on the Primary Therapy of Early Breast Cancer 2013. *Ann Oncol*. 2013;24(9):2206–2223.

33. Pinker K, Chin J, Melsaether AN, Morris EA, Moy L. Precision medicine and radiogenomics in breast cancer: new approaches toward diagnosis and treatment. *Radiology*. 2018;287(3):732–747.

34. Esteva FJ, Hortobagyi GN. Prognostic molecular markers in early breast cancer. *Breast Cancer Res*. 2004;6(3):109–118.

35. Reig B, Heacock L, Geras KJ, Moy L. Machine learning in breast MRI. *J Magn Reson Imaging*. 2020;52(4):998–1018.

36. Huber KE, Carey LA, Wazer DE. Breast cancer molecular subtypes in patients with locally advanced disease: impact on prognosis, patterns of recurrence, and response to therapy. *Semin Radiat Oncol*. 2009;19(4):204–210.

37. Lam SW, Jimenez CR, Boven E. Breast cancer classification by proteomic technologies: current state of knowledge. *Cancer Treat Rev*. 2014;40(1):129–138.

38. Iborra S, Stickeler E. HER2-orientated therapy in early and metastatic breast cancer. *Breast Care (Basel)*. 2016;11(6):392–397.

39. Lal S, McCart Reed AE, de Luca XM, Simpson PT. Molecular signatures in breast cancer. *Methods*. 2017;131:135–146.

40. Reis-Filho JS, Pusztai L. Gene expression profiling in breast cancer: classification, prognostication, and prediction. *Lancet*. 2011;378(9805):1812–1823.

41. Weigelt B, Baehner FL, Reis-Filho JS. The contribution of gene expression profiling to breast cancer classification, prognostication and prediction: a retrospective of the last decade. *J Pathol*. 2010;220(2):263–280.

42. Harris LN, Ismaila N, McShane LM, et al. Use of biomarkers to guide decisions on adjuvant systemic therapy for women with early-stage invasive breast cancer: American Society of Clinical Oncology clinical practice guideline. *J Clin Oncol*. 2016;34(10):1134–1150.

43. Gupta A, Mutebi M, Bardia A. Gene-expression-based predictors for breast cancer. *Ann Surg Oncol*. 2015;22(11):3418–3432.

44. Coates AS, Winer EP, Goldhirsch A, et al. Tailoring therapies: improving the management of early breast cancer: St Gallen International Expert Consensus on the Primary Therapy of Early Breast Cancer 2015. *Ann Oncol*. 2015;26(8):1533–1546.

45. Johnson KS, Conant EF, Soo MS. Molecular subtypes of breast cancer: a review for breast radiologists. *J Breast Imaging*. 2020;3(1):12–24.

46. Prat A, Perou CM. Deconstructing the molecular portraits of breast cancer. *Mol Oncol*. 2011;5(1):5–23.

47. Jatoi I, Anderson WF, Jeong JH, Redmond CK. Breast cancer adjuvant therapy: time to consider its time-dependent effects. *J Clin Oncol*. 2011;29(17):2301–2304.

48. Bare M, Tora N, Salas D, et al. Mammographic and clinical characteristics of different phenotypes of screen-detected and interval breast cancers in a nationwide screening program. *Breast Cancer Res Treat*. 2015;154(2):403–415.

49. Tamaki K, Ishida T, Miyashita M, et al. Correlation between mammographic findings and corresponding histopathology: potential predictors for biological characteristics of breast diseases. *Cancer Sci*. 2011;102(12):2179–2185.

50. Ko ES, Lee BH, Kim HA, Noh WC, Kim MS, Lee SA. Triple-negative breast cancer: correlation between imaging and pathological findings. *Eur Radiol*. 2010;20(5):1111–1117.

51. Grimm LJ, Johnson KS, Marcom PK, Baker JA, Soo MS. Can breast cancer molecular subtype help to select patients for preoperative MR imaging? *Radiology*. 2015;274(2):352–358.

52. Navarro Vilar L, Alandete German SP, Medina Garcia R, Blanc Garcia E, Camarasa Lillo N, Vilar Samper J. MR imaging findings in molecular subtypes of breast cancer according to BIRADS system. *Breast J*. 2017;23(4):421–428.

53. Uematsu T, Kasami M, Yuen S. Triple-negative breast cancer: correlation between MR imaging and pathologic findings. *Radiology*. 2009;250(3):638–647.

54. Kim EJ, Kim SH, Park GE, et al. Histogram analysis of apparent diffusion coefficient at 3.0 T: correlation with prognostic factors and subtypes of invasive ductal carcinoma. *J Magn Reson Imaging*. 2015;42(6):1666–1678.

55. Shen L, Zhou G, Tong T, et al. ADC at 3.0 T as a noninvasive biomarker for preoperative prediction of Ki67

expression in invasive ductal carcinoma of breast. *Clin Imaging.* 2018;52:16–22.

56. Liu F, Wang M, Li H. Role of perfusion parameters on DCE-MRI and ADC values on DWMRI for invasive ductal carcinoma at 3.0 tesla. *World J Surg Oncol.* 2018;16(1):239.

57. Fan M, He T, Zhang P, et al. Diffusion-weighted imaging features of breast tumours and the surrounding stroma reflect intrinsic heterogeneous characteristics of molecular subtypes in breast cancer. *NMR Biomed.* 2018;31:2.

58. Martincich L, Deantoni V, Bertotto I, et al. Correlations between diffusion-weighted imaging and breast cancer biomarkers. *Eur Radiol.* 2012;22(7):1519–1528.

59. Jeh SK, Kim SH, Kim HS, et al. Correlation of the apparent diffusion coefficient value and dynamic magnetic resonance imaging findings with prognostic factors in invasive ductal carcinoma. *J Magn Reson Imaging.* 2011;33(1):102–109.

60. Kim SH, Cha ES, Kim HS, et al. Diffusion-weighted imaging of breast cancer: correlation of the apparent diffusion coefficient value with prognostic factors. *J Magn Reson Imaging.* 2009;30(3):615–620.

61. Iima M, Kataoka M, Kanao S, et al. Intravoxel incoherent motion and quantitative non-Gaussian diffusion MR imaging: evaluation of the diagnostic and prognostic value of several markers of malignant and benign breast lesions. *Radiology.* 2018;287(2):432–441.

62. Horvat JV, Bernard-Davila B, Helbich TH, et al. Diffusion-weighted imaging (DWI) with apparent diffusion coefficient (ADC) mapping as a quantitative imaging biomarker for prediction of immunohistochemical receptor status, proliferation rate, and molecular subtypes of breast cancer. *J Magn Reson Imaging.* 2019;50(3):836–846.

63. Suo S, Zhang D, Cheng F, et al. Added value of mean and entropy of apparent diffusion coefficient values for evaluating histologic phenotypes of invasive ductal breast cancer with MR imaging. *Eur Radiol.* 2019;29(3):1425–1434.

64. Amornsiripanitch N, Nguyen VT, Rahbar H, et al. Diffusion-weighted MRI characteristics associated with prognostic pathological factors and recurrence risk in invasive ER+/HER2− breast cancers. *J Magn Reson Imaging.* 2018;48(1):226–236.

65. Kim JY, Kim JJ, Hwangbo L, Kang T, Park H. Diffusion-weighted imaging of invasive breast cancer: relationship to distant metastasisfree survival. *Radiology.* 2019;291(2):300–307.

66. Kamitani T, Matsuo Y, Yabuuchi H, et al. Correlations between apparent diffusion coefficient values and prognostic factors of breast cancer. *Magn Reson Med Sci.* 2013;12(3):193–199.

67. Choi SY, Chang YW, Park HJ, Kim HJ, Hong SS, Seo DY. Correlation of the apparent diffusion coefficiency values on diffusion-weighted imaging with prognostic factors for breast cancer. *Br J Radiol.* 2012;85(1016):e474–e479.

68. Vidic I, Egnell L, Jerome NP, et al. Support vector machine for breast cancer classification using diffusion-weighted MRI histogram features: preliminary study. *J Magn Reson Imaging.* 2018;47(5):1205–1216.

69. Suo S, Cheng F, Cao M, et al. Multiparametric diffusion-weighted imaging in breast lesions: association with pathologic diagnosis and prognostic factors. *J Magn Reson Imaging.* 2017;46(3):740–750.

70. Kawashima H, Miyati T, Ohno N, et al. Differentiation between luminal-A and luminal-B breast cancer using intravoxel incoherent motion and dynamic contrast-enhanced magnetic resonance imaging. *Acad Radiol.* 2017;24(12):1575–1581.

71. Lee YJ, Kim SH, Kang BJ, et al. Intravoxel incoherent motion (IVIM)-derived parameters in diffusion-weighted MRI:

72. Kim Y, Ko K, Kim D, et al. Intravoxel incoherent motion diffusion-weighted MR imaging of breast cancer: association with histopathological features and subtypes. *Br J Radiol.* 2016;89(1063). 20160140.

73. Cho GY, Moy L, Kim SG, et al. Evaluation of breast cancer using intravoxel incoherent motion (IVIM) histogram analysis: comparison with malignant status, histological subtype, and molecular prognostic factors. *Eur Radiol.* 2016;26(8):2547–2558.

74. Cipolla V, Santucci D, Guerrieri D, Drudi FM, Meggiorini ML, de Felice C. Correlation between 3T apparent diffusion coefficient values and grading of invasive breast carcinoma. *Eur J Radiol.* 2014;83(12):2144–2150.

75. Belli P, Costantini M, Bufi E, et al. Diffusion magnetic resonance imaging in breast cancer characterisation: correlations between the apparent diffusion coefficient and major prognostic factors. *Radiol Med.* 2015;120(3):268–276.

76. Molinari C, Clauser P, Girometti R, et al. MR mammography using diffusion-weighted imaging in evaluating breast cancer: a correlation with proliferation index. *Radiol Med.* 2015;120(10):911–918.

77. Arponen O, Sudah M, Masarwah A, et al. Diffusion-weighted imaging in 3.0 Tesla breast MRI: diagnostic performance and tumor characterization using small subregions vs. whole tumor regions of interest. *PLoS One.* 2015;10(10):e0138702.

78. Durando M, Gennaro L, Cho GY, et al. Quantitative apparent diffusion coefficient measurement obtained by 3.0 Tesla MRI as a potential noninvasive marker of tumor aggressiveness in breast cancer. *Eur J Radiol.* 2016;85(9):1651–1658.

79. Kitajima K, Yamano T, Fukushima K, et al. Correlation of the SUVmax of FDG-PET and ADC values of diffusion-weighted MR imaging with pathologic prognostic factors in breast carcinoma. *Eur J Radiol.* 2016;85(5):943–949.

80. Shin HJ, Kim SH, Lee HJ, et al. Tumor apparent diffusion coefficient as an imaging biomarker to predict tumor aggressiveness in patients with estrogen-receptor-positive breast cancer. *NMR Biomed.* 2016;29(8):1070–1078.

81. Fan M, He T, Zhang P, Zhang J, Li L. Heterogeneity of diffusion-weighted imaging in tumours and the surrounding stroma for prediction of Ki-67 proliferation status in breast cancer. *Sci Rep.* 2017;7(1):2875.

82. Fan M, He T, Zhang P, et al. Diffusion-weighted imaging features of breast tumours and the surrounding stroma reflect intrinsic heterogeneous characteristics of molecular subtypes in breast cancer. *NMR Biomed.* 2018;31(2):e3869.

83. Zhuang Z, Zhang Q, Zhang D, et al. Utility of apparent diffusion coefficient as an imaging biomarker for assessing the proliferative potential of invasive ductal breast cancer. *Clin Radiol.* 2018;73(5):473–478.

84. Surov A, Clauser P, Chang YW, et al. Can diffusion-weighted imaging predict tumor grade and expression of Ki-67 in breast cancer? A multicenter analysis. *Breast Cancer Res.* 2018;20(1):58.

85. Thakur SB, Durando M, Milans S, et al. Apparent diffusion coefficient in estrogen receptor-positive and lymph node-negative invasive breast cancers at 3.0 T DW-MRI: a potential predictor for an oncotype Dx test recurrence score. *J Magn Reson Imaging.* 2018;47(2):401–409.

86. Igarashi T, Furube H, Ashida H, Ojiri H. Breast MRI for prediction of lymphovascular invasion in breast cancer patients with clinically negative axillary lymph nodes. *Eur J Radiol.* 2018;107:111–118.

87. Park SH, Choi HY, Hahn SY. Correlations between apparent diffusion coefficient values of invasive ductal carcinoma and pathologic factors on diffusion-weighted MRI at 3.0 tesla. *J Magn Reson Imaging.* 2015;41(1):175–182.

88. Fogante M, Tagliati C, De Lisa M, Berardi R, Giuseppetti GM, Giovagnoni A. Correlation between apparent diffusion coefficient of magnetic resonance imaging and tumor-infiltrating lymphocytes in breast cancer. *Radiol Med.* 2019;124(7):581–587.

89. Tang WJ, Jin Z, Zhang YL, et al. Whole-lesion histogram analysis of the apparent diffusion coefficient as a quantitative imaging biomarker for assessing the level of tumor-infiltrating lymphocytes: value in molecular subtypes of breast cancer. *Front Oncol.* 2020;10:611571.

90. Springer CS Jr. Using ^{1}H$_2$O MR to measure and map sodium pump activity in vivo. *J Magn Reson.* 2018;291:110–126.

91. Kato F, Kudo K, Yamashita H, et al. Differences in morphological features and minimum apparent diffusion coefficient values among breast cancer subtypes using 3-tesla MRI. *Eur J Radiol.* 2016;85(1):96–102.

92. Hyder SM, Murthy L, Stancel GM. Progestin regulation of vascular endothelial growth factor in human breast cancer cells. *Cancer Res.* 1998;58(3):392–395.

93. Heacock L, Lewin AA, Gao Y, et al. Feasibility analysis of early temporal kinetics as a surrogate marker for breast tumor type, grade, and aggressiveness. *J Magn Reson Imaging.* 2018;47(6):1692–1700.

94. Parekh VS, Jacobs MA. Integrated radiomic framework for breast cancer and tumor biology using advanced machine learning and multiparametric MRI. *NPJ Breast Cancer.* 2017;3:43.

95. Turashvili G, Brogi E. Tumor heterogeneity in breast cancer. *Front Med (Lausanne).* 2017; 4:227.

96. Youk JH, Son EJ, Chung J, Kim J-A, Kim E-k. Triple-negative invasive breast cancer on dynamic contrast-enhanced and diffusion-weighted MR imaging: comparison with other breast cancer subtypes. *Eur Radiol.* 2012;22(8):1724–1734.

97. Hwang ES, Hyslop T, Lynch T, et al. The COMET (Comparison of Operative versus Monitoring and Endocrine Therapy) trial: a phase III randomised controlled clinical trial for low-risk ductal carcinoma in situ (DCIS). *BMJ Open.* 2019;9(3):e026797.

98. Bickel H, Pinker-Domenig K, Bogner W, et al. Quantitative apparent diffusion coefficient as a noninvasive imaging biomarker for the differentiation of invasive breast cancer and ductal carcinoma in situ. *Invest Radiol.* 2015;50(2):95–100.

99. Hussein H, Chung C, Moshonov H, Miller N, Kulkarni SR, Scaranelo AM. Evaluation of apparent diffusion coefficient to predict grade, microinvasion, and invasion in ductal carcinoma in situ of the breast. *Acad Radiol.* 2015;22(12):1483–1488.

100. Mori N, Ota H, Mugikura S, et al. Detection of invasive components in cases of breast ductal carcinoma in situ on biopsy by using apparent diffusion coefficient MR parameters. *Eur Radiol.* 2013;23(10):2705–2712.

101. Iima M, Le Bihan D, Okumura R, et al. Apparent diffusion coefficient as an MR imaging biomarker of low-risk ductal carcinoma in situ: a pilot study. *Radiology.* 2011;260(2):364–372.

102. Kim JY, Kim JJ, Lee JW, et al. Risk stratification of ductal carcinoma in situ using whole-lesion histogram analysis of the apparent diffusion coefficient. *Eur Radiol.* 2019;29(2):485–493.

103. Rahbar H, Partridge SC, Eby PR, et al. Characterization of ductal carcinoma in situ on diffusion weighted breast MRI. *Eur Radiol.* 2011;21(9):2011–2019.

104. Mori N, Ota H, Mugikura S, et al. Luminal-type breast cancer: correlation of apparent diffusion coefficients with the Ki-67 labeling index. *Radiology.* 2015;275(1):66–73. doi:10.1148/radiol.14140283

105. Okuma H, Sudah M, Kettunen T, et al. Peritumor to tumor apparent diffusion coefficient ratio is associated with biologically more aggressive breast cancer features and correlates with the prognostication tools. *PLoS One.* 2020;15(6):e0235278.

106. Celebi F, Agacayak F, Ozturk A, et al. Usefulness of imaging findings in predicting tumor-infiltrating lymphocytes in patients with breast cancer. *Eur Radiol.* 2020;30(4):2049–2057.

107. Shin HJ, Park JY, Shin KC, et al. Characterization of tumor and adjacent peritumoral stroma in patients with breast cancer using high-resolution diffusion-weighted imaging: correlation with pathologic biomarkers. *Eur J Radiol.* 2016;85(5):1004–1011.

108. Chen Q, Fan M, Zhang P, Li L, Xu M. Heterogeneity of tumor and its surrounding stroma on DCE-MRI and diffusion weighted imaging in predicting histological grade and lymph node status of breast cancer. SPIE; 2019.

109. Song SE, Park EK, Cho KR, et al. Additional value of diffusion-weighted imaging to evaluate multifocal and multicentric breast cancer detected using pre-operative breast MRI. *Eur Radiol.* 2017;27(11):4819–4827.

110. Park VY, Kim SG, Kim EK, Moon HJ, Yoon JH, Kim MJ. Diffusional kurtosis imaging for differentiation of additional suspicious lesions on preoperative breast MRI of patients with known breast cancer. *Magn Reson Imaging.* 2019;62:199–208.

111. Nakajo M, Kajiya Y, Kaneko T, et al. FDG PET/CT and diffusion-weighted imaging for breast cancer: prognostic value of maximum standardized uptake values and apparent diffusion coefficient values of the primary lesion. *Eur J Nucl Med Mol Imaging.* 2010;37(11):2011–2020.

112. Choi EJ, Youk JH, Choi H, Song JS. Dynamic contrast-enhanced and diffusion-weighted MRI of invasive breast cancer for the prediction of sentinel lymph node status. *J Magn Reson Imaging.* 2020;51(2):615–626.

113. Surov A, Chang Y-W, Li L, et al. Apparent diffusion coefficient cannot predict molecular subtype and lymph node metastases in invasive breast cancer: a multicenter analysis. *BMC Cancer.* 2019;19(1):1043.

114. Xing H, Song CL, Li WJ. Meta analysis of lymph node metastasis of breast cancer patients: Clinical value of DWI and ADC value. *Eur J Radiol.* 2016;85(6):1132–1137.

115. Iima M, Kataoka M, Okumura R, Togashi K. Detection of axillary lymph node metastasis with diffusion-weighted MR imaging. *Clin Imaging.* 2014;38(5):633–636.

116. Scaranelo AM, Eiada R, Jacks LM, Kulkarni SR, Crystal P. Accuracy of unenhanced MR imaging in the detection of axillary lymph node metastasis: study of reproducibility and reliability. *Radiology.* 2012;262(2):425–434.

117. Fornasa F, Nesoti MV, Bovo C, Bonavina MG. Diffusion-weighted magnetic resonance imaging in the characterization of axillary lymph nodes in patients with breast cancer. *J Magn Reson Imaging.* 2012;36(4):858–864.

118. Rahbar H, Conlin JL, Parsian S, et al. Suspicious axillary lymph nodes identified on clinical breast MRI in patients newly diagnosed with breast cancer: can quantitative features improve discrimination of malignant from benign? *Acad Radiol.* 2015;22(4):430–438.

119. Dong Y, Feng Q, Yang W, et al. Preoperative prediction of sentinel lymph node metastasis in breast cancer based on radiomics of T2-weighted fat-suppression and diffusion-weighted MRI. *Eur Radiol.* 2018;28(2):582–591.

120. Jiang X, Xie F, Liu L, Peng Y, Cai H, Li L. Discrimination of malignant and benign breast masses using automatic segmentation and features extracted from dynamic contrast-enhanced and diffusion-weighted MRI. *Oncol Lett.* 2018;16(2):1521–1528.

121. Bickelhaupt S, Paech D, Kickingereder P, et al. Prediction of malignancy by a radiomic signature from contrast agent-free diffusion MRI in suspicious breast lesions found on screening mammography. *J Magn Reson Imaging.* 2017;46(2):604–616.

122. Liu Z, Li Z, Qu J, et al. Radiomics of multiparametric MRI for pretreatment prediction of pathologic complete response to neoadjuvant chemotherapy in breast cancer: a multicenter study. *Clin Cancer Res.* 2019;25(12):3538–3547.

123. Tahmassebi A, Wengert GJ, Helbich TH, et al. Impact of machine learning with multiparametric magnetic resonance imaging of the breast for early prediction of response to neoadjuvant chemotherapy and survival outcomes in breast cancer patients. *Invest Radiol.* 2019;54(2):110–117.

Chapter 5

Disease and Treatment Monitoring

Wen Li, PhD, David C. Newitt, PhD, Savannah C. Partridge, PhD, and Nola M. Hylton, PhD

Preoperative, or neoadjuvant chemotherapy (NAC), in which systemic therapy is administered before surgery, is used to downstage primary breast cancers while reducing the risk of recurrence.[1-4] NAC often results in complete eradication of tumor at the time of surgery (pathological complete response [pCR]), and it is well established that pCR confers excellent survival outcomes.[5-8] The US Food and Drug Administration (FDA) now accepts pCR as an endpoint in clinical trials to support accelerated drug approval for high-risk early-stage breast cancer.[9]

Among breast imaging methods, dynamic contrast-enhanced magnetic resonance imaging (DCE MRI) is particularly effective for visualizing the effects of neoadjuvant treatment on breast tumors. DCE MRI has been found to be more effective than clinical examination and other routine imaging modalities (mammography and ultrasound) for detecting residual disease and defining its extent.[10,11] In addition to its high sensitivity, DCE MRI noninvasively provides information about breast tumor biology that can be used to predict response.[12-14]

Although DCE is the standard MRI method for evaluating breast cancer, diffusion-weighted imaging (DWI) has been shown to provide additional and complementary information about tissue cellularity and microstructure of the tumor and surrounding tissue environment, which can also be used to characterize breast tumors and to monitor their response to treatment.[15-23] In fact, several studies have suggested that changes in quantitative diffusion measurements from DWI can be detectable earlier in the course of NAC than changes in tumor size or vascularity measured by DCE MRI.[17,22] This is because effective drugs induce apoptosis and/or necrosis in the tumor, which alters the cell density and reduces barriers to water diffusion. Before the cell death associated with NAC, cell swelling or damage to membrane integrity can occur, which may also affect the water diffusion in the tumor. For this reason, many studies have evaluated DWI for prediction of breast cancer treatment response.[18-22,24-36]

Diffusion-Weighted Magnetic Resonance Imaging Approaches for Treatment Monitoring

Three primary requirements common to almost all studies investigating quantitative DWI for treatment outcome prediction are DWI acquisition; image analysis, in particular the selection of regions of interest (ROIs) for quantitation; and statistical analysis for prediction of a clinically useful patient outcome. In the setting of neoadjuvant treatment of invasive breast cancer, the outcome of interest is generally the pathological response at surgery or disease-free survival at 3 to 5 years following treatment—both short-term endpoints commonly used as surrogates of overall survival.

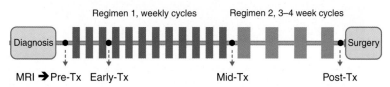

Fig. 5.1 Illustration of a typical multiregimen neoadjuvant chemotherapy (NAC) treatment plan for invasive breast cancer. For a treatment monitoring clinical trial magnetic resonance imaging (MRI) studies can be conducted at any time or times before the patient going to surgery. In this illustration, modeled after the I-SPY 2 TRIAL, MRI are acquired at four time points: pretreatment, after three weekly cycles of the first regimen, midtreatment between the two regimens, and posttreatment before surgery. *Tx*: treatment.

Fig. 5.1 illustrates a typical multiregimen NAC treatment timeline, showing sequential MRI examinations at baseline (pretreatment), early in the first drug regimen, between the first and second regimens, and posttreatment before surgery, similar to that used in the I-SPY 2 TRIAL. Timing of the early treatment MRI varies among published studies and is generally between 1 and 6 weeks of treatment. Fig. 5.2 illustrates serial DWI acquisitions for a patient undergoing NAC. In this example, multiparametric MRI examinations including DCE MRI and DWI acquisitions were conducted at fixed time points before, during (early and midtreatment), and after the full course of NAC treatment (see Fig. 5.1). The patient showed a positive but incomplete response to treatment with both MRI modalities.

DCE MRI showed a large reduction in tumor volume but residual enhancing tumor following treatment. On DWI, tumor apparent diffusion coefficient (ADC) increased steadily with treatment but remained lower than that of normal fibroglandular tissue.

DWI ACQUISITION AND ADC MAPPING

For DWI acquisition, the most common sequence is a 2D, fat-suppressed single-shot echo-planar imaging (SS-EPI) using a single low b value (generally 0) and a single high b value applied in three gradient directions (isotropic acquisition). This sequence has the advantages of simplicity and speed, with reasonably good signal-to-noise ratio (SNR). There is currently no consensus on the optimum high b value for

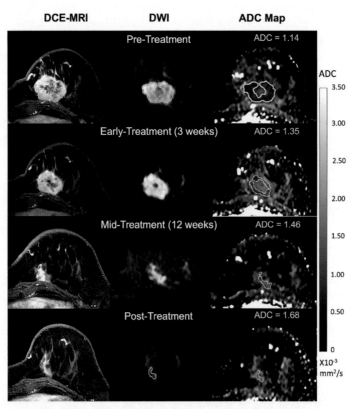

Fig. 5.2 Illustration of diffusion-weighted imaging (DWI) monitoring of treatment response for a patient undergoing neoadjuvant chemotherapy (NAC). Treatment consisted of a paclitaxel-based chemotherapy for 12 weekly cycles followed by four 2- to 3-week cycles of anthracycline-cyclophosphamide (AC). Magnetic resonance imaging (MRI) was conducted at four time points, as indicated in the center column. Shown are three representative axial images from each of the MRI studies: dynamic contrast-enhanced (DCE) MRI subtraction image *(left)*, b = 800 s/mm² DWI *(middle)*, and apparent diffusion coefficient (ADC) map *(right)*. Yellow contours on the DWI and ADC map illustrate typical manually delineated tumor regions of interest (ROIs). As seen in the right column, mean tumor ADC for this patient increased steadily over the course of NAC but did not regain the full value of normal tissue. (This figure was originally published in the ACRIN 6698 primary aim paper.[33])

evaluating therapeutic effects, with a range of at least 600 to 1500 s/mm² reported in the majority of treatment response studies. The primary disadvantages of the two *b* value SS-EPI DWI approach are the limitation to monoexponential modeling (yielding a single ADC metric) and image quality issues common to EPI-based acquisitions including distortions, ghosting, and incomplete fat suppression. These issues are of particular concern in treatment monitoring as they can be inconsistent over the course of multiple longitudinal examinations, contributing errors to the measurement of changes in diffusion parameters.

IMAGE ANALYSIS

For image analysis, a particular challenge of DWI treatment response studies is appropriate definition of ROIs. Tumor localization and delineation on breast DWI can be difficult or even impossible in this setting. As opposed to DCE MRI, which is generally obtained with relatively high spatial resolution and high SNR, DWI scans are typically of lower resolution and poorer

SNR. Furthermore, spatial resolution differences and geometrical distortions that are common in DWI also make it difficult to transfer tumor ROIs directly from DCE MRI, where they can be more accurately defined.

Currently, most breast DWI studies employ manually drawn ROIs done either on a picture archiving and communication system (PACS) workstation (where ROI geometries may be limited) or on a dedicated research workstation. It is a common practice to avoid necrotic and cystic areas and clip artifacts so that only viable tissues are included. Fig. 5.3 illustrates some challenges of ROI definition by contrasting a single mass lesion with a diffusely enhancing tumor being evaluated for ADC before treatment. The guideline applied in these examples was to identify the lesion on a DCE MRI image and then manually delineate the ROI at the corresponding locations on the diffusion scan, referencing the high *b* value DWI (e.g., b = 800 s/mm²), the ADC map, or a combination thereof, selecting regions hyperintense on DWI and hypointense on ADC. The challenge of getting a true

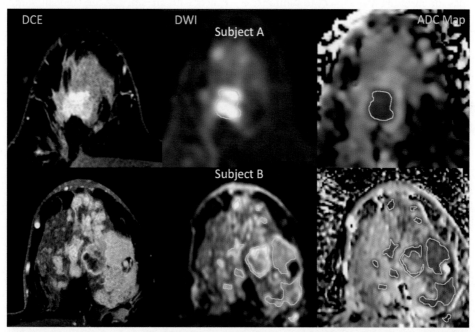

Fig. 5.3 Two examples of diffusion-weighted imaging (DWI) manual region of interest (ROI) complexity showing image planes with the largest tumor area for each subject. Images in each row are postcontrast dynamic contrast enhanced (DCE) *(left)*, b = 800 s/mm² DWI *(middle)*, and apparent diffusion coefficient (ADC) map *(right)*. Subject A *(top)* had a single mass breast tumor that was conspicuous on both DCE and DWI allowing quick and accurate delineation of the ROI. For this case, seven 2D ROI were defined on 6 planes to capture the entire DWI tumor volume of 5.53 cc. Subject B *(bottom)* had diffuse enhancement throughout much of the breast, requiring much more attention and time to ROI definition to accurately quantify the whole-tumor diffusion characteristics like mean tumor ADC. Sixty-six regions on 13 planes were used for this whole tumor segmentation with a volume of 53.9 cc.

whole-tumor segmentation in diffuse or multifocal disease is clearly illustrated by the number of individual contours seen in the second example in Fig. 5.3. In a consensus publication by Padhani and colleagues, the recommendation was made that ROIs be drawn to completely delineate lesions on images that have the highest contrast between lesion and normal tissue and to avoid defining smaller ROIs within lesions, which is considered more subjective and not recommended for assessing treatment response.[37]

It is common to define "pseudo-3D" regions by selecting tumor on multiple planes to reduce sampling errors inherent with single-plane definitions. However, this can greatly increase the skilled-operator time required for analysis, and there are some indications there may be no benefit over single-slice ROIs.[38] Studies with multiple readers, unless explicitly investigating interreader reproducibility, generally use consensus ROIs from multiple radiologists or trained researchers. For longitudinal trials, most commonly a single operator or consensus team would evaluate all DWI studies for an individual subject to minimize errors from interoperator variability. We also note that in longitudinal studies, the challenge of defining reproducible tumor ROIs tends to increase in difficulty over the course of NAC, as the contrast between tumor and normal fibroglandular tissue decreases, particularly in good responders. This may be less of a concern in studies investigating the early-treatment prediction of patient outcome; however, even as early as 3 weeks into NAC, there are examples of excellent responders where the tumor is no longer discernable on MRI (Fig. 5.4).

STATISTICAL ANALYSIS FOR RESPONSE PREDICTION

Selection of outcome variable(s) and methods for evaluation of predictive capability of the predictor variable(s) can vary between treatment response trials. As mentioned earlier, the most common outcome variable across studies is pCR, defined as the absence of residual invasive cancer in the breast and all sampled axillary lymph nodes. The FDA also allows a stricter guideline requiring absence of both residual invasive cancer and in situ cancer, and all sampled axillary

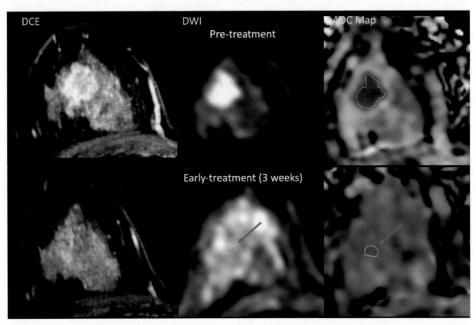

Fig. 5.4 An example case of an excellent response by 3 weeks after the therapy initiation. Images are postcontrast dynamic contrast enhanced (DCE) *(left)*, $b = 800\,s/mm^2$ diffusion weighted imaging (DWI) *(middle)*, and apparent diffusion coefficient (ADC) map *(right)* at pretreatment *(top)* and after 3 weeks of neoadjuvant chemotherapy (NAC) *(bottom)*. Both DCE and DWI/ADC show minimal or no residual tumor at the 3-week treatment. One option for obtaining a usable ADC measure for such cases is to define a small region of interest (ROI) *(red arrow)* in normal appearing breast tissue located either in a region of residual enhancement on the DCE or located anatomically in the region of the original tumor imaged at baseline.

lymph nodes.[9] For binary endpoints like pCR predictive ability is generally evaluated using receiver operating characteristic (ROC) analysis with area under the receiver-operator curve (AUC) as the primary metric. In some studies, response is defined by clinical or imaging measurements by applying the response evaluation criteria in solid tumor (RECIST) definition of less than 30% reduction to identify nonresponders.

Tumor Mean ADC for Predicting Response

The most common diffusion measurement for NAC monitoring and outcome prediction is the mean ADC value within the tumor. ADC is typically calculated pixel-wise by fitting a monoexponential function to all b values acquired in the DWI sequence (or directly if there are only two b values) and then taking the mean over the region representing some or all of the cancerous lesion. Alternatively, mean ADC can be calculated using the average DWI signal intensities (e.g., b = 0, 800 s/mm^2) over the region. Iima and colleagues demonstrated that the second approach is less affected by noise than the first approach and thus is more accurate.[39] As mentioned earlier, the region is generally delineated by user-defined ROIs. Numerous studies have investigated the value of tumor mean ADC measures before, during and after NAC, as well as ADC changes from pretreatment values to later time points during NAC, for the prediction of response to treatment.

PRETREATMENT ADC: CORRELATION WITH TREATMENT OUTCOME

Although the major focus of monitoring treatment response is on assessing the disease state during the course of NAC, the pretreatment determination of tumor ADC may be helpful for categorizing tumors, especially when combined with tumor subtype information, and may help in assignment of treatment. Several studies have found lower pretreatment tumor ADC to be associated with positive treatment response.[21,24–28,40] A retrospective study by Park and colleagues looked at 53 consecutive women with invasive breast cancer who had MRI examinations with DCE and DWI (b = 0, 750 s/mm^2, 1.5T) before and after NAC. Pretreatment ADC was significantly lower in clinical responders (based on RECIST criteria) than

ADC in nonresponders.[21] Richard and colleagues performed a similar study in a larger cohort of 118 women who had DWI (b = 50, 700 s/mm^2, 1.5T) performed less than 15 days before chemotherapy. In this study, pretreatment ADC was also found to be significantly lower in complete responders but only in an $n = 37$ subgroup with triple negative tumors (ADC = $1.060 \pm 0.143 \times 10^{-3}$ mm^2/s vs. $1.227 \pm 0.271 \times 10^{-3}$ mm^2/s, $P = .047$).[25] In this analysis, pathological response were classified according to the Chevallier and Sataloff classifications.[41,42] However, in a 2018 report on 142 women, Yuan and colleagues found small but significant differences in baseline ADC value between pCR and non-pCR groups within all genomic subtypes.[40] This result was part of a broader investigation of optimum time points for DWI evaluation, described in more detail later. A possible explanation for an inverse relationship between pretreatment ADC and response could be that high ADCs may be due to local necrosis or fibrosis, which indicate more poorly perfused tumors and relative difficulty in delivering chemotherapy agents into the tumor.[24] Other studies failed to find statistical difference of pretreatment tumor ADC values between responders and nonresponders.[16,19,43,44]

CHANGE IN ADC WITH NEOADJUVANT TREATMENT

Tumor ADC tends to increase with treatment, approaching the higher values typical of healthy fibroglandular tissue. Several animal studies demonstrated that DWI-detected cellular changes are associated with treatment-induced cell death.[45–48] For example, Cheng and colleagues observed ADC values increased on day 3 after chemotherapy, and further showed that these changes preceded measurable tumor volume changes in a gastric cancer mouse model.[45] In a preclinical study of a breast cancer mouse model treated by anti-DR5 antibody, Kim and colleagues found ADC values increased on day 3 with the amount of increased dose level dependent, and ADC increases were inversely proportional to the density of cells showing Ki67 expression.[46]

A number of clinical studies have also reported that an increase in tumor ADC can be detected early in the course of the treatment (e.g., after one cycle of NAC),[11,13,14,26,29–32,34] in some instances before the tumor shows any significant decrease in size.[11,13,29,30,34] In a prospective study of 62 patients, both DCE MRI and DWI (b = 0, 750 s/mm^2, 1.5T) were acquired at pretreatment, after one cycle (3–4 weeks, anthracycline- and cyclophosphamide-based NAC), and posttreatment.[29] The study found that the percent increase in mean ADC after one cycle of NAC was significantly higher in the pCR group ($P <$ .001). The longest diameter was also measured from DCE MRI, but no significant differences were found between pCR and non-pCR groups after one cycle of NAC. Similar results were also seen in studies with smaller cohorts,[30,34] using different methodologies to measure tumor size before and after one cycle of NAC.

MRI TIME POINT SELECTION FOR RESPONSE

Selecting the most effective timings and frequency for DWI assessment in NAC treatment outcome prediction is a challenge. Many factors weigh into the optimum time point or points, including treatment regimens, tumor subtypes, drugs administered, and possibly technical aspects such as the typical SNR and b value selection, which may affect the magnitude of ADC changes that can be detected. Yuan and colleagues systematically studied ADC and change in ADC from pretreatment (ΔADC) in the prediction of pCR in 142 patients, using DWI (b = 0, 300, 600, and 1000 s/mm^2, 3.0T) at pretreatment and after the first, second, third, fourth, sixth, and eighth cycles of NAC.[40] Each cycle of therapy in this study was 3 weeks long, in contrast to weekly cycles commonly used in other treatment regimens. The study cohort included patients in three different treatment regimens and included analysis by genomic subtype. The study found first that ΔADC was generally better for pCR prediction than absolute ADC measures. This was generally true across subtypes; for example, for luminal B subtype in one treatment regimen, the best AUC for ΔADC was 0.865 versus only 0.602 for the best single time point ADC. Similar results were seen in other subtypes and treatment arms, though not all showed as strong predictive performance. The optimal timing window during NAC for ADC measurement for prediction of pCR was found to vary by subtype and treatment, but in all cases was either after the first or second 3-week cycle of NAC. By contrast, in the prospective ACRIN-6698 study (discussed in the next section), Partridge and colleagues did not find significant predictive power of ADC for pCR after 3 weekly cycles of NAC but did find significance at 12-week and later time points.[33]

MULTICENTER CLINICAL TRIALS USING DWI FOR OUTCOME PREDICTION

Given the heterogeneity of breast DWI protocols across institutions and the differences in DWI implementations across scanner platforms, well-controlled multicenter, multivendor trials are essential for establishing the efficacy of DWI-based biomarkers for treatment response. In a multicenter study of 39 patients enrolling in three different prospective clinical trials at separate sites, Galban and colleagues tested ADC metrics for assessing response to NAC.[49] All patients had invasive breast cancer and were treated with NAC. MRI examinations with DWI (b = 0, 800 s/mm^2, 1.5T, and 3T) were performed at pretreatment and 3 to 7 days, 8 to 11 days, and 35 days after treatment was initiated, respectively, for the three trials. Treatment outcome was assessed either by palpation after the first cycle of NAC (one site) or by RECIST 1.1 evaluated on DCE MRI (two sites). Assessment of treatment response on DWI scans was done using ADC both with the standard ROI-based mean analysis and the parametric response map (PRM) technique. The PRM technique involves intervisit image registration, using a combination of rigid registration and manually assisted nonrigid registration, allowing calculation of voxel-wise maps for change in diffusion parameters. Applied to the ADC maps, volumetric parameters PRM_{ADC-}, PRM_{ADC0}, and PRM_{ADC+} were calculated as the fractional tumor volumes with decreasing, stable, and increasing ADC values, respectively. Due to the small numbers in each trial and different methods applied for determining response, two patient groups were defined: (1) responders and stable disease (R/SD); and (2) progressive disease (PD). Change of mean ADC was found to be significantly predictive of outcome ($P = 0.012$) at the 35-day time point, although the sample size was small ($n = 14$). PRM_{ADC+} was also found to be significantly higher in the R/SD group than the PD group both at the 8- to 11-day time point ($P = .006$) and the 35-day time point ($P = .004$).

A larger multicenter study was the American College of Radiology Imaging Network (ACRIN) trial 6698, a multicenter prospective study to evaluate DWI for prediction of pathological response (ClinicalTrials. gov Identifier: NCT01564368), performed as a substudy of I-SPY 2 (Investigation of Serial Studies to Predict Your Therapeutic Response through Imaging and Molecular Analysis 2, ClinicalTrials.gov Identifier: NCT01042379).[33,50] The primary objective of ACRIN 6698 was to test whole-tumor ADC for prediction of pCR in women undergoing NAC for breast cancer.[33] A secondary aim was to evaluate repeatability of ADC measurements.[51] ACRIN 6698 used a standardized DWI acquisition ($b = 0, 100, 600, 800 \, s/mm^2$, 1.5T, or 3.0T) optimized for breast scanning, along with a QA/QC program for DWI-specific site qualification and image quality review.[52] DWI was performed within the same examinations as DCE MRI at 4 time points during NAC: pretreatment, early treatment (typically after 3 weekly cycles), interregimen/midtreatment, and posttreatment/presurgery (see Fig. 5.1 for the study schema). Ten I-SPY 2 sites that completed DWI qualification enrolled patients to ACRIN 6698 between August 2012 and January 2015. The study used manually delimited whole-tumor ROIs.

The trial reported primary results in 242 patients, in which the change of tumor ADC was found to be predictive of pCR at midtreatment (between regimen) and before surgery.[33] The change of ADC at the early treatment time point did not show a statistically significant difference between pCR and non-pCR groups. Repeatability of tumor ADC measures was assessed in a subset of 71 subjects who underwent "coffee-break" style repeat DWI scans, with inter- and intra-reader reproducibility also assessed in a 20-subject subgroup.[51] Overall, the results showed that excellent repeatability and reproducibility of breast tumor ADC

measures could be achieved in a multiinstitution setting using a standardized protocol and QA procedure (e.g., repeatability within subject coefficient of variation [wCV] = 4.8%). This study is discussed further in Chapter 14. In regard to treatment response monitoring, we note that these repeatability and reproducibility results only pertain directly to ADC measures taken pretreatment or within the first few cycles of NAC treatment. Reproducibility may be poorer at later time points due to increased challenges in defining tumor ROIs after significant treatment response.

Alternative DWI Metrics to Mean ADC

HISTOGRAM AND TEXTURE-BASED DWI PARAMETERS FOR TREATMENT RESPONSE

Mean tumor ADC is the most commonly used metric for quantitative measurement in DWI and it has demonstrated predictive value for patients undergoing NAC, as described earlier. However, it is an average measurement of water diffusivity for the entire tumor and does not reflect the spatial heterogeneity of the tumor microenvironment. Analysis of ADC histograms may provide additional information for characterizing changes with treatment (Fig. 5.5). Several studies found lower percentiles of tumor ADC histograms to be most predictive of treatment response in breast and other cancers.[32,53,54] In a study of glioblastoma treated with concurrent chemotherapy and temozolomide, the fifth percentile of the cumulative

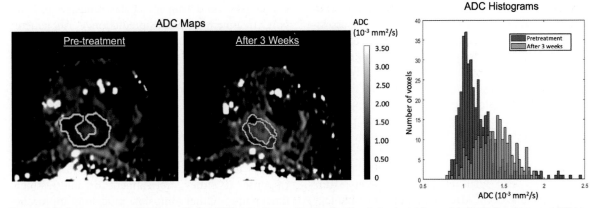

Fig. 5.5 Quantitative apparent diffusion coefficient (ADC) maps from pretreatment and early-treatment time points illustrating changes of ADC histograms after 3 weeks of neoadjuvant therapy (see Fig. 6.2 for further images of this subject). Representative ADC map images are *(left, center)* shown with typical manually drawn tumor ROIs for the displayed slices. Histograms are shown *(right)* for the full 3D tumor regions of interest (ROIs) drawn on multiple slices at each time point. We see both a strong increase in mean ADC value and a broadening of the ADC histogram with treatment in this case.

histogram differentiated between true progression and pseudoprogression.[53] The study of Kyriazi and colleagues found that percentage change of the 25th percentile of the ADC histogram was most predictive of treatment response after the first and third cycles for patients with advanced ovarian cancer.[54] Wilmes and colleagues found strongest correlations between early treatment increase of lower (15th or 25th) ADC percentile and posttreatment tumor volume change in patients with breast cancer.[32] However, other studies found median or higher ADC percentiles to be more predictive of pCR. For example, in a multiparametric 3T MRI study of breast cancer with 42 patients, the highest AUC using DWI was for median ADC after 2 cycles of NAC.[35]

Histogram shape descriptors can give more detail on how intensities distribute within a tumor ROI. In a retrospective study of 46 patients, Kim and colleagues observed lower skewness of ADC in good responders after NAC.[55] In another retrospective study including 31 women who underwent NAC followed by surgery, 22 image features were extracted from each pretreatment MRI, and Gallivanone and colleagues found statistical correlation between histogram skewness and entropy with pCR outcome ($P < .05$ and $P = .05$, respectively).[56] In studies applying radiomic methods, second order (gray-level co-occurrence matrix [GLCM]) and higher-order structural texture features can characterize spatial gray-level intensity distribution and capture image patterns that may not be recognizable to the human eye and may potentially be predictive of treatment response. Most radiomic studies applied to breast cancer treatment response assessment have analyzed texture features extracted from DCE MRI and/or T_2-weighted MRI.[57] Few included DWI probably due to insufficient image quality or lack of clinical standardization of DWI protocols. Yoon and colleagues investigated a cohort of 83 patients and a total of 46 ADC texture features, also from pretreatment DWI examinations. They found second angular moment and entropy to be statistically different between pCR and non-pCR groups ($P = .033$ and $P = .025$, respectively).[58] The relationship between texture analysis parameters of ADC maps and histopathology was demonstrated using breast cancer xenograft models.[59] In that study, the first- and second-order texture analysis of ADC maps was performed on DWIs

obtained on a 9.4T scanner. Several texture analysis parameters were found to be correlated with histopathologic features of breast cancer xenograft models, such as proportion and pattern of necrosis, cell proliferation marker, and vascularity. Yoon and colleagues found that histogram-derived features and a parent matrix that indicates global and local heterogeneity showed significant differences between responders and nonresponders.[58] Recently, a study conducted by Eun and colleagues with a large patient cohort ($n = 136$) from a single institute found that the change of texture features of ADC maps at midtreatment were associated with pCR, analyzed by a random forest method.[60] However, texture analysis is only possible for larger lesions with at least 1 cm^3 in size.[57] It is not suitable for analysis at later treatment time points.

ADVANCED DWI MODELING

Advanced DWI modeling approaches that go beyond the Gaussian, monoexponential decay model (yielding standard ADC measures) may provide additional biological insights in evaluating therapies. There is emerging data exploring several advanced approaches to identify and differentiate treatment effects on tissue perfusion and microstructural characteristics. Intravoxel incoherent motion (IVIM; see Chapters 1 and 8) biexponential modeling in particular has been investigated for prediction of pathological outcomes in breast cancer.[28,61,62] In a study of 36 breast cancer patients, Che and colleagues investigated IVIM metrics (perfusion fraction [f], perfusion-related diffusion [D*], and true molecular diffusion [D]) for NAC treatment response prediction.[62] All patients underwent a pretreatment IVIM DWI (12 b values, 0–1000 s/mm^2, 3T) and 28 also had a midtreatment IVIM scan after 2 cycles of NAC (given every 3 weeks). Their study showed compelling evidence that pretreatment f could significantly distinguish responders (pCR) from nonresponders ($P = .034$), and that midtreatment changes in both D and f were strongly predictive ($P < .001$). On the other hand, D* was not significantly associated with treatment response at either pretreatment or midtreatment time points. Other diffusion modeling approaches including diffusion tensor imaging (DTI) to probe microstructural organization (see Chapter 9), and non-Gaussian diffusion modeling (see Chapter 8) to evaluate tissue complexity/heterogeneity, such as kurtosis and stretched-exponential models, are also being investigated for monitoring therapy.[63]

However, at the current time, the value of advanced approaches for use in treatment prediction for breast cancer remains inconclusive due to the small patient numbers in existing studies and further investigation is warranted.

Combined DCE and DWI Approaches to Outcome Prediction

Whereas DCE MRI can detect changes in the contrast uptake affected by tumor angiogenesis and microcirculation, DWI detects changes in tumor microstructure, membrane integrity, and cell density caused by treatment-induced cell death that could precede changes detected in DCE MRI. Although DCE MRI is considered as the standard tool in response assessment for breast cancer treated by NAC, DWI can be added to the imaging protocol with little extra acquisition time. Furthermore, the combination of quantitative parameters of these two modalities may outperform metrics derived from either modality individually for the early prediction of treatment response.

Li and colleagues tested the combination of kinetic parameters from high temporal resolution DCE MRI (16 s per phase) with DWI ADC, obtained before and after the first cycle of NAC.[64] They found that after the first cycle of NAC a hybrid variable ($\frac{k_{ep}}{ADC}$, where k_{ep} is the efflux rate constant derived from the extended Tofts-Kety [ETK] model for DCE MRI) achieved higher AUC (0.86) than either k_{ep} (AUC = 0.77) or ADC (AUC = 0.81) alone for predicting pCR, though only the difference with k_{ep} achieved statistical significance. Although this was a relatively small study ($n = 33$ at the later time point), it supports the hypothesis that combining kinetic and diffusion metrics may yield improved predictive performance for treatment response.

An interesting alternative approach to logistic regression modeling for combining DWI with other metrics from multiparametric MRI examinations is to use machine learning techniques. In a recent study Tahmassebi and colleagues examined a suite of 23 features, including three DWI ADC features (minimum, mean, and maximum), along with multiple qualitative and quantitative parameters from DCE MRI and T_2w

images for prediction of several pathological and survival outcome variables (residual cancer burden [RCB] class, recurrence-free survival [RFS], and disease-specific survival [DSS]).[65] After recursive feature elimination, DWI-derived features were among the most relevant for prediction of all outcomes, though the highest-ranked DWI metric varied by outcome (minimum ADC for RCB, mean ADC for RFS, and maximum ADC for DSS). Although this was a relatively small study ($n = 38$) and did not directly address the question of additive value of DWI, it shows promise for future larger-scale studies investigating machine learning techniques for outcome prediction.

The multicenter ACRIN 6698 study also included an exploratory analysis of pCR prediction combining data from DWI and DCE, with tumor subtype.[33] A subset of 207 patients was split into a training set (60%) and a validation set (40%). A model combining pretreatment to midtreatment percent change of ADC (from DWI) and functional tumor volume (FTV) (from DCE), along with HR/HER2 subtype, resulted in an AUC of 0.71 (95% CI: 0.59, 0.84), whereas the AUC for percent change of ADC and subtype was 0.72 (95% CI: 0.61, 0.83). This exploratory study showed that the predictive value of ADC may be comparable to or higher than that of FTV at the midtreatment time point. However, it did not show improvement of predictive performance by adding ADC to the model with FTV and subtype.

A subsequent study by Li and colleagues investigated the additive value of ADC to FTV in a larger I-SPY 2 TRIAL cohort that included two- and four-*b* value DWI data from all I-SPY2 sites.[44] The analysis included 354 patients enrolled in I-SPY 2 between 2010 and 2014, including 95 in the ACRIN 6698 substudy. This study analysis also used whole-tumor ADC from manually delimited ROIs but was restricted to two *b* values (0 and 800 s/mm²). The study investigated both pretreatment ADC and FTV and percent change in ADC and FTV from baseline to the later time points, starting with an "FTV-only" logistic regression model and then evaluating the added benefit of the ADC measures. Results were presented for both the full cohort and for subcohorts defined by HR/HER2 subtype. Example ROC curves for the full cohort and selected subtypes are shown in Fig. 5.6. There were small but statistically significant increases in AUC with the addition of ADC in the full cohort at later time

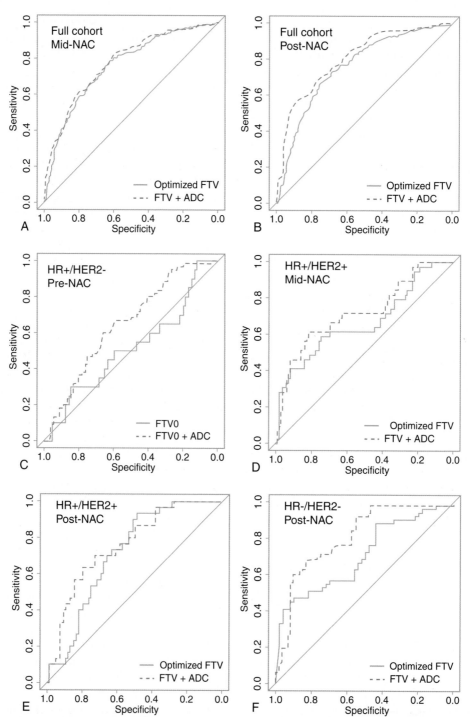

Fig. 5.6 Region of interest (ROC) curves for logistic regression models for FTV measures with versus without apparent diffusion coefficient (ADC) for different subtype cohorts. In each plot ROC curves are shown for a model with FTV predictors only ("Optimized FTV" or "FTV0," *solid lines*) and a model with FTV and ADC predictors ("FTV+ADC," *dotted lines*). Shown are subtype and time point combinations that showed a statistically significant increase in area under curve (AUC) with the addition of ADC predictors. Subtype was included in the model for the full cohort analysis. No significant increase was observed at any time. Point for the HR−/HER2+subtype. *HR*: hormone receptor. *HER2*: human epidermal growth factor receptor 2. (This figure was originally published by Li et al.[44] and the permission to reuse was granted from the publisher.)

points (e.g., midtreatment AUC increased from 0.76–0.78). More interestingly, larger increases in AUC were observed in some subtype analyses; for example, at pretreatment the HR+/HER2− group AUC increased from 0.52 to 0.65, and at posttreatment the triple negative HR−/HER2− group AUC increased from 0.71 to 0.81, but no additive value was observed in the HR−/HER2+ subtype (not shown).

Fig. 5.7 shows examples of how the addition of ADC affects prediction at the individual case level. Results from two patients with triple negative tumors are shown: Patient A, who achieved pCR, and Patient B, who did not. Using the DCE data up through the posttreatment visit gave indeterminate results in the logistic regression model with predicted probabilities of pCR for the two patients (52.4% and 56.2%, respectively). When DWI metrics were added to the model, these probabilities shifted to 87.5% and 10.0% for Patient A (pCR) and B (non-pCR), respectively.

Subtype Dependency of ADC Prediction

Breast cancer is now recognized as a spectrum of diseases that is heterogeneous in both prognosis and treatment outcomes.[66,67] Perou and colleagues originally classified breast tumors by gene expression patterns using cDNA microarrays as luminal, ErbB2 overexpressing, basal-like, and normal breast.[68] Clinically, tumors can be categorized into molecular subtypes by expression of the estrogen (ER) or progesterone (PR) hormone receptor (HR) and the human epidermal growth factor receptor 2 (HER2) using immunohistochemistry (IHC). The IHC subtypes triple negative (i.e., ER-negative, PR-negative, and HER2-negative), HER2-positive (i.e., ER- and PR-positive or negative), and ER-positive (i.e., HER2-negative, PR-positive or negative) correspond roughly to the intrinsic subtypes basal-like, HER2-positive and luminal, respectively (see Chapter 4). Differences in response rates to NAC among breast cancer subtypes have been reported in many studies, with highest rates of pCR in HER2-positive and triple negative breast cancers.[69,70]

Studies examining agreement between DCE MRI and residual disease size on histopathology have found agreement to be variable by subtype, with higher

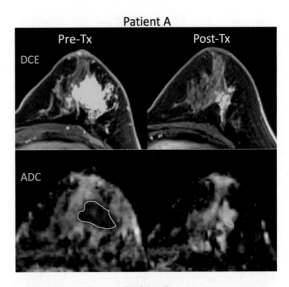

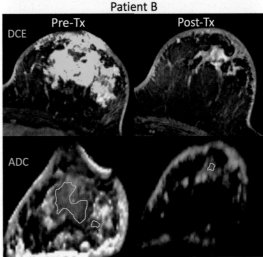

Fig. 5.7 Two patient examples showing additive benefit of apparent diffusion coefficient (ADC) measures over FTV alone in the I-SPY 2 Trial. Both patients had triple negative (HR−/HER2−) cancers and Patient A achieved pathological complete response (pCR), whereas Patient B did not. Shown are the dynamic contrast-enhanced (DCE) postcontrast images with an overlaid color mask of the voxels included in the FTV calculation *(top rows)* and the ADC map with manually drawn regions of interest (ROIs) *(bottom rows)*. Only pretreatment *(left)* and posttreatment *(right)* time points are shown, but data from all four study magnetic resonance imaging (MRI) visits was included in analysis. Using all available FTV information in a logistic model, the prediction for pCR was indeterminant in both cases: 52.4% and 56.2% probability of pCR for Patients A and B, respectively. When ADC metrics were added to the model, these probabilities went to 87.5% for Patient A (pCR) and 10.0% for Patient B (non-pCR).

agreement reported among HER2+ and triple negative tumors.[71] The systematic reviews by Marinovich and colleagues and Graeser and colleagues examining the accuracy of DCE MRI for early prediction of pathological response found that the large heterogeneity of methodological approaches made comparison of results difficult and precluded definitive conclusions.[11,12] Fewer studies have evaluated the subtype dependence of DWI for predicting response to treatment, which have a greater extent of methodological heterogeneity and limited subgroup sample sizes. In the study by Richard and colleagues, significant difference of pretreatment ADC between complete responders and noncomplete responders was found in triple negative tumors only, with a sample size of 37 and ADC maps generated from two-b DWI (50, 700 s/mm²).[25] Similar findings were reported by Liu and colleagues, in which 35 patients were included and DWI was acquired with two b values (0, 800 s/mm²); lower pretreatment ADC was found in responders with only triple negative breast cancer.[72] ACRIN 6698 found higher association between percent change of mean ADC and pCR in HR+/HER2− tumors than other subtypes at midtreatment, although the study was not adequately powered to evaluate differences by subtype.[33] The subsequent multicenter study conducted by Li and colleagues included a larger cohort ($n = 354$) and was better powered for subcohort analysis.[44] Even so, no significant differences in mean ADC were found between pCR and non-pCR groups at pretreatment in any subtype. At midtreatment, significant differences were found in HR+/HER2−, HR+/HER2+, and triple negative subtypes. Furthermore, the combination of DWI and DCE metrics achieved higher AUCs than DWI or DCE alone in the HR+/HER2− group at pretreatment, HR+/HER2+ at midtreatment and before surgery, and triple negatives before surgery.

Current Challenges and Future Directions

With growing evidence of the unique potential of DWI to provide early indication of treatment efficacy, there is increasing interest to incorporate DWI into clinical trials and practice. Additional advantages of DWI as an imaging biomarker include lack of need for exogenous contrast agents, short acquisition time, wide availability on most commercial MR scanners, and robust reproducibility and repeatability of ADC measurements.[51] However, there remain obstacles to routine clinical implementation of breast DWI for therapeutic monitoring related to technical challenges and the lack of standardization of imaging protocols.

Although multicenter trials have validated promising smaller single-center studies showing predictive value of ADC in breast cancer treatment,[33,44] they also highlighted a need for further technical developments to address persistent image quality issues. For example, Li and colleagues found it necessary to exclude 51 of 415 cases (12%) due to poor image quality of the DWI acquisition that prevented serial ADC assessment.[44] Low resolution, geometrical distortion, and frequent artifacts are current challenges of breast DWI[73] that are particularly detrimental for precise serial quantitative assessment, potentially limiting its utility as a reliable clinical biomarker. Partial volume averaging in particular is an issue with DWI that compromises assessment of important features such as tumor margins and intralesion heterogeneity. Furthermore, across studies to date, there has been wide variation in DWI acquisition and analysis approaches, including the choice of b values and tumor ROI quantitation method, as well as treatment time points for imaging. As a result, there is considerable variability in reported ADC values for similar breast pathologies and the magnitude of ADC change indicating response. This lack of standardization has hampered definition of generalizable guidelines for using ADC as a biomarker in prospective trials.

Future studies aimed to improve the standardization of approach and consistency of image quality in multicenter trials are essential for further advancement of breast DW MRI biomarkers (see Chapter 14). Toward these goals, the Radiological Society of North America (RSNA) Quantitative Imaging Biomarkers Alliance (QIBA) recently put forth a DWI profile detailing acquisition and analysis specifications to support use of ADC as a robust quantitative biomarker for breast cancer,[74] with a breast claim based primarily on repeatability data from the ACRIN 6698 multicenter trial. Consensus recommendations were also recently proposed by the European Society of Breast Imaging (EUSOBI) International Breast Diffusion-Weighted Imaging working group[75] to facilitate standardization and to provide best practices for general clinical breast DWI acquisition and interpretation.

Toward improving image quality, several emerging DWI acquisition strategies hold potential to overcome the technical issues inherent to standard EPI for breast imaging. These include multishot (e.g., readout-segmented[76] and multiplexed sensitivity encoding[77]) and reduced field-of-view[32] EPI techniques, each of which shorten echo spacing and/or echo train lengths to allow for improved spatial resolution and reduced susceptibility artifacts. Preliminary data comparing reduced field-of-view and standard DWI approaches for longitudinal assessment shows high-resolution DWI may improve ability to precisely characterize breast tumor ADC and predict NAC treatment response.[32] However, these advanced acquisition methods require trade-offs of longer scan times and/or reduced coverage and are not yet widely implemented across different vendor platforms. New simultaneous multislice (SMS) approaches, which accelerate acquisitions in the slice dimension, show promise to reduce breast DWI acquisition times and have been used in conjunction with readout-segmented EPI in the breast to leverage benefits of both techniques.[78] Postprocessing techniques have also been developed to mitigate EPI distortions from magnetic field inhomogeneity[79,80] and correct b value inaccuracies due to gradient nonlinearities,[81] which can further improve diffusion image quality and ADC accuracy.

Although ADC has been by far the most widely studied DWI metric as an imaging biomarker in breast cancer, advanced modeling techniques may provide more specific characterization of therapeutic effects.[82,83] IVIM modeling could allow characterization of treatment effects on microcirculation in addition to tissue diffusivity. Diffusion kurtosis imaging, which provides measures of structural complexity, may reflect early treatment-induced microstructural alterations such as intracellular nuclear-cytoplasmic ratio. Further exploration of these and other advanced diffusion models may enhance the value of diffusion-weighted MRI for biological characterization in future breast cancer clinical trials.

In summary, both single-center and multicenter studies demonstrate the value of DWI for early response assessment in breast cancer treatment, which could allow for improved tailoring of therapeutic regimens. Specifically, growing evidence supports ADC as a quantitative imaging biomarker in breast cancer therapy. Improved standardization of the assay for serial breast tumor ADC assessment is still needed to support wide clinical implementation, with important efforts already underway through QIBA and EUSOBI in support of this goal. Furthermore, more investigations are warranted to refine optimal imaging treatment time points and interpretation criteria. Novel acquisition techniques are under development to overcome commonly encountered image quality issues, which would improve clinical utility for serial assessment, and advanced modeling approaches hold potential to further expand the capabilities of DWI as an imaging biomarker.

REFERENCES

1. Fisher B, et al. Effect of preoperative chemotherapy on the outcome of women with operable breast cancer. *J Clin Oncol.* 1998;16:2672–2685.
2. Bear HD, et al. Sequential preoperative or postoperative docetaxel added to preoperative doxorubicin plus cyclophosphamide for operable breast cancer: National Surgical Adjuvant Breast and Bowel Project Protocol B-27. *J Clin Oncol.* 2006;24:2019–2027.
3. Wolmark N, et al. Preoperative chemotherapy in patients with operable breast cancer: nine-year results from National Surgical Adjuvant Breast and Bowel Project B-18. *J Natl Cancer Inst Monogr.* 2001;96–102.
4. Rastogi P, et al. Preoperative chemotherapy: updates of National Surgical Adjuvant Breast and Bowel Project Protocols B-18 and B-27. *J Clin Oncol.* 2008;26:778–785.
5. Peintinger F, et al. Reproducibility of residual cancer burden for prognostic assessment of breast cancer after neoadjuvant chemotherapy. *Mod Pathol.* 2015;28:913–920.
6. Esserman LJ, et al. Pathologic complete response predicts recurrence-free survival more effectively by cancer subset: results from the I-SPY 1 TRIAL-CALGB 150007/150012, ACRIN 6657. *J Clin Oncol.* 2012;30:3242–3249.
7. Sheri A, et al. Residual proliferative cancer burden to predict long-term outcome following neoadjuvant chemotherapy. *Ann Oncol.* 2015;26:75–80.
8. Cortazar P, et al. Pathological complete response and long-term clinical benefit in breast cancer: the CTNeoBC pooled analysis. *Lancet.* 2014;384:164–172.
9. U.S. Department of Health and Human Service, Food and Drug Administration and Center for Drug Evaluation and Research (CDER). Pathological complete response in neoadjuvant treatment of high-risk early-stage breast cancer: use as an endpoint to support accelerated approval. 2020.
10. Lobbes MBI, et al. The role of magnetic resonance imaging in assessing residual disease and pathologic complete response in breast cancer patients receiving neoadjuvant chemotherapy: a systematic review. *Insights Imaging.* 2013;4:163–175.
11. Marinovich ML, et al. Agreement between MRI and pathologic breast tumor size after neoadjuvant chemotherapy, and comparison with alternative tests: individual patient data meta-analysis. *BMC Cancer.* 2015;15:662.
12. Graeser M, et al. Early response by MR imaging and ultrasound as predictor of pathologic complete response to 12-week

neoadjuvant therapy for different early breast cancer subtypes: combined analysis from the WSG ADAPT subtrials. *Int J Cancer*. 2021;148(10):2614–2627.

13. Marinovich ML, et al. Early prediction of pathologic response to neoadjuvant therapy in breast cancer: systematic review of the accuracy of MRI. *Breast*. 2012;21:669–677.

14. Granzier RWY, et al. Exploring breast cancer response prediction to neoadjuvant systemic therapy using MRI-based radiomics: a systematic review. *Eur J Radiol*. 2019;121:108736.

15. Partridge SC, et al. Quantitative diffusion-weighted imaging as an adjunct to conventional breast MRI for improved positive predictive value. *Am J Roentgenol*. 2009;193:1716–1722.

16. Woodhams R, et al. Identification of residual breast carcinoma following neoadjuvant chemotherapy: diffusion-weighted imaging: comparison with contrast-enhanced MR imaging and pathologic findings. *Radiology*. 2010;254:357–366.

17. Pickles MD. Diffusion changes precede size reduction in neoadjuvant treatment of breast cancer. *Magn Reson Imaging*. 2006;24:843–847.

18. Nilsen L, et al. Diffusion-weighted magnetic resonance imaging for pretreatment prediction and monitoring of treatment response of patients with locally advanced breast cancer undergoing neoadjuvant chemotherapy. *Acta Oncol*. 2010;49:354–360.

19. Fangberget A, et al. Neoadjuvant chemotherapy in breast cancer-response evaluation and prediction of response to treatment using dynamic contrast-enhanced and diffusion-weighted MR imaging. *Eur Radiol*. 2011;21:1188–1199.

20. Iacconi C, et al. The role of mean diffusivity (MD) as a predictive index of the response to chemotherapy in locally advanced breast cancer: a preliminary study. *Eur Radiol*. 2010;20:303–308.

21. Park SH, et al. Diffusion-weighted MR imaging: pretreatment prediction of response to neoadjuvant chemotherapy in patients with breast cancer. *Radiology*. 2010;257:56–63.

22. Sharma U, et al. Longitudinal study of the assessment by MRI and diffusion-weighted imaging of tumor response in patients with locally advanced breast cancer undergoing neoadjuvant chemotherapy. *NMR Biomed*. 2009;22:104–113.

23. Partridge SC, et al. Apparent diffusion coefficient values for discriminating benign and malignant breast MRI lesions: effects of lesion type and size. *Am J Roentgenol*. 2010;194:1664–1673.

24. Tsukada H, et al. Accuracy of multi-parametric breast MR imaging for predicting pathological complete response of operable breast cancer prior to neoadjuvant systemic therapy. *Magn Reson Imaging*. 2019;62:242–248.

25. Richard R, et al. Diffusion-weighted MRI in pretreatment prediction of response to neoadjuvant chemotherapy in patients with breast cancer. *Eur Radiol*. 2013;23:2420–2431.

26. Li X-R, et al. DW-MRI ADC values can predict treatment response in patients with locally advanced breast cancer undergoing neoadjuvant chemotherapy. *Med Oncol*. 2012;29:425–431.

27. Shin HJ, et al. Prediction of pathologic response to neoadjuvant chemotherapy in patients with breast cancer using diffusion-weighted imaging and MRS. *NMR Biomed*. 2012;25:1349–1359.

28. Bedair R, et al. Assessment of early treatment response to neoadjuvant chemotherapy in breast cancer using non-mono-exponential diffusion models: a feasibility study comparing the baseline and mid-treatment MRI examinations. *Eur Radiol*. 2017;27:2726–2736.

29. Pereira NP, et al. Diffusion-weighted magnetic resonance imaging of patients with breast cancer following neoadjuvant chemotherapy provides early prediction of pathological response: a prospective study. *Sci Rep*. 2019;9:16372.

30. Iwasa H, et al. Early prediction of response to neoadjuvant chemotherapy in patients with breast cancer using diffusion-weighted imaging and gray-scale ultrasonography. *Oncol Rep*. 2014;31:1555–1560.

31. Jensen LR, et al. Diffusion-weighted and dynamic contrast-enhanced MRI in evaluation of early treatment effects during neoadjuvant chemotherapy in breast cancer patients. *J Magn Reson Imaging*. 2011;34:1099–1109.

32. Wilmes LJ, et al. High-resolution diffusion-weighted imaging for monitoring breast cancer treatment response. *Acad Radiol*. 2013;20:581–589.

33. Partridge SC, et al. Diffusion-weighted MRI findings predict pathologic response in neoadjuvant treatment of breast cancer: the ACRIN 6698 Multicenter Trial. *Radiology*. 2018; 289:618–627.

34. El Bakoury EAEM, et al. Diffusion weighted imaging in early prediction of neoadjuvant chemotherapy response in breast cancer. *Egypt J Radiol Nucl Med*. 2017;48:529–535.

35. Minarikova L, et al. Investigating the prediction value of multiparametric magnetic resonance imaging at 3 T in response to neoadjuvant chemotherapy in breast cancer. *Eur Radiol*. 2017;27:1901–1911.

36. Manton DJ, et al. Neoadjuvant chemotherapy in breast cancer: early response prediction with quantitative MR imaging and spectroscopy. *Br J Cancer*. 2006;94:427–435.

37. Padhani AR, et al. Diffusion-weighted magnetic resonance imaging as a cancer biomarker: consensus and recommendations. *Neoplasia*. 2009;11:102–125.

38. Belli P, et al. Diffusion-weighted imaging in evaluating the response to neoadjuvant breast cancer treatment. *Breast J*. 2011;17:610–619.

39. Iima M, et al. Six DWI questions you always wanted to know but were afraid to ask: clinical relevance for breast diffusion MRI. *Eur Radiol*. 2020;30:2561–2570.

40. Yuan L, et al. Diffusion-weighted MR imaging of locally advanced breast carcinoma: the optimal time window of predicting the early response to neoadjuvant chemotherapy. *Cancer Imaging*. 2018;18:38.

41. Chevallier B, et al. Inflammatory breast cancer. Pilot study of intensive induction chemotherapy (FEC-HD) results in a high histologic response rate. *Am J Clin Oncol*. 1993;16:223–228.

42. Sataloff DM, et al. Pathologic response to induction chemotherapy in locally advanced carcinoma of the breast: a determinant of outcome. *J Am Coll Surg*. 1995;180:297–306.

43. Bufi E, et al. Role of the apparent diffusion coefficient in the prediction of response to neoadjuvant chemotherapy in patients with locally advanced breast cancer. *Clin Breast Cancer*. 2015;15:370–380.

44. Li W, et al. Additive value of diffusion-weighted MRI in the I-SPY 2 TRIAL. *J Magn Reson Imaging*. 2019;50(6):1742–1753.

45. Cheng J, et al. Chemotherapy response evaluation in a mouse model of gastric cancer using intravoxel incoherent motion diffusion-weighted MRI and histopathology. *World J Gastroenterol*. 2017;23:1990–2001.

46. Kim H, et al. Breast tumor xenografts: diffusion-weighted MR imaging to assess early therapy with novel apoptosis-inducing anti-DR5 antibody. *Radiology*. 2008;248:844–851.

47. Baboli M, et al. Evaluation of metronomic chemotherapy response using diffusion and dynamic contrast-enhanced MRI. *PLoS One*. 2020;15:e0241916.

48. Chenevert TL, et al. Diffusion magnetic resonance imaging: an early surrogate marker of therapeutic efficacy in brain tumors. *J Natl Cancer Inst*. 2000;92:2029–2036.

49. Galbán CJ, et al. Multi-site clinical evaluation of DW-MRI as a treatment response metric for breast cancer patients undergoing neoadjuvant chemotherapy. *PLoS One*. 2015;10:e0122151.

50. Newitt DC, et al. ACRIN 6698/I-SPY 2 Breast DWI [Data set]. *The Cancer Imaging Archive*. 2021. https://doi.org/10.7937/tcia.kk02-6d95.

51. Newitt DC, et al. Test-retest repeatability and reproducibility of ADC measures by breast DWI: results from the ACRIN 6698 trial. *J Magn Reson Imaging*. 2018;49(6):1617–1628.

52. Hylton N, et al. ACRIN 6698 trial protocol. *American College of Radiology Imaging Network*. 2012.

53. Song YS, et al. True progression versus pseudoprogression in the treatment of glioblastomas: a comparison study of normalized cerebral blood volume and apparent diffusion coefficient by histogram analysis. *Korean J Radiol*. 2013;14:662–672.

54. Kyriazi S, et al. Metastatic ovarian and primary peritoneal cancer: assessing chemotherapy response with diffusion-weighted MR imaging: value of histogram analysis of apparent diffusion coefficients. *Radiology*. 2011;261:182–192.

55. Kim Y, et al. Intravoxel incoherent motion diffusion-weighted MRI for predicting response to neoadjuvant chemotherapy in breast cancer. *Magn Reson Imaging*. 2018;48:27–33.

56. Gallivanone F, et al. Biomarkers from in vivo molecular imaging of breast cancer: pretreatment (18)F-FDG PET predicts patient prognosis, and pretreatment DWI-MR predicts response to neoadjuvant chemotherapy. *MAGMA*. 2017;30:359–373.

57. Reig B, et al. Machine learning in breast MRI. *J Magn Reson Imaging*. 2019;52(4):998–1018.

58. Yoon H-J, et al. Predicting neo-adjuvant chemotherapy response and progression-free survival of locally advanced breast cancer using textural features of intratumoral heterogeneity on F-18 FDG PET/CT and diffusion-weighted MR imaging. *Breast J*. 2019;25:373–380.

59. La Yun B, et al. Intratumoral heterogeneity of breast cancer xenograft models: texture analysis of diffusion-weighted MR imaging. *Korean J Radiol*. 2014;15:591–604.

60. Eun NL, et al. Texture analysis with 3.0-T MRI for association of response to neoadjuvant chemotherapy in breast cancer. *Radiology*. 2020;294:31–41.

61. Cho GY, et al. Intravoxel incoherent motion (IVIM) histogram biomarkers for prediction of neoadjuvant treatment response in breast cancer patients. *Eur J Radiol Open*. 2017;4:101–107.

62. Che S, et al. Role of the intravoxel incoherent motion diffusion weighted imaging in the pre-treatment prediction and early response monitoring to neoadjuvant chemotherapy in locally advanced breast cancer. *Medicine (Baltimore)*. 2016;95(4):e2420.

63. Furman-Haran E, et al. Quantitative evaluation of breast cancer response to neoadjuvant chemotherapy by diffusion tensor imaging: initial results. *J Magn Reson Imaging*. 2018;47:1080–1090.

64. Li X, et al. Multiparametric magnetic resonance imaging for predicting pathological response after the first cycle of neoadjuvant chemotherapy in breast cancer. *Invest Radiol*. 2015;50:195–204.

65. Tahmassebi A, et al. Impact of machine learning with multiparametric magnetic resonance imaging of the breast for early prediction of response to neoadjuvant chemotherapy and survival outcomes in breast cancer patients. *Invest Radiol*. 2019;54:110–117.

66. Polyak K. Heterogeneity in breast cancer. *J Clin Invest*. 2011;121:3786–3788.

67. Zardavas D, et al. Clinical management of breast cancer heterogeneity. *Nat Rev Clin Oncol*. 2015;12:381–394.

68. Perou CM, et al. Molecular portraits of human breast tumours. *Nature*. 2000;406:747–752.

69. de Ronde JJ, et al. Concordance of clinical and molecular breast cancer subtyping in the context of preoperative chemotherapy response. *Breast Cancer Res Treat*. 2010;119:119–126.

70. Houssami N, et al. Meta-analysis of the association of breast cancer subtype and pathologic complete response to neoadjuvant chemotherapy. *Eur J Cancer*. 2012;48:3342–3354.

71. Fukuda T, et al. Accuracy of magnetic resonance imaging for predicting pathological complete response of breast cancer after neoadjuvant chemotherapy: association with breast cancer subtype. *Springerplus*. 2016;5:152.

72. Liu S, et al. Diffusion-weighted imaging in assessing pathological response of tumor in breast cancer subtype to neoadjuvant chemotherapy. *J Magn Reson Imaging*. 2015;42:779–787.

73. Iima M, et al. Diffusion MRI of the breast: current status and future directions. *J Magn Reson Imaging*. 2020;52:70–90.

74. Quantitative Imaging Biomarkers Alliance QIBA profile: diffusion-weighted magnetic resonance imaging (DWI). *RSNA*. 2017;1:45.

75. Baltzer P, et al. Diffusion-weighted imaging of the breast: a consensus and mission statement from the EUSOBI International Breast Diffusion-Weighted Imaging working group. *Eur Radiol*. 2020;30:1436–1450.

76. Bogner W, et al. Readout-segmented echo-planar imaging improves the diagnostic performance of diffusion-weighted MR breast examinations at 3.0 T. *Radiology*. 2012;263:64–76.

77. Daimiel Naranjo I, et al. High-spatial-resolution multishot multiplexed sensitivity-encoding diffusion-weighted imaging for improved quality of breast images and differentiation of breast lesions: a feasibility study. *Radiol Imaging Cancer*. 2020;2:e190076.

78. Filli L, et al. Simultaneous multi-slice readout-segmented echo planar imaging for accelerated diffusion-weighted imaging of the breast. *Eur J Radiol*. 2016;85:274–278.

79. Hancu I, et al. Distortion correction in diffusion-weighted imaging of the breast: performance assessment of prospective, retrospective, and combined (prospective + retrospective) approaches. *Magn Reson Med*. 2017;78:247–253.

80. Teruel JR, et al. Inhomogeneous static magnetic field-induced distortion correction applied to diffusion weighted MRI of the breast at 3T. *Magn Reson Med*. 2015;74:1138–1144.

81. Newitt DC, et al. Gradient nonlinearity correction to improve apparent diffusion coefficient accuracy and standardization in the American College of Radiology Imaging Network 6698 Breast Cancer Trial. *J Magn Reson Imaging*. 2015;42:908–919.

82. Le Bihan D. Apparent diffusion coefficient and beyond: what diffusion MR imaging can tell us about tissue. *Radiology*. 2013;268(2):318–322.

83. Tang L, Zhou XJ. Diffusion MRI of cancer: from low to high b-values. *J Magn Reson Imaging*. 2019;49:23–40.

Chapter 6

Diffusion MRI as a Stand-Alone Unenhanced Approach for Breast Imaging and Screening

Hee Jung Shin, MD, Woo Kyung Moon, MD, Nita Amornsiripanitch, MD, and Savannah C. Partridge, PhD

List of Abbreviations

ADC—apparent diffusion coefficient
BI-RADS—Breast Imaging Reporting and Data System
BPS—background parenchymal signal
DCE—dynamic contrast-enhanced
DCIS—ductal carcinoma in situ
DWIST—Diffusion-Weighted Magnetic Resonance Imaging Screening Trial
DW MRI—diffusion-weighted MRI
EPI—echo-planar imaging
MIP—maximum intensity projection

Although dynamic contrast-enhanced magnetic resonance imaging (DCE MRI) is highly sensitive and endorsed by multinational organizations as a supplemental screening tool for high-risk women,[1–3] widespread implementation of DCE MRI is limited by high cost and uncertain long-term effects of gadolinium retention from contrast administration.[4,5] In addition, the cost-effectiveness of DCE MRI in intermediate risk patients, such as those with history of breast cancer and dense breasts, remains unclear.[3] Therefore there is great interest in identifying an affordable, unenhanced imaging modality suitable for breast cancer screening. Diffusion-weighted (DW) MRI has emerged as one of the leading options, owing to its short scan time, relative availability and promising sensitivity for identifying breast cancer. DW MRI enables detection of breast malignancies without the need for administering a contrast agent, based instead on microstructural characteristics (e.g., cellular density), as reflected by endogenous diffusional water movement[6] (Fig. 6.1). To date, most

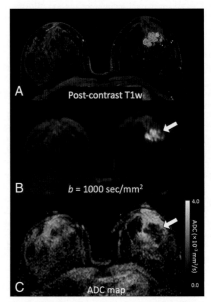

Fig. 6.1 Invasive breast cancer detectable at DW MRI. Postcontrast T1-weighted image (A) in a 37-year-old woman demonstrates a 33-mm irregular mass in the anterior left breast, corresponding to biopsy-proven invasive lobular carcinoma. On DW MRI, the lesion exhibits reduced diffusivity compared with normal breast parenchyma, appearing hyperintense on $b = 1000$ s/mm² diffusion-weighted image (B, *arrow*) and hypointense on the ADC_{0-800} map (calculated from $b = 0, 800$ s/mm²) (C, *arrow*). *ADC*, Apparent diffusion coefficient; *DW*, diffusion weighted; *MRI*, magnetic resonance imaging. (Reprinted with permission from Partridge SC, Amornsiripanitch N. The role of DWI in the assessment of breast lesions. *Top Magn Reson Imaging*. 2017;26(5):201–209.)

experimental and clinical uses of DW MRI have been as an adjunct to DCE MRI in lesion assessment,[7–12] for preoperative staging of ipsilateral and contralateral breasts,[13,14] and for evaluating the response to neoadjuvant chemotherapy.[15,16] However, there is increasing interest in exploring the use of DW MRI as a stand-alone tool for breast cancer detection.[17–24]

This chapter summarizes the evidence for DW MRI in cancer detection and describes the optimal unenhanced breast cancer screening methods. In addition, the chapter discusses ongoing multicenter DW MRI screening trials and issues associated with clinical implementation.

Current Evidence for DW MRI as a Stand-Alone Modality

Real-world performance of DW MRI for noncontrast cancer detection in the clinical screening setting has been investigated in a variety of reader studies, most of which were performed retrospectively.[13,14,17,18,20–22,24–34] The readers in these studies assessed only unenhanced MRI sequences (i.e., DW MRI with or without anatomical nonenhanced T1- or T2-weighted sequences) for suspicious findings and were blinded to DCE MRI. They assigned either a binary category (suspicious vs. benign/negative) or a number on a scale corresponding to the level of suspicion, similar to the Breast Imaging Reporting and Data System (BI-RADS) categories. Study designs ranged from inclusion of only asymptomatic intermediate- to high-risk patients,[27,29,34] patients with suspicious imaging or clinical symptoms,[20–22,24–26,30] to those with known malignancy;[13,14,17,18] some studies included a combination of more than one of the above.[23,31–33]

DW MRI cancer detection performance across these various studies is summarized in Table 6.1. The mean sensitivity was 81% (range 44%–97%), and the mean specificity was 88% (range 73%–96%). However, among studies that simulated clinical screening experience by including negative/benign cases,[14,27–29,31,34] mean sensitivity was 76% (range 45%–100%), and the mean specificity was 89% (range 79%–95%). Variation in the reported sensitivities is likely due to the inclusion criteria, imaging, and interpretation protocol. The study with the lowest sensitivity included only mammographically occult cancer and used relatively low maximum b values (600–800 s/mm^2),[29] whereas some studies with higher sensitivities evaluated only (previously biopsied) known malignancy,[17,18] used advanced imaging acquisition techniques,[22,27,32] or performed double reading.[31]

Some previous studies have reported on the performance of DW MRI versus other imaging modalities, including mammography,[18,26,29,34] DCE MRI,[14,20,22,24,27,30,32,34] abbreviated breast MRI,[13,22] and ultrasound.[35] Compared with mammography, DW MRI was found to be more sensitive (mean sensitivity across studies 78% vs. 59% for DW MRI vs. mammogram, respectively).[18,26,28,34] Compared with DCE MRI, DW MRI was found to be less sensitive (mean sensitivity across studies 81% vs. 95% for DW MRI vs. DCE MRI, respectively).[14,20,22,24–27,30,32,34] No studies directly compared blinded DW MRI performance with that of screening whole-breast ultrasonography; however, a nonblinded study of 60 mammographically occult cancers showed that more cancers were detectable on DW MRI (78%) compared with MRI-guided focused ultrasound (63%).[35] In another study of 1146 women with newly diagnosed breast cancer, DW MRI of the contralateral breast showed higher sensitivity than mammography (77% and 30%, respectively) or combined mammography and ultrasound (40%) in detecting clinically occult cancer.[36] The cancer detection rate (20 per 1000 examinations) and positive predictive value (42%) for biopsy recommendation of DW MRI was also higher compared with combined mammography and ultrasound (10 per 1000 examinations and 19%, respectively; Fig. 6.2)[36].

Common false-negative lesions in DW MRI include ductal carcinoma in situ (DCIS), mucinous carcinomas, and cancers presenting as nonmass enhancement and small masses. DCIS was more likely to be missed by DW MRI than invasive ductal carcinoma.[10,14,17–20,22–24,29,31–33] DCIS commonly presents as a nonmass enhancement on DCE MRI[37] with higher apparent diffusion coefficient (ADC) than invasive carcinomas,[40] making it difficult to detect (Fig. 6.3), with false-negative rates reported as high as 86% using this technique.[24,31,33,38] Tumors with high liquid content, such as mucinous cancers and necrotic triple-negative cancers, can also exhibit a high ADC.[39,40] Mucinous carcinoma was frequently missed on DW MRI[10,17,24,32] (Fig. 6.4), with a false-negative rate as high as 100%.[24,32] Finally, small cancers (<10–12 mm) and invasive lobular cancer were also frequently missed[23,24,28,31,33] (Fig. 6.5). This was due to the low spatial resolution of conventional DW MRI techniques, which may lead to partial volume

TABLE 6.1   Blinded Reader Studies Evaluating DW MRI Performance for Breast Cancer Detection

Study	Total Women	Cancer Prevalence[†]	Field Strength (tesla)	Max b Value (s/mm^2)	MRI Sequences Evaluated	Study Population	Sensitivity	Specificity
Kuroki-Suzuki et al., 2007	70	100%[a] (70/70)	1.5	1000	ssEPI, STIR, ADC	Known malignancy	97	N/A
Yoshikawa et al., 2007	48	100%[a] (48/48)	1.5	800	ssEPI, T1WI, T2WI	Known malignancy	94	N/A
Baltzer et al., 2010	80	67%[b] (54/81)	1.5	1000	ssEPI, T2WI, ADC[‡]	Suspicious mammographic or ultrasound findings and/or clinical symptoms	91* (87–94)	85* (85–85)
Yabuuchi et al., 2011	63	67%[a] (42/63)	1.5	1000	ssEPI, T2WI	DCE MRI detected asymptomatic malignancy + negative controls	50	95
Kazama et al., 2012	46	27%[c] (25/92)	1.5	800	ssEPI, T2WI ADC[‡]	Under 50 years of age with known malignancy + negative controls	74	93
Wu et al., 2014	58	45%[b] (29/65)	3	750	ssEPI, T2WI	Suspicious mammographic or ultrasound findings of <2 cm	90* (86–93)	88* (81–94)
Trimboli et al., 2014	67	32%[c] (37/116)	1.5	1000	ssEPI, T1WI, STIR, ADC	Known malignancy, patients with suspicious mammographic or ultrasound findings, and intermediate- to high-risk screening	77* (76–78)	90* (90–90)
Telegrafo et al., 2015	280	46%[a] (129/280)	1.5	1000	DWIBS, T2WI, STIR, ADC[‡]	Suspicious mammographic or ultrasound findings and high-risk screening	94	79
Bickelhaupt et al., 2016	50	48%[a] (24/50)	1.5	1500	DWIBS MIP, T2WI	Suspicious mammographic or ultrasound findings	92	94
Belli et al., 2016	118	45%[c] (104/233)	1.5	1000	ssEPI, STIR, ADC[‡]	Known malignancy and patients with suspicious mammographic or ultrasound findings	77* (77–78)	96* (96–96)
O'Flynn et al., 2016	61	44%[a] (27/61)	1.5	1150	ss-EPI	Suspected breast pathology	44	-

(continued)

TABLE 6.1   Blinded Reader Studies Evaluating DW MRI Performance for Breast Cancer Detection (continued)

Study	Total Women	Cancer Prevalence[†]	Field Strength (tesla)	Max b Value (s/mm^2)	MRI Sequences Evaluated	Study Population	Sensitivity	Specificity
Shin et al., 2016	87	83%[b] (107/129)	3	1000	rs-EPI, T1WI, rs-EPI fused to T1WI, ADC[‡]	Known malignancy	89* (85–92)	88* (82–96)
McDonald et al., 2016	48	25%[c] (24/95)	1.5, 3	600, 800	ssEPI, T2WI, T1WI, ADC	Asymptomatic high-risk with dense breast tissue with mammographically occult cancer + negative controls	45	91
Kang et al., 2017	343	2.5%[d] (9/358)	3	1000	rs-EPI MIP, rs-EPI fused to T1WI	Asymptomatic with history of breast cancer and no known active malignancy	93* (89–100)	94* (93–95)
Baltzer et al., 2018	113	59%[a] (67/113)	3	850	rs-EPI, ADC[‡]	Suspicious mammographic or ultrasound findings	91* (91–91)	73* (71–75)
Pinker et al., 2018	106	63%[b] (69/110)	3	850	ss-EPI, ADC[‡]	Suspicious mammographic or ultrasound findings	82* (78–84)	87* (85–90)
Bu et al., 2019	166	54%[b] (95/176)	3	800	ss-EPI, TIRM, ADC[‡]	Dense breast and suspicious mammographic and/or MRI findings	94	84
Rotili et al., 2020	378	25%[a] (96/378)	1.5	1000	ss-EPI, ADC	Known malignancy, suspicious mammographic or ultrasound findings and/or clinical symptoms, and intermediate- to high-risk screening	93§	86§
Ha et al., 2020	1130	1.9%[c] (21/1130)	3.0	1000	ss-EPI, ADC[‡]	Contralateral breast of women with newly diagnosed unilateral breast cancer	77.8	87.3

*Mean sensitivity and specificity for multiple readers was not reported in the original article and was calculated by the authors.
[†]Cancer prevalence calculations vary by study based on per [a]patient, [b]lesion, [c]breast, or [d]examination (as indicated) in order to match the performance metrics reported in the study.
[‡]Quantitative ADC measurement was used as part of noncontrast imaging analysis.
§Calculated from double reading.
ADC, Apparent diffusion coefficient; DWIBS, diffusion-weighted MRI with background suppression; MIP, maximum intensity projection; rs-EPI, readout-segmented echo-planar diffusion-weighted imaging; ssEPI, single-shot echo planar imaging; STIR, short TI inversion recovery; T2WI, T2-weighted imaging; T1WI, T1-weighted imaging; N/A, not available.

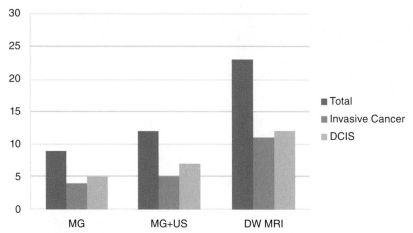

Fig. 6.2 Cancer yield of different imaging methods. Of the 30 contralateral breast cancers, DW MRI detected 23 (76.7%) cancers (11 invasive and 12 DCIS), whereas mammography combined with ultrasound detected 12 (40.0%) cancers (five invasive and seven DCIS; $P = .009$). The bar graph shows the number of clinically occult contralateral cancers detected in 1146 women. *DCIS,* Ductal carcinoma in situ; *DW,* diffusion weighted; *MRI,* magnetic resonance imaging. MG, mammography; US, ultrasound. (Reprinted with permission from Ha SM, Chang JM, Lee SH, et al. Detection of contralateral breast cancer using diffusion-weighted magnetic resonance imaging in women with newly diagnosed breast cancer: comparison with combined mammography and whole-breast ultrasound. Korean J Radiol. 2021;22(6):867–879.)

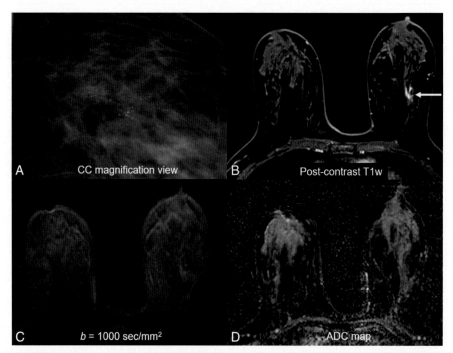

Fig. 6.3 Microinvasive ductal carcinoma not detectable at DW MRI. (A) Left craniocaudal magnification mammography in a 67-year-old woman shows 25-mm segmental pleomorphic calcifications in the left outer breast. DCE MR image (B) shows a 20-mm nonmass-enhancing lesion in the 3 o'clock position of the left breast *(arrow),* which is not detected on either DW MRI at $b = 1000$ s/mm² (C) or ADC_{0-1000} map (D). This was proven to be a 17-mm microinvasive ductal carcinoma. *ADC,* Apparent diffusion coefficient; *DCE,* dynamic-contrast enhanced; *DW,* diffusion weighted; *MRI,* magnetic resonance imaging.

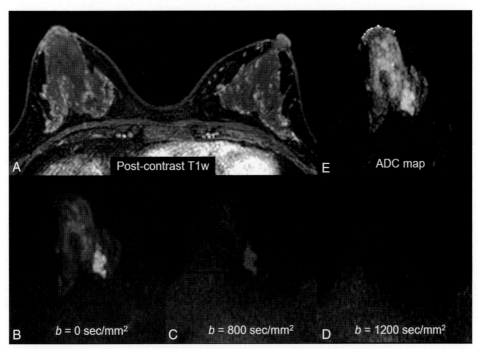

Fig. 6.4 A 45-year-old woman with mucinous carcinoma. (A) DCE MRI shows marked diffuse background parenchymal enhancement, and there was no abnormal focal-enhancing lesion in the right breast. (B)–(D) DW MRI shows an irregular, not circumscribed, heterogeneous high signal intensity mass in the right breast, in which signals gradually decrease with increasing b values from 0 to 1200 s/mm^2. (E) The diffusion level of this mass is very high on the ADC$_{0-800}$ map (calculated from $b = 0$, 800 s/mm^2), and the ADC value was 2.35×10^{-3} mm^2/s. This was proven to be a 20-mm mucinous carcinoma with nuclear and histological grade 1. *ADC,* Apparent diffusion coefficient; *DCE,* dynamic-contrast enhanced; *DW,* diffusion weighted; *MRI,* magnetic resonance imaging.

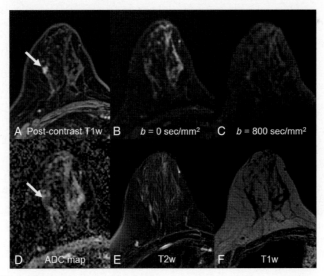

Fig. 6.5 A 61-year-old woman with a small invasive cancer. (A) DCE MR image shows a 7-mm irregular enhancing mass *(arrow)* in the right breast. (B)–(D) There is no abnormal focal lesion visible in the corresponding area on either the $b = 0$ (B) or 800 s/mm^2 (C) DW MR images (B, C, respectively), although there is subtle diffusion restriction on the ADC$_{0-800}$ map (ADC = 0.86×10^{-3} mm^2/s, *arrow*) calculated from $b = 0$ and 800 s/mm^2 (D). (E) and (F) This small mass is also not detected on the precontrast T2- or T1-weighted images, respectively. This lesion was proven to be 10-mm mixed invasive ductal and lobular carcinoma, which was considered a false negative. *ADC,* Apparent diffusion coefficient; *DCE,* dynamic-contrast enhanced; *DW,* diffusion weighted; *MR,* magnetic resonance.

averaging, producing results that are not significantly better than the standard in-plane resolution and slice thickness (commonly 2 × 2 mm² and 3–5 mm, respectively). Expected false negative lesions on DW MRI also could include tumors with a low water content (e.g., low cellularity cancers with extensive desmoplastic stromal fibrosis).[38]

The notable false positives using DW MRI included complicated/proteinaceous cysts, fibroadenomas, and artifactual "lesions."[23,28,29,32,33] Complicated/proteinaceous cysts, which are known to exhibit restricted diffusion (Fig. 6.6), represent the majority of DW MRI false positives in some settings.[32] Similarly, fibroadenomas may be mistaken as a suspicious finding due to the wide range of possible ADC values. More than a third of fibroadenomas have ADCs in the same range as those of malignancies.[41] Finally, false positives can be produced by artifactual signal, such as near the nipple-areolar complex, an area known to be prone to susceptibility-based distortion in DW MRI.[28,29]

Technical Requirements as an Unenhanced Screening Modality

Expert consensus from the European Society of Breast Imaging (EUSOBI) recommended standardized parameters for high-quality breast DW MRI,[38] which were extended specifically for the application of unenhanced breast cancer screening in a DW trial protocol[42] (Table 6.2).

Given that *b* values are known to directly affect the image's signal-to-noise ratio, lesion contrast-to-noise ratio, and ADC values, selecting an optimal *b* value may improve cancer detection. As the maximum *b* value increases, the contrast-to-noise ratio and the differences in signal decay between cancer and normal/benign tissues increase, improving cancer visibility and specificity.[43–45] On the other hand, as *b* value increases, the signal-to-noise ratio decreases. Furthermore, image acquisition at high *b* values is lengthy and prone to distortions due to increased

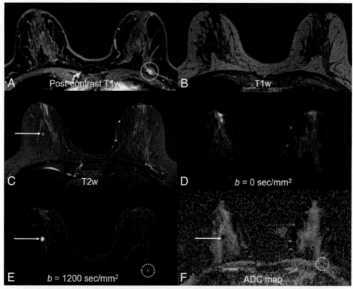

Fig. 6.6 A 59-year-old woman with an invasive cancer in the left breast and a complicated cyst in the right breast. (A) DCE MRI shows a 15-mm irregular enhancing mass in the posterior left breast. (B) T1-weighted image shows no abnormal focal lesion in either breast. (C) T2-weighted image shows a small intermediate signal intensity lesion in the right central breast *(arrow)*, which is considered a complicated cyst on ultrasound and did not change over 18 months. (D) DW MRI for *b* = 0 s/mm² shows no abnormal focal lesion in either breast. (E) On DW MRI for *b* = 1200 s/mm², there is a small oval, circumscribed, homogeneous signal intensity mass with very low diffusion level in the right breast *(arrow)* and a round, not circumscribed, homogeneous mass with low diffusion level in the left breast *(circle)*. (F) ADC$_{0-800}$ map (calculated from *b* = 0 and 800 s/mm²) shows both lesions exhibit diffusion restriction; ADC values are 0.64 × 10⁻³ mm²/s for the right breast lesion and 1.25 × 10⁻³ mm²/s for the left breast lesion. The small mass in the right breast was considered a false positive, and a mass in the left breast was proven to be a 15-mm invasive ductal carcinoma. *ADC,* Apparent diffusion coefficient; *DCE,* dynamic-contrast enhanced; *DW,* diffusion weighted; *MRI,* magnetic resonance imaging.

TABLE 6.2 Standardized Breast DW MRI Acquisition Parameters		
	Minimum Requirement From EUSOBI	**Acquisition Parameter From DWIST**
Study Purpose	**Tumor Characterization**	**Cancer Detection**
Equipment		
Magnet field strength	$\geq$1.5 T	3.0 T
Type of coil	Dedicated breast coil with $\geq$4 channels	16 or 18 channels
Timing of acquisition	Before contrast injection, when possible	Before contrast injection
Acquisition Parameter		
Type of sequence	EPI based	EPI based
Orientation	Axial	Axial
Field of view	Both breasts with or without covering the axillary region	Both breasts with covering the axillary region
In-plane resolution	$\leq$2 × 2 mm^2	$\leq$1.3 × 1.3 mm^2
Slice thickness	$\leq$4 mm	$\leq$3 mm
Number of b values	2	3
Lowest b value	0 s/mm^2 (not exceeding 50 s/mm^2)	0 s/mm^2
High b value	800 s/mm^2	800 s/mm^2 and additional acquisition of 1200 s/mm^2
Fat saturation	SPAIR	SPAIR or STIR
Echo time (ms)	Minimum possible	Minimum possible
Repetition time (ms)	$\geq$3000	$\geq$6000
Acceleration factor	$\geq$2	$\geq$2
Postprocessing	Generation of ADC maps	Generation of computed multiple b values MIP series and ADC map

ADC, Apparent diffusion coefficient; *DWIST,* Diffusion-Weighted Imaging Screening Trial; *DW MRI,* diffusion-weighted magnetic resonance imaging; *EPI,* echo-planar imaging; *EUSOBI,* European Society of Breast Imaging; *MIP,* maximum intensity projection image; *SPAIR,* spectral attenuated inversion recovery; *STIR,* short tau inversion recovery.

susceptibility and eddy currents.[46] Based on the data and expert consensus, an optimal maximum b value of 800 s/mm^2 is recommended for generalizable quantitative ADC mapping.[38,47,48] In a screening setting, evidence suggests using a higher b value of 1200 to 1500 s/mm^2 to maximize lesion contrast and visibility,[5,49,50] although this may result in longer acquisition times. Computed DW MRI, a technique that synthesizes higher b value images from images acquired at lower b values, could provide higher image quality and lesion conspicuity compared with those acquired directly[30,49] (Fig. 6.7). However, one should remain cautious that extrapolation from lower b value images by assuming diffusion is monoexponential (Gaussian) may result in interpretation errors of some findings[51] (see Chapter 1).

DW MRI's performance as a screening tool could be further enhanced by advanced techniques.[5] High-resolution acquisition techniques including multishot (e.g., readout-segmented and simultaneous multislice read-out segmented)[52–55] and reduced field-of-view echo-planar imaging (EPI)[56–58] could improve lesion conspicuity and produce sharper images, which would enable better assessment of tumor shape and margin. Image registration algorithms can reduce magnetic field inhomogeneity-related EPI distortions as well as spatial inaccuracies and artifacts caused by eddy currents and motion.[59,60] Postprocessing techniques can also correct b value inaccuracies due to gradient nonlinearities.[61,62] Display-enhancing techniques can also be used to improve cancer detection accuracy and reduce reading time.[13,27,63] These

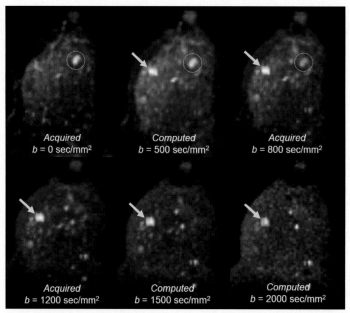

Fig. 6.7 **A 47-year-old woman with an invasive cancer in the left inner breast and a benign mass in the left outer breast.** DW MRI shows a 6-mm high signal intensity mass for $b = 0 \, s/mm^2$ in the lower outer quadrant of the left breast *(circle)*, which shows a gradually decreased signal from lower to higher b value DW images on computed DW MRI. The ADC_{0-800} value (calculated from acquired $b = 0$ and $800 \, s/mm^2$) of this lesion was $1.95 \times 10^{-3} \, mm^2/s$ and was considered a probably benign mass. On the other hand, an 8-mm mass was detected on the inner portion of the left breast *(arrow)*, which shows a gradually increasing signal intensity from lower to higher b values on computed DW MRI series. The ADC_{0-800} value was $0.88 \times 10^{-3} \, mm^2/s$, and it was proven to be a 9-mm invasive ductal carcinoma. *ADC*, Apparent diffusion coefficient; *DW*, diffusion weighted; *MRI*, magnetic resonance imaging.

methods include maximum intensity projections (MIPs), which render a 3D display of DW MRI, and the fusion of DW images to nonenhanced anatomical T1- or T2-weighted images.[13,27,63]

Image Interpretation Strategies

Standardized terminology is needed to describe unenhanced DW MRI findings, interpretation, and management recommendations, similar to the standardized classification for other breast imaging modalities. A variety of interpretation strategies for noncontrast breast screening with DW MRI have been implemented in prior reader studies, with a common approach to first identify unique areas of signal hyperintensity on diffusion-weighted images but varying reliance on quantitative ADC assessment, morphology, and appearance on other unenhanced sequences (T1 and T2 weighted).[14,27–29,31–34] Based on the prior work, a standardized lexicon and interpretation criteria for DW MRI and precontrast T1- and T2-weighted

sequences (Tables 6.3 and 6.4) was proposed by the Diffusion-Weighted MRI Screening Trial (DWIST) group in 2019,[42] which has been used in over 1200 patients in the stand-alone DW MRI program at Seoul National University Hospital since January 2020. The approach is summarized in Fig. 6.8, and the interpretation algorithms for unique findings on DW MRI are outlined in Fig. 6.9. In this guideline, an ADC cutoff value of $1.3 \times 10^{-3} \, mm^2/s$ was determined based on a diffusion level lexicon from EUSOBI guidelines[39] in order to decrease false positives and increase cancer detection.

ASSESSMENT OF IMAGE QUALITY

As with DCE MRI interpretation, the first step in unenhanced breast MRI interpretation is to assess image quality. This includes evaluating for adequate positioning, optimal technique, and motion artifact. The image quality of DW MRI could affect lesion visibility and ADC evaluation. In the A6702 study, the qualitative assessment of the imaging data determined

MRI Sequence	Classification	Terms	Description
TABLE 6.3 Unenhanced Breast MRI With DWI: Definitions for the Interpretation Lexicon			
High-*b* value DWI	Background parenchymal signal (BPS)	*Level*	
		Minimal	A few punctate foci (<25% of fibroglandular tissue)
		Mild	Several punctate foci (25%–50% of fibroglandular tissue)
		Moderate	Several foci and patch areas (50%–75% of fibroglandular tissue)
		Marked	Multiple patchy areas (>75% of fibroglandular tissue)
		Symmetry	
		Symmetrical	Mirror-image patterns bilaterally
		Asymmetrical	More foci or patch areas in one breast than in the other
	Focus	Focus (Solitary)	Punctate and too small to characterize (≤4 mm)
		Foci (Multiple)	Two or more foci adjacent to each other (only if they are not BPS)
	Mass	*Shape*	
		Oval	Elliptical or egg-shaped, may include two or three undulations
		Round	Spherical, ball-shaped, circular, or globular in shape
		Irregular	Uneven shape neither round or oval shape
		Margin	
		Circumscribed	Sharply demarcated
		Not circumscribed	Irregular or spiculated
		Internal signal characteristics	
		Homogeneous	Uniform
		Heterogeneous	Not uniform
		Rim	More intense at the periphery of the mass
	Nonmass	*Distribution*	
		Focal	In a confined area, <25% of quadrant
		Linear	Arrayed in a line toward nipple or a line that branches
		Segmental	Triangular or cone shaped with the apex at the nipple
		Regional	Geographical, ≥25% of quadrant
		Diffuse	Distributed uniformly and evenly throughout breast
		Internal signal characteristics	
		Homogeneous	Uniform
		Heterogeneous	Not uniform, clumped
	Other findings	Intramammary lymph node	Oval/round mass with hilar fat and near vessel
		Skin lesions	Lesions within the skin
DWI of multiple *b* values	Signal intensity change with increasing *b* value	Decrease	Signal intensity decreases with increasing *b* value
		No change	No significant change of signal intensity with increasing *b* value
		Increase	Signal intensity increases with increasing *b* value

(continued)

TABLE 6.3 Unenhanced Breast MRI With DWI: Definitions for the Interpretation Lexicon (continued)

MRI Sequence	Classification	Terms	Description
ADC map	Signal intensity	Hyperintense	Brighter than the adjacent breast parenchyma
		Isointense	Similar brightness as the adjacent breast parenchyma
		Mildly hypointense	Mildly darker than the adjacent breast parenchyma
		Moderately hypointense	Moderately darker than the adjacent breast parenchyma
		Markedly hypointense	Markedly darker than the adjacent breast parenchyma
	ADC value		Values in mm²/s by drawing a small ROI on the lesion
	Diffusion level	Very high	Hyperintense on ADC map or ADC value range, $>2.1 \times 10^{-3}$ mm²/s
		High	Isointense on ADC map or ADC value range, $1.7–2.1 \times 10^{-3}$ mm²/s
		Intermediate	Mildly hypointense on ADC map or ADC value range, $1.3–1.7 \times 10^{-3}$ mm²/s
		Low	Moderately hypointense on ADC map or ADC value range, $0.9–1.3 \times 10^{-3}$ mm²/s
		Very low	Markedly hypointense on ADC map or ADC value range, $<0.9 \times 10^{-3}$ mm²/s
T1-/T2-weighted images	Amount of fibroglandular tissue (FGT)	A	Almost entirely fat
		B	Scattered fibroglandular tissue
		C	Heterogeneous fibroglandular tissue
		D	Extreme fibroglandular tissue
	Mass	*Shape*	
		Oval	Elliptical or egg-shaped, includes two or three undulations
		Round	Spherical, ball-shaped, circular, or globular in shape
		Irregular	Uneven shape, neither round or oval-shaped
		Margin	
		Circumscribed	Sharply demarcated
		Not circumscribed	Irregular or spiculated
		Signal intensity on T1WI	
		High	Bright signal suggesting blood or proteinaceous contents
		Intermediate	Same brightness as the adjacent breast parenchyma
		Low	Dark signal
		Signal intensity on T2WI	
		High	Bright signal suggesting cysts, mucin content or necrosis
		Intermediate	Same brightness as the adjacent breast parenchyma
		Low	Dark signal

(continued)

TABLE 6.3	Unenhanced Breast MRI With DWI: Definitions for the Interpretation Lexicon (continued)		
MRI Sequence	**Classification**	**Terms**	**Description**
	Other findings	Intramammary lymph node	Circumscribed reniform mass that has hilar fat
		Solitary or multiple cysts	Circumscribed oval or round mass with T2 high signal intensity
		Ductal high signal on T1WI	Proteinaceous or bloody discharge filled duct with T1 high signal intensity
		Skin lesion	Lesions within the skin
		Postoperative findings	Hematoma, seroma, fat necrosis, or scar at the surgical site
		Architectural distortion	Distorted breast parenchyma without discernible mass
		Foreign body	Clips, injections granulomas, etc.
		Fat-containing lesions	Hamartoma, fat necrosis, lymph node
		Implant complication	Peri-implant fluid collection, rupture, etc.
	Associated findings	Nipple retraction	Pulling-in portion of the nipple
		Skin retraction	Skin abnormally pulled in
		Skin thickening	>2 mm in thickness, focal or diffuse
		Trabecular thickening	Widening of fibrous septa due to fluid-filled lymphatics
		Axillary adenopathy	Abnormal appearing axillary lymph nodes
Location of lesion	Location		Laterality, quadrants/clock face, distance from the nipple
	Depth		Anterior, middle, posterior
Assessment categories	Category 0		Incomplete assessment, additional imaging needed
	Category 1		Negative, routine follow-up
	Category 2		Benign, routine follow-up
	Category 3		Probably benign, short-interval (6 months) follow-up
	Category 4		Suspicious, biopsy recommended
	Category 5		Highly suggestive of malignancy, biopsy recommended
	Category 6		Known malignancy, appropriate action should be taken

ADC, Apparent diffusion coefficient; *DWI*, diffusion-weighted imaging; *MRI*, magnetic resonance imaging; *ROI*, region of interest; *T1WI*, T1-weighted imaging; *T2WI*, T2-weighted imaging.

that 30% (42/142) of MRI-detected breast lesions were deemed nonevaluable due to technical issues relating to both image quality and spatial resolution on DW MRI.[64] Misregistration of images due to patient motion and/or eddy-current effects was the factor most commonly associated with lesion nonevaluability. Thus every scan should be reviewed for multiple quality factors including artifacts, signal-to-noise ratio, misregistration, and fat suppression. Any image quality factors that affect interpretation should be described.

GLOBAL ASSESSMENT OF BACKGROUND PARENCHYMAL SIGNAL

To establish a standardized interpretation, it is necessary to understand the appearance of normal breast parenchyma on DW MRI. The signal intensity of normal breast parenchyma is typically high for low b value DW MRI, and as the b value increases, the signal intensity of normal breast tissue is suppressed. However, the amount and degree of background parenchymal signal (BPS) in high b value DW MRI varies among women. BPS can be visually

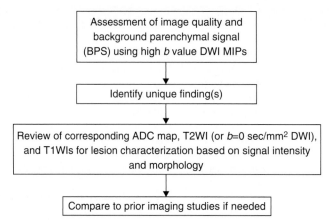

Fig. 6.8 **Approach to unenhanced breast MRI interpretations.** *ADC,* Apparent diffusion coefficient; *BPS,* background parenchymal signal; *DWI,* diffusion-weighted imaging; *MRI,* magnetic resonance imaging; *T1 or T2WI,* T1 or T2-weighted imaging.

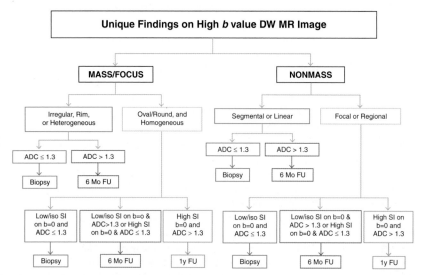

Fig. 6.9 **Interpretation algorithms for unique findings in baseline DW MRI.** ADC map is calculated from *b* = 0 and 800 s/mm2 DW image, and the unit for the ADC value is 10^{-3} mm2/s. An ADC cutoff of 1.3 was determined based on a diffusion level lexicon from EUSOBI guidelines[39] in order to decrease false positive and increase cancer detection. These algorithms are not meant to dictate individual case management decisions. The ultimate decision regarding DW MRI interpretation must be made by the interpreting radiologist, taking into consideration all of the circumstances presented in an individual examination. *ADC,* Apparent diffusion coefficient; *DW,* diffusion-weighted; *FU,* follow-up; *SI,* signal intensity. (Reprinted with permission from Lee SH, Shin HJ, Moon WK. Diffusion-weighted magnetic resonance imaging of the breast: standardization of image acquisition and interpretation. *Korean J Radiol.* 2021;22(1):9–22. doi:10.3348/kjr.2020.0093.)

assessed according to a four-point scale of minimal, mild, moderate, and marked (Fig. 6.10), similar to background parenchymal enhancement (BPE) of DCE MRI.[65] In a study of women with known breast cancer, younger age, premenopausal status, mammographically dense breasts, and high BPE on DCE MRI were associated with increased BPS.[66] The BPS

level could affect the visibility of breast lesions in DW MRI[66] and thus should be documented in each MRI report.

IDENTIFYING UNIQUE FINDINGS

Once the BPS has been assessed, the next step is to identify lesions that are unique or distinct from the

BPS. The use of MIP of high b value DW MRI enables a quick overview of the entire breast volume, determines the absence or presence of abnormal findings, and shortens the reading time for lesion detection (Fig. 6.11), similar to the use of MIPs for DCE MRI.[22] An MIP is also helpful to determine the symmetry versus asymmetry of findings and unifocality versus multiplicity of lesions. Areas of high signal intensity on the high b value sequence indicate possible restricted diffusion and require further evaluation. Characterization of these lesions is based on a combination of lesion morphology and diffusion level on the DW images as well as the ADC maps and internal signal characteristics on the noncontrast T1- and T2-weighted images (see Table 6.4). The window level should also be adjusted so that the differences in signal intensity between fat, tissue, and fluid can be seen. If the window and level range are set too narrowly, areas may falsely appear as being bright on DW and T2-weighted images.

QUALITATIVE ASSESSMENT FOR DW MRI

Assessment of the location, size, and morphology of lesions is possible for DW images, although this is limited by its spatial resolution, which is inferior to the resolution in anatomical T1- and T2-weighted sequences. When available, these should be interpreted together. As with DCE MRI interpretation, high-signal lesions on DW MRI can be classified into three categories: focus, mass, and nonmass lesions. For masses, the shape (round/oval, irregular) and internal signal pattern (homogeneous, heterogeneous, rim) can be reported, and for nonmass lesions, the distribution (focal, regional, linear, segmental) and internal signal pattern (homogeneous, heterogeneous) can be documented.[38] Qualitative evaluation of lesion morphology could help avoid misclassification of false-positive benign lesions such as intramammary lymph nodes (Fig. 6.12) and complicated cysts or fibroadenomas; it could also help avoid misdiagnosis of false-negative malignant lesions, such as mucinous carcinoma or invasive breast cancer with extensive necrosis.[65,67]

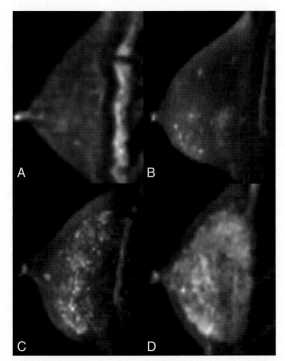

Fig. 6.10 Examples of different levels of BPS on high b value DW MR image ($b = 1200\,\text{s/mm}^2$). (A) Minimal BPS in a 62-year-old woman. (B) Mild BPS in a 50-year-old woman. (C) Moderate BPS in a 52-year-old woman. (D) Marked BPS in a 37-year-old woman. *BPS,* Background parenchymal signal; *DW,* diffusion weighted; *MR,* magnetic resonance.

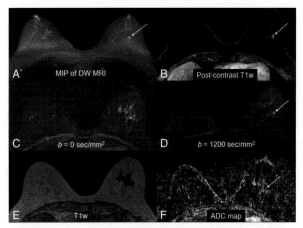

Fig. 6.11 A 69-year-old woman with a small invasive cancer. (A) MIP of DW MRI shows a small, high signal intensity mass *(arrow)* in the left breast. (B) DCE MRI shows a 7-mm enhancing mass *(arrow)* in the left breast. (C) and (D) DW MRIs at $b = 0$ and $1200\,\text{s/mm}^2$ show a small, high signal intensity mass in the left breast, which was proven to be a 7-mm invasive ductal carcinoma. (E) T1-weighted image shows an intermediate signal intensity in the corresponding area. (F) This mass shows a very low diffusion level, and the ADC_{0-800} value is $0.63 \times 10^{-3}\,\text{mm}^2/\text{s}$ (calculated from $b = 0$ and $800\,\text{s/mm}^2$). *ADC,* Apparent diffusion coefficient; *DCE,* dynamic-contrast enhanced; *DW,* diffusion weighted; *MIP,* maximum intensity projection; *MRI,* magnetic resonance imaging.

TABLE 6.4	Unenhanced Breast MRI With DWI: Interpretation Criteria			
Sequence	Criteria	Suspicious	Not Suspicious	
DW MRI	Morphology: shape/distribution	Irregular/segmental, linear	Oval, round/focal, regional, diffuse	
DWI, T1 or T2WI	Morphology: margin	Not circumscribed	Circumscribed	
DW MRI	Morphology: internal signal characteristics	Heterogeneous, rim	Homogeneous	
ADC map	Diffusion level	Low or very low	Intermediate, high, or very high	
T1 or T2WI	Signal intensity	Low to intermediate	High	

ADC, Apparent diffusion coefficient; *DWI*, diffusion-weighted imaging; *DW MRI*, diffusion-weighted magnetic resonance imaging; *T1WI*, T1-weighted image; *T2WI*, T2-weighted image.

QUANTITATIVE ASSESSMENT OF APPARENT DIFFUSION COEFFICIENT MAP

Lesions detected on high b value DW MRI need to be cross-correlated with the ADC map to rule out "T2 shine-through." Because DW MR images are fundamentally T2-weighted, lesions that are intrinsically T2-hyperintense may retain a high signal on high b value DW MRI regardless of the true diffusion impedance. Because areas of T2 shine-through do not have a low ADC, cross-referencing these lesions on the quantitative ADC map would help avoid falsely interpreting the finding as suspicious.[67-69] The EUSOBI proposed the use of ADC values measured at a maximum b value of 800 s/mm^2 for standardization, and they proposed the classification of diffusion level in lesions as follows: very low (range of ADC, $\leq 0.9 \times 10^{-3}$ mm^2/s), low ($0.9-1.3 \times 10^{-3}$ mm^2/s), intermediate ($1.3-1.7 \times 10^{-3}$ mm^2/s), high ($1.7-2.1 \times 10^{-3}$ mm^2/s), and very high ($>2.1 \times 10^{-3}$ mm^2/s).[38] Lesions with low or very low diffusion levels suggest cancer, whereas high or very high diffusion levels are benign. However, lesion classification should not be based on diffusion level alone but should also take into account all of the anatomical and functional information available from the imaging data.

ASSESSMENT OF NONENHANCED T1- AND T2-WEIGHTED SEQUENCES

MRI signal characteristics can provide important information about lesion components. On the T1-weighted sequence, the bright signal suggests fat, blood, or proteinaceous contents, whereas on the T2-weighted sequence, the bright signal indicates cysts, necrosis, or mucin content.[38] When evaluating the T2 signal intensity, it is important to define a high T2 signal intensity as higher than that of the normal glandular tissue and equivalent to the signal of cyst fluid or normal lymph nodes.[70] High signal intensity on the T1- or T2-weighted sequence usually suggests a benign lesion and is helpful to reduce recalls and biopsies for benign lesions. However, the previously mentioned benign findings can often be accompanied by a malignant case, so caution should be taken when interpreting the results. It should also be noted that high-resolution anatomical T1-weighted sequences can provide information regarding the shape and margins of the lesion. Lesions with spiculated margins suggest cancer (Fig. 6.13), whereas circumscribed margins are benign.

COMPARISON TO PREVIOUS IMAGING STUDIES

Unenhanced MRI scans must be interpreted together with mammography, other current or prior breast imaging, and relevant patient history. When interpreting MRI scans, sensitivity and specificity are improved when they are compared with conventional breast imaging, such as mammographic and ultrasound examinations. Notably, some DCIS or small invasive cancers that are not well seen on DW MRI can be detected in conventional imaging.[28] Typical benign findings on conventional imaging, such as intramammary lymph nodes, fibroadenomas, complicated cysts, and fat necrosis, can show diffusion restriction in DW MRI. As with DCE MRI, comparing the scan with previous DW MRI examinations could help interpret diffusion restriction lesions.

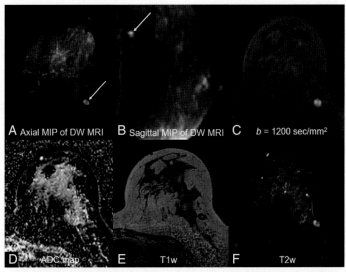

Fig. 6.12 A 41-year-old woman with an intramammary lymph node in the left breast. (A) Axial and (B) sagittal DW MIP images clearly show a high signal intensity mass in the upper outer quadrant of the left breast. (C) DW MRI for $b = 1200$ s/mm^2 and (D) ADC map show a 10-mm oval, circumscribed, reniform high signal intensity mass in the corresponding area, which shows a low diffusion level on the ADC map. The ADC_{0-800} value was 0.947×10^{-3} mm^2/s (calculated from $b = 0$ and 800 s/mm^2). (E) and (F) T1- and T2-weighted images show an oval mass with hilar fat, with an intermediate signal intensity on the T1-weighted image and a high signal intensity on the T2-weighted image, which was determined to be an intramammary lymph node. *ADC*, Apparent diffusion coefficient; *DW*, diffusion weighted; *MIP*, maximum intensity projection.

ASSESSMENT AND MANAGEMENT OF LESIONS

An assessment should be rendered that includes the degree of concern and any recommendations. The assessment categories based on BI-RADS should be used for the unenhanced MRI report. Recommendations for management include a 1-year follow-up for category 1 and 2 assessments, incomplete/need additional imaging evaluation for category 0 assessment, short-term follow-up for category 3 assessment, and biopsy for category 4 and 5 assessments.[71] Further workup for lesions detected by unenhanced breast MRI could be performed with MRI-directed targeted ultrasound if there is no mammographic correlate. Although a screening whole breast ultrasound may be negative, an MRI-directed targeted ultrasound may be able to detect the lesion, especially masses larger than 5 mm.

DW MRI-guided biopsy is another potential option.[72] Biopsy and short-term follow-up should be reserved for lesions greater than 4 mm on the baseline MRI. However, biopsy should be recommended for any discrete, unique findings that are new or increasing in size on an unenhanced MRI scan. The threshold for recommending a biopsy or follow-up depends on the patient's risk for breast cancer. Caution should be taken when applying a BI-RADS 3 lesion assessment to high-risk women in an MR screening program, because the malignancy risk in this cohort may be higher than 2%.[73]

Target Population for Unenhanced MRI Screening

As of now, most experts have concluded that the benefit of using contrast agents for breast MRIs in high-risk (≥20%–25% lifetime risk) women, including *BRCA* or other deleterious mutation carriers, outweighs the small risks associated with repeated exposure to contrast agents.[74] Thus full standard DCE MRI protocol is currently recommended, and further research is needed before unenhanced MRI can also be used for high-risk women. Some institutions have considered use of abbreviated protocols during incidence screening rounds subsequent to the first (prevalent) MRI examination conducted with a full protocol.

Unenhanced MRI can be a valuable alternative option for high-risk women with contraindications to gadolinium-based contrast agents, such as patients with severe kidney dysfunction who are at risk for

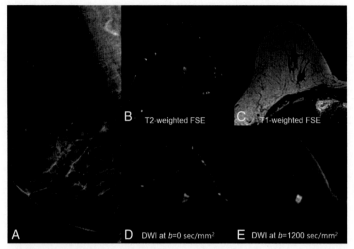

Fig. 6.13 A 68-year-old woman with an invasive cancer in the right breast. (A) Right mammography shows a 12-mm irregular isodense mass with a spiculated margin in the right upper breast. (B) T2-weighted image shows an 11-mm irregular intermediate signal intensity mass in the corresponding area and (C) a low signal intensity mass with a spiculated margin on the T1-weighted image. (D) and (E) DW MR images show an irregular, not circumscribed, heterogeneous mass for both $b = 0$ and $1200\,s/mm^2$. The ADC_{0-800} value of this lesion was $0.758 \times 10^{-3}\ mm^2/s$ (calculated from $b = 0$ and $800\,s/mm^2$). This was proven to be a 12-mm invasive ductal carcinoma with nuclear and histological grade 2, positive estrogen and progesterone receptor, and negative HER2 status. *ADC,* Apparent diffusion coefficient; *HER2,* human epidermal growth factor receptor 2; *DW,* diffusion weighted; *MR,* magnetic resonance.

nephrogenic systemic fibrosis and patients with a previous acute reaction to a gadolinium-based contrast agent.[4,5] Another target patient population for unenhanced MRI is intermediate-risk women, such as those with personal history of breast cancer, dense breast tissue, and those with a lifetime risk of breast cancer between 15% and 20%.[75]

Other Issues in Clinical Implementation

Steps to consider when implementing an unenhanced MRI program include protocol selection and execution, scheduling, and billing. Because there is no standardized protocol, one of the first steps to introducing an unenhanced MRI program is determining and implementing a protocol. An unenhanced breast MRI program was introduced at Seoul National University Hospital in January 2020, and the MRI protocol included an anatomical T1-weighted sequence and a DW sequence with b values of 0, 800, and $1200\,s/mm$. The T2-weighted sequence was not acquired because the DW MRI $b = 0$ images provide nearly identical T2-weighted weighted image contrast. The unenhanced protocol takes about 10 minutes compared with 35 minutes for a full standard protocol.

Adjusting the MRI scheduling templates to accommodate the 15-minute unenhanced MRI examination is helpful and enables efficient throughput compared with the standard 40-minute MRI examination. With the shorter examination period, four unenhanced MRI examinations can be performed per hour. There are medical codes for an unenhanced MRI in most countries, so a self-pay charge is not needed in most cases. In the United States, current procedural terminology codes 77046 (unilateral) and 77047 (bilateral) are reported for breast MRI without contrast. The 2019 national Medicare reimbursement for DCE MRI is 58% higher compared with a noncontrast breast MRI ($403.84 vs. $255.51).[76]

The development and success of an unenhanced breast MRI program require collaboration and communication between the breast radiologists and the staff and stakeholders from multiple sites. Quality control for unenhanced MRI should include appropriate protocols for image acquisition and image interpretation and for the management of lesions identified by unenhanced MRI. As the unenhanced MRI program is incorporated into clinical practice, auditing routine screening outcomes quarterly is critical for the program's continued success.

Ongoing Prospective Trials

Several prospective single-center or multicenter DW MRI studies are underway (as currently listed on http://clinicaltrials.gov), and the study designs are summarized in Table 6.5. DWIST is a multicenter, intraindividual comparative cohort study designed to compare the performance of mammography, ultrasound, DCE MRI, and DW MRI screening for women at a high risk of developing breast cancer.[42] The primary DWIST study is in progress targeting a total of 890 women with the *BRCA* mutation or a family history of breast cancer and a lifetime risk greater than 20%. The patients are enrolled from eight academic medical centers in South Korea, and the participants undergo two annual breast screenings with digital mammography, ultrasound, DCE MRI, and DW MRI at 3.0 T. The images are independently interpreted by trained radiologists. The reference standard is a combination of pathology and a 12-month follow-up. Each image modality and their combination will be compared in terms of sensitivity, specificity, accuracy, positive predictive value, rate of invasive cancer detection, abnormal interpretation rate, and characteristics of detected cancers. For this study, we hypothesize that the sensitivity of current high-resolution DW MRI in 3.0 T scanners is higher than that of mammography or ultrasound but lower than that of DCE MRI. However, because DW MRI is safer and less expensive, it could be used as an alternative to DCE MRI for breast cancer screening in high-risk women, provided there are no significant differences between DCE MRI and DW MRI in their invasive cancer detection rates. The first participant was enrolled in April 2019, and active enrollment of patients is ongoing. Enrollment completion is expected in 2022, and the study results are expected to be presented in 2025.

TABLE 6.5	Ongoing Prospective Studies for Noncontrast DW MRI Screening			
Title	DW MRI Breast Cancer Screening (DWIST–01)	DW MRI Breast Cancer Screening (DWIST–02)	Noncontrast DWI for Supplemental Screening	DWI for Staging and Screening Contralateral Breast Cancer (DWIST–03)
Identifier	NCT03835897	NCT04619186	NCT03607552	NCT04656639
Country	South Korea	South Korea	United States	South Korea
Study type	Prospective cohort, multicenter	Prospective cohort, single-center	Prospective cohort, single-center	Prospective cohort, multicenter
Study population	Women aged 30–75 years at high risk for breast cancer	Women with a personal history of breast cancer	Women with dense breasts, referred for clinical breast MRI	Newly diagnosed breast cancer patients planning for breast conservation surgery
Estimated enrollment	890	1694	275	685
Comparison	DW MRI vs. DCE MRI vs. mammography vs. ultrasound	DW MRI vs. combined mammography and ultrasound	DW MRI vs. DCE MRI	1. Conventional (mammography and ultrasound) vs. conventional + DW MRI 2. DCE vs. DCE + DWI
Outcome	Sensitivity, invasive cancer detection rate, specificity, accuracy	Interval cancer rate, characteristics of detected cancers	Sensitivity, specificity	Sensitivity, specificity, accuracy, surgical management change, axillary nodal tumor burden
Estimated study completion date	December 2023	December 2025	July 2023	December 2024

DCE, Dynamic contrast enhanced; *DW MRI,* diffusion-weighted magnetic resonance imaging.

Other ongoing prospective clinical trials identified in http://clinicaltrials.gov are investigating the role of DW MRI in screening women with a personal history of breast cancer (NCT04619186), women with dense breast tissue (NCT03607552), and screening the contralateral breast in women with newly diagnosed breast cancers (NCT04656639). Further research is needed to investigate more specific and customized strategies for screening, diagnosing, staging, and monitoring treatment using DW MRI as a stand-alone unenhanced imaging modality.

SUMMARY

Current evidence suggests that DW MRI combined with anatomical T1- and T2-weighted sequences has a sensitivity that is lower than DCE MRI but superior to mammography. However, advances in DW MRI acquisition, postprocessing, and standardized interpretation can further improve the performance of DW MRI in breast cancer detection. In addition, DW MRI has a shorter scan time and does not require intravenous contrast materials, which could increase the availability and cost-effectiveness of breast MRI scans and enable a faster throughput. The technique has potential to benefit high-risk women with contraindications to gadolinium-based contrast agents, but indications may be expanded to women of intermediate risk factors such as personal history of breast cancer or dense breast tissue. The results of ongoing prospective clinical trials are expected to provide the evidence necessary to implement DW MRI as a stand-alone modality in a diverse patient population.

REFERENCES

1. Mann RM, Kuhl CK, Kinkel K, Boetes C. Breast MRI: guidelines from the European Society of Breast Imaging. *Eur Radiol.* 2008;18(7):1307–1318. doi:10.1007/s00330-008-0863-7.
2. Monticciolo DL, Newell MS, Moy L, Niell B, Monsees B, Sickles EA. Breast cancer screening in women at higher-than-average risk: recommendations from the ACR. *J Am Coll Radiol.* 2018;15(3 Pt A):408–414. doi:10.1016/j.jacr.2017.11.034.
3. Saslow D, Boetes C, Burke W, et al.; American Cancer Society Breast Cancer Advisory Group. American Cancer Society guidelines for breast screening with MRI as an adjunct to mammography. *CA Cancer J Clin.* 2007;57(2):75–89. doi:10.3322/canjclin.57.2.75
4. Gulani V, Calamante F, Shellock FG, Kanal E, Reeder SB; International Society for Magnetic Resonance in Medicine. Gadolinium deposition in the brain: summary of evidence and recommendations. *Lancet Neurol.* 2017;16(7):564–570. doi:10.1016/S1474-4422(17)30158-8
5. Amornsiripanitch N, Bickelhaupt S, Shin HJ, et al. Diffusion-weighted MRI for unenhanced breast cancer screening. *Radiology.* 2019;293(3):504–520. doi:10.1148/radiol.2019182789.
6. Partridge SC, Nissan N, Rahbar H, Kitsch AE, Sigmund EE. Diffusion-weighted breast MRI: clinical applications and emerging techniques. *J Magn Reson Imaging.* 2017;45(2):337–355. doi:10.1002/jmri.25479.
7. Le Bihan D, Breton E, Lallemand D, Grenier P, Cabanis E, Laval-Jeantet M. MR imaging of intravoxel incoherent motions: application to diffusion and perfusion in neurologic disorders. *Radiology.* 1986;161(2):401–407. doi:10.1148/radiology.161.2.3763909.
8. Partridge SC, DeMartini WB, Kurland BF, Eby PR, White SW, Lehman CD. Quantitative diffusion-weighted imaging as an adjunct to conventional breast MRI for improved positive predictive value. *Am J Roentgenol.* 2009;193(6):1716–1722. doi:10.2214/AJR.08.2139.
9. Ei Khouli RH, Jacobs MA, Mezban SD, et al. Diffusion-weighted imaging improves the diagnostic accuracy of conventional 3.0-T breast MR imaging. *Radiology.* 2010;256(1):64–73. doi:10.1148/radiol.10091367.
10. Zhang L, Tang M, Min Z, Lu J, Lei X, Zhang X. Accuracy of combined dynamic contrast-enhanced magnetic resonance imaging and diffusion-weighted imaging for breast cancer detection: a meta-analysis. *Acta Radiol.* 2016;57(6):651–660. doi:10.1177/0284185115597265.
11. Spick C, Pinker-Domenig K, Rudas M, Helbich TH, Baltzer PA. MRI-only lesions: application of diffusion-weighted imaging obviates unnecessary MR-guided breast biopsies. *Eur Radiol.* 2014;24(6):1204–1210. doi:10.1007/s00330-014-3153-6.
12. Rahbar H, Zhang Z, Chenevert TL, et al. Utility of diffusion-weighted Imaging to decrease unnecessary biopsies prompted by breast MRI: a trial of the ECOG-ACRIN Cancer Research Group (A6702). *Clin Cancer Res.* 2019;25(6):1756–1765. doi:10.1158/1078-0432.CCR-18-2967.
13. Shin HJ, Chae EY, Choi WJ, et al. Diagnostic performance of fused diffusion-weighted imaging using unenhanced or post-contrast T1-weighted MR imaging in patients with breast cancer. *Medicine (Baltimore).* 2016;95(17):e3502. doi:10.1097/MD.0000000000003502.
14. Ha SM, Chang JM, Lee SH, et al. Diffusion-weighted MRI at 3.0 T for detection of occult disease in the contralateral breast in women with newly diagnosed breast cancer. *Breast Cancer Res Treat.* 2020;182(2):283–297. doi:10.1007/s10549-020-05697-0.
15. Partridge SC, Zhang Z, Newitt DC, et al.; ACRIN 6698 Trial Team, I-SPY 2 Trial Investigators. Diffusion-weighted MRI findings predict pathologic response in neoadjuvant treatment of breast cancer: the ACRIN 6698 multicenter trial. *Radiology.* 2018;289(3):618–627. doi:10.1148/radiol.2018180273.
16. Cavallo Marincola B, Telesca M, Zaccagna F, et al. Can unenhanced MRI of the breast replace contrast-enhanced MRI in assessing response to neoadjuvant chemotherapy? *Acta Radiol.* 2019;60(1):35–44. doi:10.1177/0284185118773512.
17. Kuroki-Suzuki S, Kuroki Y, Nasu K, Nawano S, Moriyama N, Okazaki M. Detecting breast cancer with non-contrast MR imaging: combining diffusion-weighted and STIR imaging. *Magn Reson Med Sci.* 2007;6(1):21–27. doi:10.2463/mrms.6.21.
18. Yoshikawa MI, Ohsumi S, Sugata S, et al. Comparison of breast cancer detection by diffusion-weighted magnetic resonance

imaging and mammography. *Radiat Med.* 2007;25(5):218–223. doi:10.1007/s11604-007-0128-4.

19. Partridge SC, Demartini WB, Kurland BF, Eby PR, White SW, Lehman CD. Differential diagnosis of mammographically and clinically occult breast lesions on diffusion-weighted MRI. *J Magn Reson Imaging.* 2010;31(3):562–570. doi:10.1002/jmri.22078.

20. Baltzer PAT, Benndorf M, Dietzel M, Gajda M, Camara O, Kaiser WA. Sensitivity and specificity of unenhanced MR mammography (DWI combined with T2-weighted TSE imaging, ueMRM) for the differentiation of mass lesions. *Eur Radiol.* 2010;20(5):1101–1110. doi:10.1007/s00330-009-1654-5.

21. Wu LM, Chen J, Hu J, Gu HY, Xu JR, Hua J. Diffusion-weighted magnetic resonance imaging combined with T2-weighted images in the detection of small breast cancer: a single-center multi-observer study. *Acta Radiol.* 2014;55(1):24–31. doi:10.1177/0284185113492458.

22. Bickelhaupt S, Laun FB, Tesdorff J, et al. Fast and noninvasive characterization of suspicious lesions detected at breast cancer x-ray screening: capability of diffusion-weighted MR imaging with MIPs. *Radiology.* 2016;278(3):689–697. doi:10.1148/radiol.2015150425.

23. Belli P, Bufi E, Bonatesta A, et al. Unenhanced breast magnetic resonance imaging: detection of breast cancer. *Eur Rev Med Pharmacol Sci.* 2016;20(20):4220–4229.

24. Pinker K, Moy L, Sutton EJ, et al. Diffusion-weighted imaging with apparent diffusion coefficient mapping for breast cancer detection as a stand-alone parameter: comparison with dynamic contrast-enhanced and multiparametric magnetic resonance imaging. *Invest Radiol.* 2018;53(10):587–595. doi:10.1097/RLI.0000000000000465.

25. Baltzer PAT, Bickel H, Spick C, et al. Potential of noncontrast magnetic resonance imaging with diffusion-weighted imaging in characterization of breast lesions: intraindividual comparison with dynamic contrast-enhanced magnetic resonance imaging. *Invest Radiol.* 2018;53(4):229–235. doi:10.1097/RLI.0000000000000433.

26. Bu Y, Xia J, Joseph B, et al. Non-contrast MRI for breast screening: preliminary study on detectability of benign and malignant lesions in women with dense breasts. *Breast Cancer Res Treat.* 2019;177(3):629–639. doi:10.1007/s10549-019-05342-5.

27. Kang JW, Shin HJ, Shin KC, et al. Unenhanced magnetic resonance screening using fused diffusion-weighted imaging and maximum-intensity projection in patients with a personal history of breast cancer: role of fused DWI for postoperative screening. *Breast Cancer Res Treat.* 2017;165(1):119–128. doi:10.1007/s10549-017-4322-5.

28. Kazama T, Kuroki Y, Kikuchi M, et al. Diffusion-weighted MRI as an adjunct to mammography in women under 50 years of age: an initial study. *J Magn Reson Imaging.* 2012;36(1):139–144. doi:10.1002/jmri.23626.

29. McDonald ES, Hammersley JA, Chou SH, et al. Performance of DWI as a rapid unenhanced technique for detecting mammographically occult breast cancer in elevated-risk women with dense breasts. *Am J Roentgenol.* 2016;207(1):205–216. doi:10.2214/AJR.15.15873.

30. O'Flynn EA, Blackledge M, Collins D, et al. Evaluating the diagnostic sensitivity of computed diffusion-weighted MR imaging in the detection of breast cancer. *J Magn Reson Imaging.* 2016;44(1):130–137. doi:10.1002/jmri.25131.

31. Rotili A, Trimboli RM, Penco S, et al. Double reading of diffusion-weighted magnetic resonance imaging for breast cancer detection. *Breast Cancer Res Treat.* 2020;180(1):111–120. doi:10.1007/s10549-019-05519-y.

32. Telegrafo M, Rella L, Stabile Ianora AA, Angelelli G, Moschetta M. Unenhanced breast MRI (STIR, T2-weighted TSE, DWIBS): an accurate and alternative strategy for detecting and differentiating breast lesions. *Magn Reson Imaging.* 2015;33(8):951–955. doi:10.1016/j.mri.2015.06.002.

33. Trimboli RM, Verardi N, Cartia F, Carbonaro LA, Sardanelli F. Breast cancer detection using double reading of unenhanced MRI including T1-weighted, T2-weighted STIR, and diffusion-weighted imaging: a proof of concept study. *Am J Roentgenol.* 2014;203(3):674–681. doi:10.2214/AJR.13.11816.

34. Yabuuchi H, Matsuo Y, Sunami S, et al. Detection of non-palpable breast cancer in asymptomatic women by using unenhanced diffusion-weighted and T2-weighted MR imaging: comparison with mammography and dynamic contrast-enhanced MR imaging. *Eur Radiol.* 2011;21(1):11–17. doi:10.1007/s00330-010-1890-8.

35. Amornsiripanitch N, Rahbar H, Kitsch AE, Lam DL, Weitzel B, Partridge SC. Visibility of mammographically occult breast cancer on diffusion-weighted MRI versus ultrasound. *Clin Imaging.* 2018;49:37–43. doi:10.1016/j.clinimag.2017.10.017.

36. Ha SM, Chang JM, Lee SH, et al. Detection of contralateral breast cancer using diffusion-weighted magnetic resonance imaging in women with newly diagnosed breast cancer: comparison with combined mammography and whole-breast ultrasound. *Korean J Radiol.* 2021;22(6):867–879. doi:10.3348/kjr.2020.1183.

37. Jansen SA, Newstead GM, Abe H, Shimauchi A, Schmidt RA, Karczmar GS. Pure ductal carcinoma in situ: kinetic and morphologic MR characteristics compared with mammographic appearance and nuclear grade. *Radiology.* 2007;245(3):684–691. doi:10.1148/radiol.2453062061.

38. Baltzer P, Mann RM, Iima M, et al.; EUSOBI International Breast Diffusion-Weighted Imaging Working Group. Diffusion-weighted imaging of the breast: a consensus and mission statement from the EUSOBI International Breast Diffusion-Weighted Imaging working group. *Eur Radiol.* 2020;30(3):1436–1450. doi:10.1007/s00330-019-06510-3

39. Woodhams R, Matsunaga K, Kan S, et al. ADC mapping of benign and malignant breast tumors. *Magn Reson Med Sci.* 2005;4(1):35–42.

40. Youk JH, Son EJ, Chung J, Kim JA, Kim EK. Triple-negative invasive breast cancer on dynamic contrast-enhanced and diffusion-weighted MR imaging: comparison with other breast cancer subtypes. *Eur Radiol.* 2012;22(8):1724–1734. doi:10.1007/s00330-012-2425-2.

41. Parsian S, Rahbar H, Allison KH, et al. Nonmalignant breast lesions: ADCs of benign and high-risk subtypes assessed as false-positive at dynamic enhanced MR imaging. *Radiology.* 2012;265(3):696–706. doi:10.1148/radiol.12112672.

42. Shin HJ, Lee SH, Park VY, et al. Diffusion-weighted magnetic resonance imaging for breast cancer screening in high-risk women: design and imaging protocol of a prospective multi-center study in Korea. *J Breast Cancer.* 2021;24(2):218–228. doi:10.4048/jbc.2021.24.e19.

43. Han X, Li J, Wang X. Comparison and optimization of 3.0 T breast images quality of diffusion-weighted imaging with multiple *b*-values. *Acad Radiol.* 2017;24(4):418–425. doi:10.1016/j.acra.2016.11.006.

44. Iima M, Yano K, Kataoka M, et al. Quantitative non-Gaussian diffusion and intravoxel incoherent motion magnetic resonance imaging: differentiation of malignant and benign breast

lesions. *Invest Radiol.* 2015;50(4):205–211. doi:10.1097/RLI.0000000000000094.

45. Tamura T, Murakami S, Naito K, Yamada T, Fujimoto T, Kikkawa T. Investigation of the optimal *b*-value to detect breast tumors with diffusion weighted imaging by 1.5-T MRI. *Cancer Imaging.* 2014;14:11. doi:10.1186/1470-7330-14-11.

46. Nilsson M, Szczepankiewicz F, van Westen D, Hansson O. Extrapolation-based references improve motion and eddy-current correction of high *b*-value DWI data: application in Parkinson's disease dementia. *PLoS One.* 2015;10(11):e0141825. doi:10.1371/journal.pone.0141825.

47. Bogner W, Gruber S, Pinker K, et al. Diffusion-weighted MR for differentiation of breast lesions at 3.0 T: how does selection of diffusion protocols affect diagnosis? *Radiology.* 2009;253(2):341–351. doi:10.1148/radiol.2532081718.

48. Dorrius MD, Dijkstra H, Oudkerk M, Sijens PE. Effect of *b* value and pre-admission of contrast on diagnostic accuracy of 1.5-T breast DWI: a systematic review and meta-analysis. *Eur Radiol.* 2014;24(11):2835–2847. doi:10.1007/s00330-014-3338-z.

49. DelPriore MR, Biswas D, Hippe DS, et al. Breast cancer conspicuity on computed versus acquired high *b*-value diffusion-weighted MRI. *Acad Radiol.* 2021;28(8):1108–1117. doi:10.1016/j.acra.2020.03.011.

50. Woodhams R, Inoue Y, Ramadan S, Hata H, Ozaki M. Diffusion-weighted imaging of the breast: comparison of *b*-values 1000 s/mm^2 and 1500 s/mm^2. *Magn Reson Med Sci.* 2013;12(3):229–234. doi:10.2463/mrms.2012-0028.

51. Iima M, Partridge SC, Le Bihan D. Six DWI questions you always wanted to know but were afraid to ask: clinical relevance for breast diffusion MRI. *Eur Radiol.* 2020;30(5):2561–2570. doi:10.1007/s00330-019-06648-0.

52. Porter DA, Heidemann RM. High resolution diffusion-weighted imaging using readout-segmented echo-planar imaging, parallel imaging and a two-dimensional navigator-based reacquisition. *Magn Reson Med.* 2009;62(2):468–475. doi:10.1002/mrm.22024.

53. Filli L, Ghafoor S, Kenkel D, et al. Simultaneous multi-slice readout-segmented echo planar imaging for accelerated diffusion-weighted imaging of the breast. *Eur J Radiol.* 2016;85(1):274–278. doi:10.1016/j.ejrad.2015.10.009.

54. McKay JA, Church AL, Rubin N, et al. A comparison of methods for high-spatial-resolution diffusion-weighted imaging in breast MRI. *Radiology.* 2020;297(2):304–312. doi:10.1148/radiol.2020200221.

55. Song SE, Woo OH, Cho KR, et al. Simultaneous multislice readout-segmented echo planar imaging for diffusion-weighted MRI in patients with invasive breast cancers. *J Magn Reson Imaging.* 2021;53(4):1108–1115. doi:10.1002/jmri.27433.

56. Singer L, Wilmes LJ, Saritas EU, et al. High-resolution diffusion-weighted magnetic resonance imaging in patients with locally advanced breast cancer. *Acad Radiol.* 2012;19(5):526–534. doi:10.1016/j.acra.2011.11.003.

57. Barentsz MW, Taviani V, Chang JM, et al. Assessment of tumor morphology on diffusion-weighted (DWI) breast MRI: diagnostic value of reduced field of view DWI. *J Magn Reson Imaging.* 2015;42(6):1656–1665. doi:10.1002/jmri.24929.

58. Park JY, Shin HJ, Shin KC, et al. Comparison of readout segmented echo planar imaging (EPI) and EPI with reduced field-of-view diffusion-weighted imaging at 3t in patients with breast cancer. *J Magn Reson Imaging.* 2015;42(6):1679–1688. doi:10.1002/jmri.24940.

59. Arlinghaus LR, Welch EB, Chakravarthy AB, et al. Motion correction in diffusion-weighted MRI of the breast at 3T.

J Magn Reson Imaging. 2011;33(5):1063–1070. doi:10.1002/jmri.22562.

60. Takatsu Y, Sagawa H, Nakamura M, Suzuki Y, Miyati T. Novel distortion correction method for diffusion-weighted imaging based on non-rigid image registration between low *b* value image and anatomical image. *Magn Reson Imaging.* 2019;57:277–284. doi:10.1016/j.mri.2018.12.002.

61. Tan ET, Marinelli L, Slavens ZW, King KF, Hardy CJ. Improved correction for gradient nonlinearity effects in diffusion-weighted imaging. *J Magn Reson Imaging.* 2013;38(2):448–453. doi:10.1002/jmri.23942.

62. Newitt DC, Tan ET, Wilmes LJ, et al. Gradient nonlinearity correction to improve apparent diffusion coefficient accuracy and standardization in the American College of Radiology Imaging Network 6698 breast cancer trial. *J Magn Reson Imaging.* 2015;42(4):908–919. doi:10.1002/jmri.24883.

63. Bickelhaupt S, Tesdorff J, Laun FB, et al. Independent value of image fusion in unenhanced breast MRI using diffusion-weighted and morphological T2-weighted images for lesion characterization in patients with recently detected BI-RADS 4/5 x-ray mammography findings. *Eur Radiol.* 2017;27(2):562–569. doi:10.1007/s00330-016-4400-9.

64. Whisenant JG, Romanoff J, Rahbar H, et al. Factors affecting image quality and lesion evaluability in breast diffusion-weighted MRI: observations from the ECOG-ACRIN Cancer Research Group multisite trial (A6702). *J Breast Imaging.* 2020;3(1):44–56. doi:10.1093/jbi/wbaa103.

65. Lee SH, Shin HJ, Moon WK. Diffusion-weighted magnetic resonance imaging of the breast: standardization of image acquisition and interpretation. *Korean J Radiol.* 2021;22(1):9–22. doi:10.3348/kjr.2020.0093.

66. Hahn SY, Ko ES, Han BK, Lim Y, Gu S, Ko EY. Analysis of factors influencing the degree of detectability on diffusion-weighted MRI and diffusion background signals in patients with invasive breast cancer. *Medicine (Baltimore).* 2016;95(27):e4086. doi:10.1097/MD.0000000000004086.

67. Radovic N, Ivanac G, Divjak E, Biondic I, Bulum A, Brkljacic B. Evaluation of breast cancer morphology using diffusion-weighted and dynamic contrast-enhanced MRI: inter-method and interobserver agreement. *J Magn Reson Imaging.* 2019;49(5):1381–1390. doi:10.1002/jmri.26332.

68. Partridge SC, McDonald ES. Diffusion weighted magnetic resonance imaging of the breast: protocol optimization, interpretation, and clinical applications. *Magn Reson Imaging Clin N Am.* 2013;21(3):601–624. doi:10.1016/j.mric.2013.04.007.

69. Bickel H, Pinker K, Polanec S, et al. Diffusion-weighted imaging of breast lesions: region-of-interest placement and different ADC parameters influence apparent diffusion coefficient values. *Eur Radiol.* 2017;27(5):1883–1892. doi:10.1007/s00330-016-4564-3.

70. Sung JS, Lehman CD. Interpretation guidelines. In: Comstock CE, Khul C, eds. *Abbreviated MRI of the Breast: A Practical Guide.* Thieme; 2018:85–104.

71. D'Orsi CJ, Sickles EA, Mendelson EB, Morris EA, et al. *ACR BI-RADS® Atlas, Breast Imaging Reporting and Data System.* 5th ed : American College of Radiology; 2013.

72. Berger N, Varga Z, Frauenfelder T, Boss A. MRI-guided breast vacuum biopsy: localization of the lesion without contrast-agent application using diffusion-weighted imaging. *Magn Reson Imaging.* 2017;38:1–5. doi:10.1016/j.mri.2016.12.006.

73. Edmonds CE, Lamb LR, Mercaldo SF, Sippo DA, Burk KS, Lehman CD. Frequency and cancer yield of BI-RADS category 3 lesions detected at high-risk screening breast MRI.

Am J Roentgenol. 2020;214(2):240–248. doi:10.2214/AJR.19.21778.

74. Sardanelli F, Cozzi A, Trimboli RM, Schiaffino S. Gadolinium retention and breast MRI screening: more harm than good? *Am J Roentgenol.* 2020;214(2):324–327. doi:10.2214/AJR.19.21988.

75. IBIS Risk Assessment Tool. Version 8.0b. ikonopedia: International Breast Cancer Intervention Study. Accessed October 3, 2020. https://ibis.ikonopedia.com/.

76. Physician Fee Schedule Search. U.S. Centers for Medicare & Medicaid Services. Published 2020. Updated October 30, 2020. Accessed Feburary 7, 2021. https://www.cms.gov/medicare-coverage-database/view/article.aspx?articleid=56448&ver=15&bc=CAAAAAAAAAAA.

Chapter 7

DWI and Breast Physiology Status

Noam Nissan, MD, PhD, Debbie Anaby, PhD, Ethan Bauer, MSc, and Miri Sklair-Levy, MD

The normal breast tissue undergoes marked alterations in size, shape, and function in response to the onset of puberty, pregnancy, lactation, and menopause.[1] Both endogenous (early menarche, older age at first pregnancy, and nulliparity) and exogenous (use of hormonal replacement therapy) hormonal exposures are associated with these physiological states and were identified as risk factors for developing breast cancer.[2] Therefore recognizing the unique imaging manifestations in each physiological state is of both diagnostic and prognostic significance.

Menstrual Cycle

Upon the onset of menarche, the breast tissue fluctuates in response to the hormonal regulation throughout the menstrual cycle.[3] Several distinct microscopic characteristics have been defined for the follicular and luteal phases, which vary in the vascular and histological features of the epithelial and stromal components.[4] Dense and cellular stroma without active mammary glandular secretion are highlights of the follicular phase, whereas the luteal phase is characterized by stromal edema, basal cell vacuolization, duct distension, venous congestion, and active glandular secretion.[5] These histological differences may be reflected in imaging studies, accounting for the periodic changes of structural and perfusion measurements. Indeed, variations in fibroglandular tissue amount were around 7% in a quantitative, longitudinal T2-weighted study during the cycle.[6] Moreover, the breast's vascular network fluctuates, as an upsurge in progesterone blood levels lead to periodic vascular dilation[7] and consequently, variations in background parenchymal enhancement (BPE) appear on dynamic contrast-enhanced magnetic resonance imaging (DCE MRI) along the cycle. This less commonly occurs in the second week of menstruation,[8,9]

which is therefore the recommended timing for scan scheduling.[10]

Unlike perfusion studies, diffusion MRI of the breast is less likely to be affected by mild physiological vascular variations. In fact, the intravoxel incoherent motion (IVIM) phenomenon of the perfusion-related (see Chapter 1), fast-decaying component on the biexponent model is hardly apparent in the normal breast, as opposed to the pronounced vascular supply of locally advanced invasive carcinoma.[11] Several studies have reported on the effects of the menstrual cycle on diffusion MRI and apparent diffusion coefficient (ADC) values.[13–17] Partridge and colleagues reported a nonstatistically significant 5% variation among four weekly ADC measurements of healthy, premenopausal volunteers scanned throughout one menstrual cycle.[18] O'Flynn and colleagues[16] and Al Rashidi and colleagues[13] reported similar breast ADC values in the proliferative and secretory phases, whereas Clendenen and colleagues found up to a 14% increase in the ADC luteal phase in comparison with the follicular phase of the cycle.[14] Furthermore, Wiederer and colleagues concluded that breast diffusion tensor imaging (DTI; see Chapters 1 and 9) parameters do not depend on the menstrual cycle,[17] which is in agreement with another report on stable parametric measurements of the DTI properties during the cycle. This study reported a nonstatistically significant intraindividual coefficient of variance between 1% and 2% for the diffusion coefficients and 5% for fractional anisotropy (FA).[15] All in all, the studies varied in design, most notably in the sample size, scanning protocol, number of scans, and means of image analysis. Despite the apparent disagreement between some of these studies, from a clinical perspective, all the studies support the conclusion that the diffusivity variations along the cycle are negligible, in comparison with the more drastic diffusivity reduction, associated with malignancy.[19] From a practical radiological standpoint, unlike the effect of the different phases of the menstrual cycle on breast cancer detectability on screening mammography[20] and DCE MRI,[21] the menstrual cycle significantly affects neither tumor detectability[22] nor ADC values of the tumor and normal fibroglandular tissue among breast cancer patients.[23] Thus the utility of diffusion MRI of the breast is not dependent on menstrual cycle effects.

Pregnancy and Lactation

During pregnancy, the breast experiences unique physiological and morphological transformations until it reaches its eventual functional competence during lactation. Ultimately, the mammary gland becomes significantly larger, and the relative composition of its three fundamental elements—glandular tissue, stroma, and adipose tissue—completely changes. There is marked glandular tissue (lobules and ducts) proliferation, resulting in a prominent and distended ductal tree at the expense of stromal involution and reduced fat distribution.[24] In order to fulfill its functional role of synthesizing and secreting milk, the breast undergoes two stages of lactogenesis, which is regulated by key hormones.[25] Lactogenesis I stage (secretory initiation) begins during the second trimester of pregnancy. However, the actual secretion of milk is stimulated only within days of the postpartum period, in the so-called lactogenesis II stage (secretory activation).

Triggered by a rapid drop in progesterone,[26] the milk's volume and composition initially presents as colostrum enriched with protein and electrolytes; however, after several days of breastfeeding it changes into a mature, stable mother's milk, with increased lipid content and decreased protein, sodium, and chloride concentrations.[27] An illustration of the lactating breast microstructure and representative DTI mean diffusivity map is shown in Fig. 7.1, which highlights the prominent ductal tree during pregnancy and lactation.

The unique features of the breast during pregnancy and lactation have been characterized by several diffusion MRI studies. The diffusion tensor properties of healthy pregnant examinees were found to resemble the ones of the premenopausal, nonpregnant population, with relatively high values of diffusivity, which is typical for dense breasts.[28] On the other hand, during lactation, three independent groups reported a relative decrease in the lactating parenchyma diffusivity (compared with nonlactating controls) using three different models: the diffusion-weighted imaging (DWI),[29] IVIM,[30] and DTI[15] protocols. The marked decrease in diffusivity between pregnancy and lactation could be attributed to the viscous nature of fat-rich milk, which causes slow diffusivity.[15] Moreover, the lactating breast has been characterized by increased perfusion fraction (f) measured with the IVIM approach,[30] which is anticipated in the view of the breast's increase in vascularity,[31] which serves to meet the high metabolic demand of lactation.[32] Interestingly, when comparing

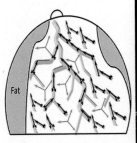 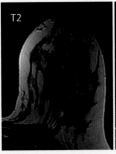 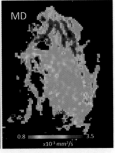

Fig. 7.1 Illustration of breast microstructural diffusivity, anatomical image, and MD map of the normal lactating breast. Illustration of the breast microstructure, showing the surrounding fat and the fibroglandular tissue. The fibroglandular tissue is composed of the ductal tree *(yellow)* and connective tissue. Anatomical T2-weighted image and DTI-derived mean diffusivity map of the normal lactating breast. On T2-weighted image, the central ducts in the nipple region are visible *(red arrows)*. This is also displayed on the MD parametric map, where increased diffusivity in a ductal-shaped configuration is exhibited in the central subareolar region and relatively decreased diffusivity is exhibited in the breast periphery, reflecting the change in the ducts' diameters in these regions. *DTI,* Diffusion tensor imaging; *MD,* mean diffusivity. (Reprinted with permission from Nissan N, Allweis T, Menes T, et al. Breast MRI during lactation: effects on tumor conspicuity using dynamic contrast-enhanced (DCE) in comparison with diffusion tensor imaging (DTI) parametric maps. *Eur Radiol.* 2020;30(2):767–777. https://doi.org/10.1007/s00330-019-06435-x.)

the intraindividual DWI IVIM properties of lactating volunteers on scans before and after milk pumping/breastfeeding, it demonstrates that the diffusivity is significantly decreased postbreastfeeding.[30] A possible clinical implication of this finding could be the recommendation to perform breast diffusion MRI scans before breastfeeding rather than the recommendation to pump milk before mammography,[33] though a comparative study is needed to confirm or deny this hypothesis. A further microstructural characterization of the lactating breast was afforded by DTI studies, which reported reduced anisotropy,[15,34] probably due to the increase in the physiological diameter of the ducts.[35] Finally, diffusion tensor MRI has also enabled probing of the underlying ductal architecture of the lactating breast, exemplified by the diffusivity with direction predominance toward the nipple and noticeable duct-like, linear appearing vectors of the first eigenvalue,[34,36] as shown in Fig. 7.2.

Involution

Upon weaning, the breast returns to its normal pre-conception, physiological condition in three gradual, overlapping steps.[27] The mammary gland undergoes dramatic involution characterized by extensive epithelial apoptosis, regrowth of the mammary adipose tissue, and tissue remodeling, which resembles the inflammatory state.[37] The size and secretory activity of the human mammary gland decline slowly as the infant begins to eat other foods, until ultimately the composition of the breast evolves, inducing withdrawal of the prominent ductal tree, which is typical of lactation and replacement with stromal and fat tissues.[25] Interestingly, after lactation and involution, breast vascularity is reset at a lower level compared with baseline.[38]

Quantitative characterization of the diffusivity and microstructural changes of the mammary gland throughout involution was represented by a recent intraindividual longitudinal study.[39] In this work, a cohort of healthy lactating volunteers were scanned twice, at the time of lactation and postweaning, using anatomical T2-weighted and DTI protocols. Anatomical comparison revealed a 42% and 41% reduction in the breast size and fibroglandular tissue percentage, respectively. Furthermore, a significant decrease in the radial diffusivity coefficients and an increase in anisotropy indices were noted postweaning, whereas axial diffusivity remained unchanged. The authors attributed these findings to the expected decrease in the mammary ductal diameter[40] in the presence of a transient, milk-like medium.[27] In another study, diffusion and IVIM parameters were

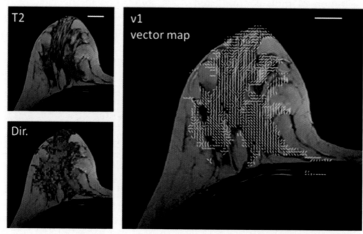

Fig. 7.2 DTI parametric mapping of lactating volunteer. Results of DTI postprocessing are shown overlaid on T2-weighted images. Dir.: direction map with red indicating left to right, green indicating anterior to posterior, and blue indicating head to feet directions. Note: direction map reveals green (posterior-anterior) predominance at the height of the nipple and vector maps of the first eigenvalue reveal linear organized vectors, which suggest ducts. This is in agreement with the visible ductal microstructure on the corresponding anatomical T2-weighted image. *DTI*, Diffusion tensor imaging. (Reprinted with permission from Nissan N, Furman-Haran E, Feinberg-Shapiro M, et al. Tracking the mammary architectural features and detecting breast cancer with magnetic resonance diffusion tensor imaging. J Vis Exp 1–18. https://doi.org/10.3791/52048. Reproduced with the permission of JoVE.)

compared between cohorts of lactating and postweaning healthy volunteers.[30] Findings revealed that ADC values tended to be higher in postweaning breasts compared with the lactation period, with significantly lower kurtosis coefficient (K). Perfusion fraction (f) significantly decreased in postweaning breasts, possibly reflecting the decreased vascularity postweaning.

Pregnancy-Associated Breast Cancer

Pregnancy-associated breast cancer (PABC) is commonly defined as breast cancer diagnosed during either pregnancy, lactation or in the first year postpartum (PABC).[41] PABC accounts for about 1% of all breast cancers; however, with the trend toward delayed parenthood, its incidence is on the rise.[42] During pregnancy and lactation, the breast is characterized with palpable nodularity, firmness, and increased mammographic density, making both clinical and radiological examination more challenging.[33] As a consequence, PABC is often a delayed diagnosis and carries a poor prognosis. It is detected only after clinical symptoms present, usually in the form of a large palpable mass.[43] Interestingly, PABC's prognosis does not differ from that of nonpregnant women when adjusted for stage and age.[44] This suggests that the delay in diagnosis, rather than the unique biological environment with overexpression of vascular, hormonal, and growth-factor mediators, is the main cause for the dismal prognosis. This demonstrates the unmet necessity for developing and using better imaging modalities for achieving early diagnosis.

During pregnancy, breast DCE MRI is contraindicated due to safety concerns related to the use of gadolinium-based contrast agents, which are known to cross the placenta.[45] Breast DCE MRI studies during pregnancy were limited to scans that were conducted immediately before planned abortion.[46] Gadolinium is considered safe during lactation,[10] yet DCE utility is hampered due to the marked BPE that is characteristic of lactation.[12,31,47,48] Consequently, annual breast MRI screening examinations for high-risk patients and MRI diagnostic workups are not performed during pregnancy and are even further postponed until weaning.[49] In the attempt to use unenhanced breast DWI as a stand-alone screening modality,[50] using diffusion MRI to achieve an early diagnosis of PABC appears to be an ideal case-study application.

Indeed, the use of breast DTI among pregnant patients at high risk or with newly diagnosed PABC was recently reported.[28] This study, with a relatively small cohort, demonstrated the feasibility and tolerability of breast MRI examination in the prone position among pregnant patients, including in the third trimester. Moreover, DTI parametric maps were found to be useful in detecting the tumor location and extent, albeit, the inability of the method to detect 7-mm tumor foci, as anticipated by the current technical drawbacks of this modality.[51] Representative cases of unenhanced DTI of PABC are shown in Fig. 7.3, highlighting the evident diagnostic capabilities of this approach.[52]

More recently, a comparative study among lactating patients with breast cancer was reported.[53] On DCE MRI, tumor conspicuity was reduced by 60% in the scans of lactating patients compared with nonlactating patients because of lactation-induced BPE. However, DTI-derived parametric maps not only detected all lesions but also provided up to an additional 138% increase in tumor conspicuity on average, compared with DCE, demonstrating a clear-cut advantage for the adjunct use of diffusion breast MRI in this setting. Further application of diffusion MRI in the setting of PABC diagnostic workup can be found in the emerging use of whole-body diffusion-weighted MRI in the evaluation of disease extent and distant metastasis. This imaging technique provides additional noninvasive diagnostic value among this distinctive population.[54–57]

Menopause

Menopause is defined as the cessation of menstruation, determined retrospectively as 12 months of amenorrhea since the last menstrual period.[58] Natural menopause occurs in the median age range of 50 to 52 years among white women from industrialized countries.[59] *BRCA1/2* gene mutation carriers are advised to undergo a premature induction of menopause via prophylactic bilateral oophorectomy, a procedure that reduces the risk of both ovarian and breast cancer.[60] Menopause reflects ovulation cessation due to a loss of ovarian follicles, which in turn results in reduced ovarian production of estrogen.[61] After the decline in hormone levels, the breast undergoes an atrophy process, resulting in replacement of

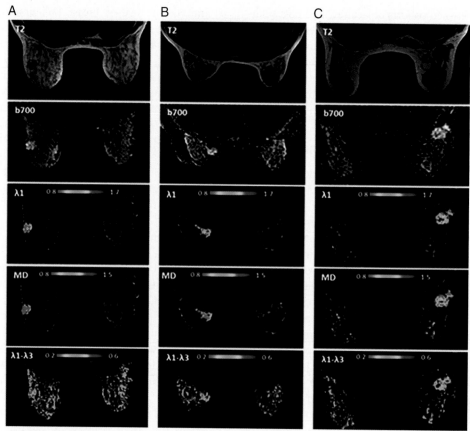

Fig. 7.3 T2, DWI, and DTI parametric maps of three PABC patients. T2-weighted, diffusion-weighted image, and DTI-derived diagnostic parametric maps of λ1, MD, and λ1–λ3 of the three patients with newly diagnosed IDC. In the three panels (A, B, and C, representing each patient) the lesion appears bright on diffusion-weighted image. Using the parametric threshold, the lesion could be easily further differentiated on the λ1 and MD maps, as well as on the λ1–λ3 map, compared with the measurements in the normal tissue. *DTI,* Diffusion tensor imaging; *DWI,* diffusion-weighted imaging; *IDC,* invasive ductal carcinoma; *MD,* mean diffusivity; *PABC,* pregnancy-associated breast cancer. (Reprinted with permission from Nissan N, Anaby D, Sklair-Levy M. Breast MRI without contrast is feasible and appropriate during pregnancy. *J Am Coll Radiol.* 2019;16(4 pt A):408–409.)

fibroglandular tissue with adipose tissue. Early postmenopausal syndrome also affects additional systems, resulting in adverse effects such as vasomotor symptoms, urogenital atrophy, osteoporosis, and further medical conditions.[62] To prevent these chronic symptoms in postmenopausal women, hormonal replacement therapy (HRT) can be administered, preferably using a low dose in selected subpopulations; however, it is important to weigh the potential benefits against the risks, such as an increased risk of breast cancer.[63]

Menopause-related breast changes are well reflected in breast imaging features, including breast density, fibroglandular tissue amount, and BPE.[64] Longitudinal studies have shown that the effects of menopause on

the decrease in mammogram density are greater than the effects of age.[63] When evaluating the diagnostic efficacy of mammography, menopausal status alone did not affect sensitivity; however, among postmenopausal women, sensitivity varied significantly with the use of HRT.[65] DCE MRI showed decreases in both BPE and fibroglandular tissue after menopause.[65] The use of HRT was found to increase the breast's BPE,[66] and therefore at least 1 month of HRT discontinuation has been recommended before MRI.[10]

Several groups have studied the effects of menopause on diffusion MRI. Age alone has not been associated with ADC values.[65,67] Yet, O'Flynn and colleagues found a decrease in breast ADC values in menopause compared with premenopausal controls.[16]

In agreement, a DTI study observed a decline in diffusivity values in postmenopausal women that were not on HRT, compared with both premenopausal women and postmenopausal women who used HRT. This suggests the preserving effect of HRT on the breast constitution and morphology, and thus on its diffusivity.[15] When evaluating the effect of menopause on the diagnostic capabilities of DWI, reports have confirmed that menstrual status affected neither tumor detectability[23] nor the differentiation between benign and malignant lesions.[68] Considering that ADC values of both invasive ductal carcinoma (IDC) lesions and normal glandular tissue were significantly reduced among postmenopausal patients,[22] it seems that the preserved proportion between the two, and not the absolute values, maintains DWI's diagnostic accuracy. This was also supported by one study showing superior diagnostic performance achieved by normalizing tumor ADC values to that of ipsilateral normal glandular tissue in the same subject,[69] although subsequent studies have not confirmed the value of this approach.[70]

Summary and Outlook

Functional diffusion activation[71] and architectural modification following a physiological challenge[72] have been mainly investigated in MRI studies of the central nervous system. Yet imaging studies in other various secreting and hormonally regulated organs, including the uterus,[73] kidney,[74] pancreas,[75] salivary glands,[76] testicles,[77] and prostate,[78] have shown how diffusivity can be modified by underlying biological processes. This thereby reflects functional and microstructural changes that go far beyond the diffusion "restriction" or "hindrance" that is often attributed to excessive cellularity in oncology studies. Likewise, diffusion MRI of the breast has been shown to transform in the different physiological stages discussed in this chapter. However, these physiologically induced changes in diffusivity seem to be negligible compared with the anticipated changes upon malignant transformation of the breast tissue, and thus stretching the robustness of this modality across variable hormonal regulation states as opposed to other imaging modalities. The safe and noninvasive nature of this technique and its advantage over the perfusion-related limitations of DCE, such as BPE induced by menstrual cycle, lactation, and HRT, suggest an opportunity for DWI to obtain a larger clinical role in these settings. Nevertheless, further large-scale studies are required to support the promising initial results of DWI as an adjunct or alternative tool to DCE in different physiological states.

REFERENCES

1. Russo J, Russo IH. Development of the human breast. *Maturitas*. 2004;49(1):2–15.
2. Kapil U, Bhadoria AS, Sareen N, et al. Reproductive factors and risk of breast cancer: a review. *Indian J Cancer*. 2014;51(4):571–576.
3. Ramakrishnan R, Khan SA, Badve S. Morphological changes in breast tissue with menstrual cycle. *Mod Pathol*. 2002;15:1348–1356. https://doi.org/10.1097/01.MP.0000039566.20817.46.
4. Vogel PM, Georgiade NG, Fetter BF, et al. *The correlation of histologic changes in the human breast with the menstrual cycle*. Am J Pathol. 1981;104(1):23–34.
5. Longacre TA, Bartow SA. A correlative morphologic study of human breast and endometrium in the menstrual cycle. *Am J Surg Pathol*. 1986;10(6):382–393. https://doi.org/10.1097/00000478-198606000-00003.
6. Chan S, Su MYL, Lei FJ, et al. Menstrual cycle-related fluctuations in breast density measured by using three-dimensional MR imaging. *Radiology*. 2011;261(3):744–751. https://doi.org/10.1148/radiol.11110506.
7. Weinstein SP, Conant EF, Sehgal CM, et al. Hormonal variations in the vascularity of breast tissue. *J Ultrasound Med*. 2005;21(1):67–72. https://doi.org/10.7863/jum.2005.24.1.67.
8. Müller-Schimpfle M, Ohmenhäuser K, Stoll P, et al. Menstrual cycle and age: influence on parenchymal contrast medium enhancement in MR imaging of the breast. *Radiology*. 1997;203:145–149. https://doi.org/10.1148/radiology.203.1.9122383.
9. Kuhl CK, Bieling HB, Gieseke J, et al. Healthy premenopausal breast parenchyma in dynamic contrast-enhanced MR imaging of the breast: normal contrast medium enhancement and cyclical-phase dependency. *Radiology*. 1997;203(1):137–144. https://doi.org/10.1148/radiology.203.1.9122382.
10. Sardanelli F, Boetes C, Borisch B, et al. Magnetic resonance imaging of the breast: Recommendations from the EUSOMA Working Group. *Eur J Cancer*. 2010;46(8):1296–1316. https://doi.org/10.1016/j.ejca.2010.02.015.
11. Sigmund EE, Cho GY, Kim S, et al. Intravoxel incoherent motion imaging of tumor microenvironment in locally advanced breast cancer. *Magn Reson Med*. 2011;65(5):1437–1447. https://doi.org/10.1002/mrm.22740.
12. Taron J, Fleischer S, Preibsch H, et al. Background parenchymal enhancement in pregnancy-associated breast cancer: a hindrance to diagnosis? *Eur Radiol*. 2019;29(3):1187–1193. https://doi.org/10.1007/s00330-018-5721-7.
13. Al Rashidi N, Waiter G, Redpath T, Gilbert FJ. Assessment of the apparent diffusion coefficient (ADC) of normal breast tissue during the menstrual cycle at 3T using image segmentation. *Eur J Radiol*. 2012;81(suppl 1):S1–S3. https://doi.org/10.1016/S0720-048X(12)70001-3.
14. Clendenen TV, Kim S, Moy L, et al. Magnetic resonance imaging (MRI) of hormone-induced breast changes in young premenopausal women. *Magn Reson Imaging*. 2013;31:1–9. https://doi.org/10.1016/j.mri.2012.06.022.

15. Nissan N, Furman-Haran E, Shapiro-Feinberg M, et al. Diffusion-tensor MR imaging of the breast: hormonal regulation. *Radiology*. 2014;271:672–680. https://doi.org/10.1148/radiol.14132084.

16. O'Flynn EAM, Morgan VA, Giles SL, DeSouza NM. Diffusion weighted imaging of the normal breast: reproducibility of apparent diffusion coefficient measurements and variation with menstrual cycle and menopausal status. *Eur Radiol*. 2012;22:1512–1518. https://doi.org/10.1007/s00330-012-2399-0.

17. Wiederer J, Pazahr S, Leo C, et al. Quantitative breast MRI: 2D histogram analysis of diffusion tensor parameters in normal tissue. *MAGMA*. 2014;27(2):185–193. https://doi.org/10.1007/s10334-013-0400-9.

18. Partridge SC, McKinnon GC, Henry RG, Hylton NM. Menstrual cycle variation of apparent diffusion coefficients measured in the normal breast using MRI. *J Magn Reson Imaging*. 2001;14:433–438. https://doi.org/10.1002/jmri.1204.

19. Partridge SC, Nissan N, Rahbar H, et al. Diffusion-weighted breast MRI: clinical applications and emerging techniques. *J Magn Reson Imaging*. 2017;45(2):337–355.

20. Miglioretti DL, Walker R, Weaver DL, et al. Accuracy of screening mammography varies by week of menstrual cycle. *Radiology*. 2011;258(2):372–379. https://doi.org/10.1148/radiol.10100974.

21. Kamitani T, Yabuuchi H, Kanemaki Y, et al. Effects of menstrual cycle on background parenchymal enhancement and detectability of breast cancer on dynamic contrast-enhanced breast MRI: a multicenter study of an Asian population. *Eur J Radiol*. 2019;110:130–135. https://doi.org/10.1016/j.ejrad.2018.11.025.

22. Shin S, Ko ES, Kim RB, et al. Effect of menstrual cycle and menopausal status on apparent diffusion coefficient values and detectability of invasive ductal carcinoma on diffusion-weighted MRI. *Breast Cancer Res Treat*. 2015;149(3):751–759. https://doi.org/10.1007/s10549-015-3278-6.

23. Kim JY, Suh HB, Kang HJ, et al. Apparent diffusion coefficient of breast cancer and normal fibroglandular tissue in diffusion-weighted imaging: the effects of menstrual cycle and menopausal status. *Breast Cancer Res Treat*. 2016;157(1):31–40. https://doi.org/10.1007/s10549-016-3793-0.

24. McManaman JL, Neville MC. Mammary physiology and milk secretion. *Adv Drug Deliv Rev*. 2003;55(5):629–641.

25. Neville MC, McFadden TB, Forsyth I. Hormonal regulation of mammary differentiation and milk secretion. *J. Mammary Gland Biol Neoplasia*. 2002;7:49–66.

26. Kent JC. How breastfeeding works. *J Midwifery Womens Health*. 2007;52(6):564–570. https://doi.org/10.1016/j.jmwh.2007.04.007.

27. Neville MC, Allen JC, Archer PC, et al. Studies in human lactation: milk volume and nutrient composition during weaning and lactogenesis. *Am J Clin Nutr*. 1991;54(1):81–92. https://doi.org/10.1093/ajcn/54.1.81.

28. Nissan N, Furman-Haran E, Allweis T, et al. Noncontrast breast MRI during pregnancy using diffusion tensor imaging: a feasibility study. *J Magn Reson Imaging*. 2018;49(2):508–517. https://doi.org/10.1002/jmri.26228.

29. Sah RG, Agarwal K, Sharma U, et al. Characterization of malignant breast tissue of breast cancer patients and the normal breast tissue of healthy lactating women volunteers using diffusion MRI and in vivo 1H MR spectroscopy. *J Magn Reson Imaging*. 2015;41:169–174. https://doi.org/10.1002/jmri.24507.

30. Iima M, Kataoka M, Sakaguchi R, et al. Intravoxel incoherent motion (IVIM) and non-Gaussian diffusion MRI of the lactating breast. *Eur J Radiol Open*. 2018;5:24–30. https://doi.org/10.1016/j.ejro.2018.01.003.

31. Espinosa LA, Daniel BL, Vidarsson L, et al. The lactating breast: contrast-enhanced MR imaging of normal tissue and cancer. *Radiology*. 2005;237:429–436. https://doi.org/10.1148/radiol.2372040837.

32. Nissan N, Sandler I, Eifer M, et al. Physiologic and hypermetabolic breast 18-F FDG uptake on PET/CT during lactation. *Eur Radiol*. 2021;31(1):163–170. https://doi.org/10.1007/s00330-020-07081-4.

33. Vashi R, Hooley R, Butler R, et al. Breast imaging of the pregnant and lactating patient: imaging modalities and pregnancy-associated breast cancer. *Am J Roentgenol*. 2013;200:321–328. https://doi.org/10.2214/AJR.12.9853.

34. Nissan N, Furman-Haran E, Feinberg-Shapiro M, et al. Tracking the mammary architectural features and detecting breast cancer with magnetic resonance diffusion tensor imaging. *J Vis Exp*. 2014;15(94):52048. https://doi.org/10.3791/52048.

35. Ramsay DT, Kent JC, Hartmann RA, Hartmann PE. Anatomy of the lactating human breast redefined with ultrasound imaging. *J Anat*. 2005;206:525–534. https://doi.org/10.1111/j.1469-7580.2005.00417.x.

36. Solomon E, Liberman G, Nissan N, Frydman L. Robust diffusion tensor imaging by spatiotemporal encoding: principles and in vivo demonstrations. *Magn Reson Med*. 2017;77(3):1124–1133.

37. Schedin P, O'Brien J, Rudolph M, et al. Microenvironment of the involuting mammary gland mediates mammary cancer progression. *J Mammary Gland Biol Neoplasia*. 2007;12(1):71–82.

38. Simpson HW, McArdle CS, George WD, et al. Pregnancy postponement and childlessness leads to chronic hypervascularity of the breasts and cancer risk. *Br J Cancer*. 2002;87(11):1246–1252. https://doi.org/10.1038/sj.bjc.6600600.

39. Nissan N, Furman-Haran E, Shapiro-Feinberg M, et al. Monitoring in-vivo the mammary gland microstructure during morphogenesis from lactation to post-weaning using diffusion tensor MRI. *J Mammary Gland Biol Neoplasia*. 2017;22(3):193–202. https://doi.org/10.1007/s10911-017-9383-x.

40. Geddes DT. Ultrasound imaging of the lactating breast: methodology and application. *Int Breastfeed J*. 4:4. https://doi.org/10.1186/1746-4358-4-4

41. Schedin P. Pregnancy-associated breast cancer and metastasis. *Nat Rev Cancer*. 2006;6(4):281–291.

42. Andersson TML, Johansson ALV, Hsieh CC, et al. Increasing incidence of pregnancy-associated breast cancer in Sweden. *Obstet Gynecol*. 2009;114(3):568–572. https://doi.org/10.1097/AOG.0b013e3181b19154.

43. Langer A, Mohallem M, Stevens D, et al. A single-institution study of 117 pregnancy-associated breast cancers (PABC): presentation, imaging, clinicopathological data and outcome. *Diagn Interv Imaging*. 2014;95(4):435–441. https://doi.org/10.1016/j.diii.2013.12.021.

44. Amant F, Von Minckwitz G, Han SN, et al. Prognosis of women with primary breast cancer diagnosed during pregnancy: results from an international collaborative study. *J Clin Oncol*. 2013;31(20):2532–2539. https://doi.org/10.1200/JCO.2012.45.6335.

45. Ray JG, Vermeulen MJ, Bharatha A, et al. Association between MRI exposure during pregnancy and fetal and childhood outcomes. *JAMA*. 2016;316(9):952–961. https://doi.org/10.1001/jama.2016.12126.

46. Myers KS, Green LA, Lebron L, Morris EA. Imaging appearance and clinical impact of preoperative breast MRI in pregnancy-associated breast cancer. *Am J Roentgenol*. 2017;209(3):W177–W183. https://doi.org/10.2214/AJR.16.17124.

47. Oh SW, Lim HS, Moon SM, et al. MR imaging characteristics of breast cancer diagnosed during lactation. *Br J Radiol.* 2017;90(1078). https://doi.org/10.1259/bjr.20170203. 20170203.

48. Nissan N, Sorin V, Bauer E, et al. MRI of the lactating breast: computer-aided diagnosis false positive rates and background parenchymal enhancement kinetic features. *Acad Radiol.* 2021;S1076-6332(21). 00529-8-8–8.

49. Johnson HM, Lewis TC, Mitchell KB. Breast cancer screening during lactation: ensuring optimal surveillance for breastfeeding women. *Obstet Gynecol.* 2020;135(1):194–198.

50. Amornsiripanitch N, Bickelhaupt S, Shin HJ, et al. Diffusion-weighted MRI for unenhanced breast cancer screening. *Radiology.* 2019;293(3):504–520. https://doi.org/10.1148/radiol.2019182789.

51. Furman-Haran E, Eyal E, Shapiro-Feinberg M, et al. Advantages and drawbacks of breast DTI. *Eur J Radiol.* 2012;81(suppl 1):S45–S47. https://doi.org/10.1016/S0720-048X(12)70017-7.

52. Nissan N, Allweis T, Menes T, et al. Breast MRI during lactation: effects on tumor conspicuity using dynamic contrast-enhanced (DCE) in comparison with diffusion tensor imaging (DTI) parametric maps. *Eur Radiol.* 2020;30(2):767–777. https://doi.org/10.1007/s00330-019-06435-x.

53. Nissan N, Anaby D, Sklair-Levy M. Breast MRI without contrast is feasible and appropriate during pregnancy. *J Am Coll Radiol.* 2019;16(4 pt A). 408–408.

54. Kosmin M, Makris A, Joshi PV, et al. The addition of whole-body magnetic resonance imaging to body computerised tomography alters treatment decisions in patients with metastatic breast cancer. *Eur J Cancer.* 2017;77:109–116. https://doi.org/10.1016/j.ejca.2017.03.001.

55. Peccatori FA, Codacci-Pisanelli G, Del Grande M, et al. Whole body MRI for systemic staging of breast cancer in pregnant women. *Breast.* 2017;35:177–181. https://doi.org/10.1016/j.breast.2017.07.014.

56. Dresen R, Han S, Michielsen K, et al. Whole-body diffusion-weighted MRI for staging of women with cancer during pregnancy: a pilot study. *Cancer Imaging.* 2015;15:P50. https://doi.org/10.1186/1470-7330-15-s1-p50.

57. Han SN, Amant F, Michielsen K, et al. Feasibility of whole-body diffusion-weighted MRI for detection of primary tumour, nodal and distant metastases in women with cancer during pregnancy: a pilot study. *Eur Radiol.* 2018;28(5):1862–1874. https://doi.org/10.1007/s00330-017-5126-z.

58. Soules MR, Sherman S, Parrott E, et al. Executive summary: Stages of Reproductive Aging Workshop (STRAW). *Climacteric.* 2001;4(4):267–272.

59. McKinlay SM. The normal menopause transition: an overview. *Maturitas.* 1996;23(2):137–145.

60. Rebbeck TR, Lynch HT, Neuhausen SL, et al. Prophylactic oophorectomy in carriers of BRCA1 or BRCA2 mutations. *N Engl J Med.* 2002;346(21):1616–1622. https://doi.org/10.1056/nejmoa012158.

61. Gold EB. The timing of the age at which natural menopause occurs. *Obstet Gynecol Clin North Am.* 2011;38(3):425–440.

62. Dalal PK, Agarwal M. Postmenopausal syndrome. *Indian J Psychiatry.* 2015; 57(suppl 2):S222–S232.

63. Rozenberg S, Vandromme J, Antoine C. Postmenopausal hormone therapy: risks and benefits. *Nat Rev Endocrinol.* 2013;9(4):216–227.

64. Heller SL, Lin LLY, Melsaether AN, et al. Hormonal effects on breast density, fibroglandular tissue, and background parenchymal enhancement. *Radiographics.* 2018;38(4):983–996. https://doi.org/10.1148/rg.2018180035.

65. King V, Gu Y, Kaplan JB, et al. Impact of menopausal status on background parenchymal enhancement and fibroglandular tissue on breast MRI. *Eur Radiol.* 2012;22(12):2641–2647. https://doi.org/10.1007/s00330-012-2553-8.

66. Delille J-P, Slanetz PJ, Yeh ED, et al. Hormone replacement therapy in postmenopausal women: breast tissue perfusion determined with MR imaging-initial observations. *Radiology.* 2005;235:36–41. https://doi.org/10.1148/radiol.2351040012.

67. Elizabeth SM, Schopp JG, Peacock S, et al. Diffusion-weighted MRI: association between patient characteristics and apparent diffusion coefficients of normal breast fibroglandular tissue at 3 T. *Am J Roentgenol.* 2014;202(5):W496–W502. https://doi.org/10.2214/AJR.13.11159.

68. Horvat JV, Durando M, Milans S, et al. Apparent diffusion coefficient mapping using diffusion-weighted MRI: impact of background parenchymal enhancement, amount of fibroglandular tissue and menopausal status on breast cancer diagnosis. *Eur Radiol.* 2018;28(6):2516–2524. https://doi.org/10.1007/s00330-017-5202-4.

69. El Khouli RH, Jacobs MA, Mezban SD, et al. Diffusion-weighted imaging improves the diagnostic accuracy of conventional 3.0-T breast MR imaging. *Radiology.* 2010;256(1):64–73. https://doi.org/10.1148/radiol.10091367.

70. McDonald ES, Romanoff J, Rahbar H, et al. Mean apparent diffusion coefficient is a sufficient conventional diffusion-weighted MRI metric to improve breast MRI diagnostic performance: results from the ECOG-ACRIN Cancer Research Group A6702 diffusion imaging trial. *Radiology.* 2021;298(1):60–70. https://doi.org/10.1148/RADIOL.2020202465.

71. Le Bihan D, Urayama SI, Aso T, et al. Direct and fast detection of neuronal activation in the human brain with diffusion MRI. *Proc Natl Acad Sci U S A.* 2006;103(21):8263–8268. https://doi.org/10.1073/pnas.0600644103.

72. Le Bihan D. Looking into the functional architecture of the brain with diffusion MRI. *Nat Rev Neurosci.* 2003;4(6):469–480. https://doi.org/10.1038/nrn1119.

73. Kido A, Kataoka M, Koyama T, et al. Changes in apparent diffusion coefficients in the normal uterus during different phases of the menstrual cycle. *Br J Radiol.* 2010;83(990):524–528. https://doi.org/10.1259/bjr/11056533.

74. Sigmund EE, Vivier PH, Sui D, et al. Intravoxel incoherent motion and diffusion-tensor imaging in renal tissue under hydration and furosemide flow challenges. *Radiology.* 2012;263(3):758–769. https://doi.org/10.1148/radiol.12111327.

75. Nissan N. Modifications of pancreatic diffusion MRI by tissue characteristics: what are we weighting for? *NMR Biomed.* 2017;30(8).

76. Chiu TW, Liu YJ, Chang HC, et al. Evaluating instantaneous perfusion responses of parotid glands to gustatory stimulation using high-temporal-resolution echo-planar diffusion-weighted imaging. *Am J Neuroradiol.* 2016;37(10):1909–1915. https://doi.org/10.3174/ajnr.A4852.

77. Nissan N, Anaby D, Tavor I, et al. The diffusion tensor imaging properties of the normal testicles at 3 tesla magnetic resonance imaging. *Acad Radiol.* 2019;26(8):1010–1016. https://doi.org/10.1016/j.acra.2018.09.019.

78. Barrett T, Tanner J, Gill AB, et al. The longitudinal effect of ejaculation on seminal vesicle fluid volume and whole-prostate ADC as measured on prostate MRI. *Eur Radiol.* 2017;27(12):5236–5243. https://doi.org/10.1007/s00330-017-4905-x.

Chapter 8

IVIM and Non-Gaussian DWI of the Breast

Mami Iima, MD, PhD, Sunitha B. Thakur, PhD, Neil Peter Jerome, PhD, Maya Honda, MD, PhD, Masako Kataoka, MD, PhD, Tone Frost Bathen, PhD, and Eric E. Sigmund, PhD

Intravoxel Incoherent Motion and Non-Gaussian Diffusion-Weighted Imaging: Introduction

The role of breast magnetic resonance imaging (MRI) has expanded into many clinical applications, including differentiation between benign and malignant breast lesions, preoperative staging, evaluation of high-risk patients, and implant assessment. For breast diffusion-weighted imaging (DWI), as described in the previous chapters, apparent diffusion coefficient (ADC) has been well investigated for differentiating malignant and benign breast tumors, although not yet incorporated into the Breast Imaging Reporting and Data System (BI-RADS) classification. ADC, calculated using the monoexponential Gaussian model, has been utilized mainly for breast tumor characterization and has revealed various meaningful results. ADC values in breast cancer often are lower than benign tumors or normal breast tissue, and international efforts are underway toward implementing diagnostic ADC thresholds and standardizing the acquisition protocol of breast DWI.

It is also known that the DWI signal contains more information to be extracted and clinically utilized. In terms of signal intensity, at low b values (around $\leq 200\,\text{s/mm}^2$) the decay of measured signal attenuation in vivo is faster than at intermediate b values, whereas it is slower at larger b values (at least $\geq 1500\,\text{s/mm}^2$; Fig. 8.1). Consequently, non-Gaussian diffusion models are proposed to better describe diffusion signal behavior, which can have a direct link with tissue physiological and pathological characteristics. Signal behavior at low/intermediate values is often characterized by the

intravoxel incoherent motion (IVIM) model, whereas departures from exponential signal decay at high b values are treated with various descriptions broadly termed non-Gaussian DWI. Non-Gaussian descriptors therefore attempt to move beyond this most simple concept of diffusion, toward a more accurate view of the underlying processes. Interpretation of observed non-Gaussian diffusion in vivo therefore requires a closer look at the process and properties of water molecule motion

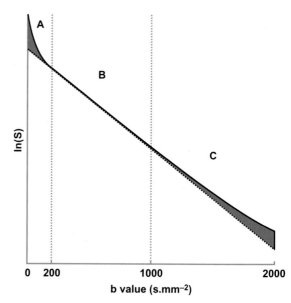

Fig. 8.1 Generalized diffusion signal decay curve, showing logarithm of signal against diffusion b value. (A) Perfusion effect (manifesting as pseudodiffusion) at low b values, followed by (B) a region of approximate Gaussian diffusion, and then (C) non-Gaussian behavior at larger b values. *Dashed line* illustrates a purely Gaussian decay curve.

within tissue and an understanding of the mechanisms of image and contrast formation in DWI.

With the increasing use of the IVIM model in clinical research, throughout the body and including the breast, the interest in more complex and extended descriptions of diffusion has become commensurately greater. Although the IVIM model has generated a great deal of interest and has been the subject of much research, it is not without its challenges.[1,2] With the advent of high performance gradient hardware systems in clinical MRI scanners, the access to high b values (beyond 1000 s/mm^2) has triggered interest in more complex and extended descriptions of diffusion beyond the standard ADC to supply new and useful information on tissue microstructure.

DWI has relatively lower sensitivity compared with dynamic contrast-enhanced (DCE) MRI, and improved diagnostic performance using a multiparametric approach combining DWI and DCE MRI has been reported by several groups. Still, although DCE MRI is a gold standard and the core of breast MRI, it requires the injection of gadolinium-based contrast agent, which is problematic for some with counterindications. Thus another benefit of IVIM and non-Gaussian DWI is that it can provide quantitative information on microcirculation and microstructure in tissues without the use of contrast agents.

This chapter introduces the methods and clinical application of IVIM and non-Gaussian DWI in the breast. First, fundamentals of Gaussian and non-Gaussian diffusion are reviewed, along with their common manifestation in clinical MRI (e.g., IVIM, diffusion kurtosis imaging [DKI]). Next, the literature of clinical applications of IVIM and non-Gaussian DWI in breast cancer is reviewed, including malignancy determination, prognostic factor correlation, and treatment response prediction. Then, methods of image acquisition of advanced breast DWI are reviewed, followed by discussion of data analysis strategies (b value choices, fitting algorithms, model comparison, and noise handling). Finally, a brief discussion is provided on the balance between microstructural characterization and clinical value, as well as the potential for wide-scale translation of IVIM and non-Gaussian DWI in the breast.

DIFFUSION IN TISSUE: FUNDAMENTALS

The term *Gaussian* relates to the distribution of the diffusion-driven molecular displacements in a free medium without borders (see Fig. 1.1), as in a glass of water or the cystic component of a lesion. This is also known as Brownian motion, "free" or "true" diffusion, in which any water molecule is free to randomly move in any direction without limit. Gaussian relates to the *normal* shape of the *diffusion propagator*, a mathematical description of the probability of finding a water molecule at a specific point away from its original position after a given time (Fig. 8.2). In bulk fluids,

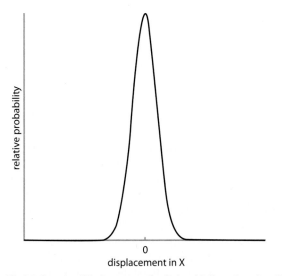

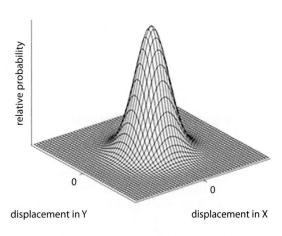

Fig. 8.2 Gaussian diffusion propagators in 1 and 2 dimensions describe the probability of finding a diffusing molecule at any new location over time.

the Gaussian diffusion coefficient is then linked to the intrinsic properties of the diffusing molecule (mass, size) and the medium (viscosity). This diffusion coefficient is independent of the choice of b values. However, in biological tissues molecular diffusion is hindered by many obstacles (e.g., cell membranes, blood vessels, fibrosis). As a result, diffusion displacements get shorter and the distribution of molecular displacement is no longer Gaussian (see Fig. 1.1). Hence diffusion coefficients, though still analyzed with a Gaussian model, are referred to as *apparent* diffusion coefficients.

Beyond the notion of restricted but Gaussian-appearing diffusion characterized by a single ADC, there are observable deviations from Gaussian behavior both at low b values and high b values. These two regimes are discussed separately later. Within this topic, the distinction between a biophysical *model* of a system and a purely mathematical *representation* is important; and we will see that some non-Gaussian descriptions are quite clearly of this latter form, and we do not attempt to explicitly describe or quantify microstructure. Two goals of performing breast DWI predominate: (1) characterization of the underlying physiology/microstructure and (2) generating biomarkers for patient management. These goals often align and are synergistic but must be appropriately prioritized. The microstructure of the breast is quite complex (comprising fibroglandular tissue [FGT] with stroma and lobular/ductal structures, adipose tissue, microvasculature, as well as possible malignant epithelium or benign hyperplasia, cysts, fibrosis, or other growths), and inferring all details of this mixture can be limited by the available data and by intravoxel heterogeneity. It is therefore pragmatic to assume that any successful description of the diffusion decay curve will be at least somewhat empirical. With this in mind, we proceed to discuss IVIM and non-Gaussian DWI contrast in general and for the particular case of breast tissue.

INTRAVOXEL INCOHERENT MOTION (IVIM)

The biophysical model of IVIM is that the DW signal originates from two compartments: molecular diffusion in tissues and microcirculation (perfusion). This is based on the assumption that the flow of blood through capillaries mimics a diffusion process due to the pseudorandom organization of capillaries in tissue. To separate the effects of diffusion and perfusion

on the DW signal, a biexponential model can be formulated as follows:

$$S_b/S_o = f\, exp(-b(Dblood + D^*)) \\ + (1 - f)\exp(-bD) \qquad [1]$$

where f is the flowing blood fraction, D^* is the pseudo-diffusion coefficient associated with blood microcirculation, D_{blood} is the water diffusion coefficient in blood (a term often omitted or absorbed into D^* in practice), and D is the apparent diffusion coefficient in the tissue space. In most cases, the pseudodiffusion coefficient associated with blood microcirculation is much larger (about 10 times larger) than the water diffusion coefficient in tissues. As depicted in Fig. 8.1, the initial slope of the diffusion decay signal observed at low b values ($b < 200\,s/mm^2$) contains a mixture of perfusion and diffusion effects, whereas diffusion effects dominate at higher b values ($200 < b < 1000\,s/mm^2$). Appropriate b value ranges for IVIM analysis are described in more detail later and depicted in Fig. 8.1 as regimes A and B.

f is sometimes called "f_{IVIM}" or "f_p," D^* is sometimes referred to as "D_p," "ADC_{fast}," or "ADC_{high}," whereas D is sometimes called "D_t," "ADC_{slow}," or "ADC_{low}," not to be confused with the standard ADC, whose calculation includes both perfusion-related and genuine diffusion effects. Regardless of nomenclature, the basic interpretation of the IVIM parameters are that (1) D reflects microstructure of the extravascular space from restricted/hindered diffusion, including cancerous cellularity; (2) f represents a blood volume marker; and (3) D^* reflects a combination of blood velocity and vascular architecture. Here we employ the (D, f, D^*) notation when summarizing the literature for consistency.

Although the biexponential model (Eq. 1) is the most commonly used form of IVIM analysis, it should be noted that it reflects only one scenario of the general case. Namely, pseudodiffusive behavior occurs in the long time limit of spins undergoing many directional changes over the echo time. In the opposite, short-time limit (also known as *ballistic regime*), where spins largely reside in one capillary segment, the signal behavior is described by a sinc-function expression. In the intermediate case, an admixture of behaviors occurs that can be teased apart with advanced methods of flow compensation and time-dependent IVIM that are beyond the scope of this chapter.[3–6] But from a fundamental point of view, the approximate nature of the common biexponential description should be kept in mind.

NON-GAUSSIAN DWI

From an empirical perspective, anything that gives rise to a diffusion signal decay as a function of the diffusion-weighting b value that deviates from a monoexponential form can be defined as non-Gaussian. This definition encompasses a variety of microstructural features, from a single restricted compartment to differently hindered compartments to multiply sized compartments; this empirical point of view leads to the creation and formulation of mathematical descriptions that are able to describe the observed decay curves. In this chapter we will review non-Gaussian MRI techniques that have been applied in breast tissue and breast cancer. Furthermore, we categorize them in two groups: those that sample non-Gaussianity as a function of diffusion weighting strength (b value) and those that sample non-Gaussianity as a function of diffusion time.

Non-Gaussianity in Spatial Scale: *b* value Dependence

Acquisition and analysis using DW images at high diffusion weighting ($b \sim 1000–2000$ s/mm^2) allow capturing such diffusion behavior beyond a single Gaussian diffusivity. A detailed description of the mathematics of every non-Gaussian approach is outside the scope of this chapter, and so later sections will focus on an illustrative few as applied to breast DWI, and discussing some of the related literature results. These techniques vary the b value as the primary contrast variable.

Diffusion Kurtosis Imaging. Diffusion kurtosis imaging (DKI), first developed by Jensen and colleagues,[7] is a mathematical representation using an extended b value range that captures the nonmonoexponential (non-Gaussian) nature of the signal decay curve at high b values. DKI includes an additional parameter K, known as the kurtosis (or mean kurtosis MK).[8,9] This parameter describes the deviation of the diffusion propagator from a normal shape, and can be thought of as the "peakedness" of the distribution function; a positive value corresponds to a more "peaky" distribution and indicates that the diffusion remains closer to the origin than would be expected for Gaussian diffusion, and so the signal decay appears slower. A K value of zero corresponds to a simple monoexponential decay, whereas a negative K would indicate faster diffusional spread (and is not expected). The kurtosis signal expression is

$$S_b = S_0 \cdot \exp\left(-b \cdot D_k + \frac{1}{6}b^2 \cdot D_k^2 \cdot K\right) \quad [2]$$

where D_k is a diffusivity coefficient. The addition of such successive terms, here in increasing powers of b, is a general strategy of *cumulant expansion*. Example signal curves are shown in Fig. 8.3, demonstrating the effect of varying both D_k and K.

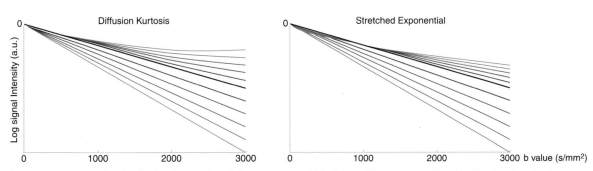

Fig. 8.3 Illustrative curves for different non-Gaussian diffusion representations, and the effect of varying model parameters. In each subplot, the *black line* represents monoexponential decay with $D = 0.001$ mm^2/s, with *blue lines* of increasing tones (dark to light), representing increases in D (or similar diffusivity parameter such as *DDC*). Increasing *red tones* (dark to light) represents (A) kurtosis K, increasing from 0; (B) Stretched α, increasing from 1. Curves are intended to illustrate the nature of the effect, and are exaggerated beyond expected values. *DDC*, Distributed diffusion coefficient.

As described earlier, the appearance of a non-Gaussian process may arise from microscopic heterogeneity or from larger-scale but subvoxel heterogeneity, and this mathematical representation may not distinguish the two. The excess kurtosis K is therefore empirical, and inferring specific biophysical properties from it usually warrants an accompanying biophysical model. Further, under certain circumstances (large K and beyond a corresponding b value), the kurtosis signal representation begins to increase, which has no physical interpretation. DKI also uses very high b values at which decreasing signal-to-noise is important, and it should be considered carefully.

Multiple Compartments: Finite and Infinite Number of Components

Bi- and Triexponentials. When b values in the higher ranges (e.g., $1000 < b < 3000 \, \text{s/mm}^2$) are acquired, it is possible to apply a biexponential representation that, although mathematically equivalent to the IVIM model, returns two diffusion components and does not attempt to capture perfusion.[10,11] Perhaps the natural extension of the IVIM model is to extend to three or more finite compartments when including an extended b value range. This approach is no less valid in theory but can fall prey to a limited amount or quality of data given the required computational task. The problem of confidently separating exponential signals that may be not sufficiently represented (from small volume fractions) or distinct enough in decay constants (diffusion coefficients) is challenging.

In general, the equation for representations with n exponential components takes the form

$$S_b = S_0 \cdot \sum_{i}^{n} C_i \cdot \exp(-b \cdot D_i) \qquad [3]$$

where each component i contributes a certain fraction C_i to the overall signal detected,[12] with a diffusion coefficient D_i (and the sum of the fractions is unity). With useful representation being essentially limited to two or three compartments, it is common to write out each term explicitly. Although there are a growing number of studies that use an explicit triexponential model for DWI in a variety of organs or contexts,[13–16] moving beyond this may introduce too many variables for the data to support.

Stretched Exponential. Another description of a multicompartmental system uses an assumed distribution of diffusion coefficients, each with their own fractional contribution, relating to a description of the system in terms of anomalous diffusion and fractal geometry. Rather than explicitly model these contributions, it is possible to summarize them using a fewer number of parameters.

In the stretched exponential representation, the monoexponential equation is modified by using a distributed diffusion coefficient (*DDC*), and the exponent itself is raised to the index α:

$$S_b = S_0 \cdot \exp(-(b \cdot DDC)^{\alpha}) \qquad [4]$$

This results in a single diffusion-coefficient *DDC*, which represents a summary of the distribution position, and α is a heterogeneity index, which represents the spread.[17] This representation therefore explicitly acknowledges the non-Gaussian nature of the curve, but conceives the system as a collection of Gaussian terms in a specific form, albeit not necessarily modeled on tissue itself, resulting in only one extra variable. Where the index α is 1, the signal curve is exponential; increasing α increases the deviation from monoexponential decay with both faster and slower diffusion features (Fig. 8.3).

Non-Gaussianity in Time: Diffusion Time Dependence

Another expression of non-Gaussian diffusion is a dependence on the observation time ("diffusion time") of the observed apparent diffusion (i.e., time-dependent diffusion). Different scenarios of water transport are conveyed by corresponding terminology, either alone or in combination. Water molecules trapped inside an impermeable cell are *restricted*, whereas those in an interstitial space are *hindered* but not ultimately limited in transport. As the total amount of diffusing time increases, molecules encountering different barrier types will be limited in displacement, and non-Gaussian effects are thus visible in the ensemble average that can be exploited for image contrast (Fig. 8.4). A practical corollary is that stating the b value is not sufficient to fully describe the experiment; the diffusion time should be provided as well. For a typical in vivo spin-echo-based diffusion-weighted MR acquisition, the diffusion time is in the

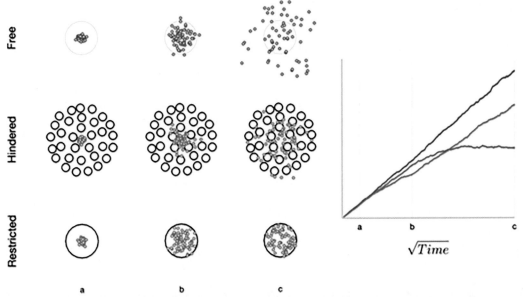

Fig. 8.4 Illustration of 2D diffusion in free *(top row)*, hindered *(middle row)*, and restricted *(bottom row)* systems. The overall average displacement at progressive timepoints (a, b, and C) show equal initial free diffusion, with hindered diffusion soon showing slower exploration. Restricted diffusion appears free, until the increasing diffusion time reflects the boundaries of the restricted molecules.

order of tens of milliseconds; for water molecules at 37°C with free diffusion coefficient of 3.0 mm²/s, the expected diffusion distance r (in 3 dimensions) after time t can be estimated from $\langle r^2 \rangle = 6Dt$. Using $t = 20$ ms, the mean expected displacement is on the order of 25 μm and thus significantly larger than typical cell diameter. We are therefore operating in the regime where apparent coefficients are sensitive to diffusion time.

COMBINED DESCRIPTIONS

The final class of representations to be considered is those that incorporate multiple contrast features (low and high b value non-Gaussianity, diffusion time, relaxation weighting) in the same analysis for a more comprehensive treatment. One example is termed non-Gaussian IVIM (NG-IVIM), which includes sampling at low (<200 s/mm²), intermediate (200–1000 s/mm²), and high (>1000 s/mm²) to measure both IVIM and kurtosis effects in the same acquisition (sampling the full behavior depicted in Fig. 8.1). This approach has been shown to deliver useful biomarkers from

both regimes and removes the bias of one on the other in curve-fitting analysis.[18–20]

Restriction spectrum imaging (RSI) is a multi-compartment tissue model that accounts for a broad range of diffusion contrast such as b value, direction, diffusion time, which has been also explored in the case of breast cancer, employing two or three components representing vascular, hindered, and restricted compartments (see Chapter 9 for more details).[15,21] The vascular, extracellular, and restricted diffusion for cytometry in tumors (VERDICT) model of diffusion also includes three components, and attempts to capture information about restricted versus hindered and pseudodiffusion by deliberately varying diffusion duration Δ, diffusion time δ, and echo time TE.[22] VERDICT has not yet been applied to breast cancer but contains many relevant aspects to its characterization that may be explored in the future. Although such acquisition strategies and corresponding analyses are not mainstream, they nevertheless illustrate the need for and potential value of full descriptions of acquisition parameters.

Clinical Application of IVIM and Non-Gaussian DWI

IVIM Differentiation of Malignant and Benign Tumors

Tumor angiogenesis and cellular proliferation are important processes in breast cancer growth and metastasis.[23] In terms of clinical application, the IVIM approach can separately reflect tissue diffusivity and tissue microcapillary perfusion in tissues without the need for contrast agents, with the advantage especially for patients contraindicated for contrast agents. Example IVIM signal decays from patients with breast lesions are shown in Fig. 8.5.[24]

Many studies have reported the utility of IVIM for differentiating malignant from benign breast tumors, with higher f values in malignant compared with benign breast tumors. IVIM or combination of IVIM and non-Gaussian DWI parameters were reported to improve diagnostic accuracy over ADC alone,[25] and the approach of combining parameters of IVIM, or IVIM and non-Gaussian (NG)–DWI to improve diagnostic accuracy, has been also explored.[18,26–28]

Many of these studies are illustrated in Fig. 8.6, and a formal meta-analysis by Liang and colleagues[25] summarized their collective implications as follows. In an analysis of 16 studies encompassing 1717 lesions, the diagnostic performance of IVIM and ADC parameters was considered in distinguishing benign from malignant lesions in terms of area under the curve (AUC), finding 0.85, 0.91, 0.85, and 0.81 for *ADC, D, f,* and *D**, respectively. Thus the individual diagnostic performance of f or D met or exceeded that of

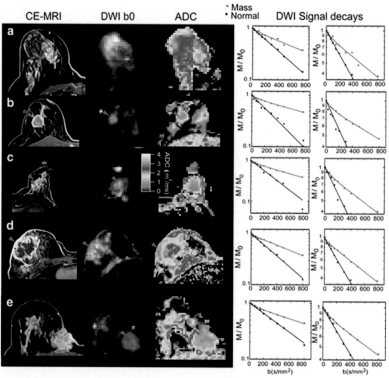

Fig. 8.5 (a) DCIS lesion and (b–e) IDC lesions. From left to right: postcontrast T1 images showing lesion location *(red arrowheads);* DWI unweighted (b0) images in which lesion is also hyperintense; ADC map showing lower values in lesions than in FG tissue; DWI signal intensity profiles on a logarithmic scale from the lesion area and normal tissue. The enlarged scale view highlights the nonexponential response (i.e., nonlinear on logarithmic scale) of the lesion tissue in comparison with the monoexponential behavior of FG tissue. *ADC,* Apparent diffusion coefficient; *DCIS,* ductal carcinoma in situ; *DWI,* diffusion-weighted imaging; *FG,* fibroglandular; *IDC,* invasive ductal carcinoma. M is a bicompartmental model defined by four parameters: total magnetization M_0, perfusion fraction f, pseudo-diffusivity D*, and tissue diffusivity D. (Reprinted with permission from Sigmund EE, Cho GY, Kim S, et al. Intravoxel incoherent motion imaging of tumor microenvironment in locally advanced breast cancer. *Magn Reson Med.* 2011;65(5):1437–1447.)

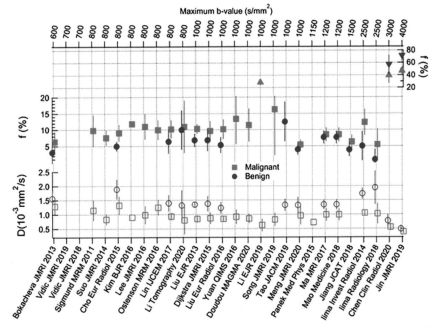

Fig. 8.6 Literature survey of two breast cancer IVIM metrics (IVIM tissue diffusivity *D* and perfusion fraction, *f*) listed in order of the maximum *b* value sampled. Right axis of the upper panel applies to values shown in triangle symbols. *IVIM*, Intravoxel incoherent motion.

ADC. Furthermore, the pooled analysis also showed IVIM parameters differentiated lesion histological subtype, grade, ER/PR/HER2/Ki-67 expression levels, and lymph node status, whereas ADC only differentiated histological subtype. This combined analysis, which incorporated studies with variable technical protocols, highlights the broad potential utility of IVIM. Detailed findings of individual studies are discussed further later.

IVIM Tumor Characterization: Subtypes, Molecular Prognostic Factors

Many IVIM studies have investigated the relationship between IVIM parameters and the hormone receptor status, HER2, and Ki-67 expression levels or molecular subtypes (luminal A, luminal B, HER2-positive, triple negative) of breast cancer.[18,26,28–32] The IVIM parameters showing significant associations with the molecular prognostic factors or subtypes are shown in Table 8.1.

A small number of studies reported that *D** decreased with ER positive or PR positive tumors[31,33] and correlated with HER2 status.[25] In one study, IVIM histogram analysis revealed that *f* and *D** histogram parameters and their histogram metrics differed depending on

ER or PR expression status.[3] In contrast, many other papers have reported no significant differences of *D** across molecular prognostic factors or subtypes.

The association between *ADC, D,* or *f* and ER or PR expression was also reported.[25] Furthermore, some studies showed that higher *f* values were found in HER2-positive compared with HER2-negative cancers, and a lower *D* value was shown in tumors with high Ki-67 expression compared with low Ki-67 expression.[25] Several IVIM parameters were found to be significantly linked to different tumor subtypes.[25] Luminal B cancers were found to have significantly lower *D* and *ADC* values compared with other tumor subtypes.[31,32] Although a number of IVIM studies have shown promising association with prognostic factors for breast cancer, they are still sporadic compared with *ADC* in part due to a lower number of published studies. Further investigation is required to validate these results.

IVIM Within Multiparametric Breast MRI

The current standard method for assessing breast lesions in MRI is morphological and semiquantitative kinetic assessments using DCE MRI, which provides

TABLE 8.1   Summary of IVIM Parameters According to Molecular Prognostic Factors and Subtypes

Investigator	Study Design	Year	Patients (n)	Field Strength	b values (s/mm²)	ER	PR	HER2	Ki-67	Molecular Subtype
IVIM and non-Gaussian DWI models										
Vidić et al.[28]	Prospective	2018	51	3T	0, 10, 20, 30, 40, 50, 70, 90, 120, 150, 200, 400, 700	n/a	n/a	See subtype	n/a	Combined model distinguished ER+ HER2− from ER+ HER2+ with high accuracy (0.90)
Zhao et al.[33]	Retrospective	2018	119	3T	0, 50, 100, 150, 200, 400, 500, 1000, 1500	$D^*\downarrow$	$D^*\downarrow$			Fraction of $D^*\downarrow$ in luminal B (HER2−) D^*; fraction of $D^*\uparrow$; $D\downarrow$ in triple negative
Suo et al.[30]	Retrospective	2017	101	3T	0, 10, 30, 50, 100, 150, 200, 500, 800, 1000, 1500, 2000, 2500	D, f, DDC, MD↓	–	–	$D^*\uparrow$, $\alpha\downarrow$	
Lee et al.[29]	Retrospective	2017	72	3T	0, 25, 50, 75, 100, 150, 200, 300, 500,800	D 50%, 75%, 90% skewness↓, ADC 50%, mean, 75%, 90% skewness↓-	ADC 75%↓	D skewness↓	f skewness↑	Luminal < HER2-positive (D 75th percentile, ADC 50%, ADC mean); luminal < triple negative < HER2-positive (ADC 75%, ADC 90%) Difference in subtypes (D skewness)
Kawashima et al.[32]	Retrospective	2017	134	3T	0, 20, 40, 80, 120, 200, 400, 600, 800	–	–	–	–	D and ADC lower;
Kim et al.[31]	Prospective	2016	275	3T	0, 30, 70,100, 150, 200, 300, 400, 500, 800	$D^*\downarrow$	$D^*\downarrow$, ADC↓,	–	$D\downarrow$	Luminal A > other subtypes (D); Luminal A < other subtypes (D^*); luminal B (HER2−) < other subtypes (ADC); HER2-positive > other subtypes (D^*)

Study	Type	Year	No.	Field	b-Values	Benign vs. Malignant	Subtypes
Cho et al.[26]	Retrospective	2016	50	3T	0, 30, 70, 100, 150, 200, 300, 400, 500, 800	$ADC_{max}\downarrow$, $D_{max}\downarrow$, DSD$\downarrow$, D^* kurtosis$\downarrow$, D^* skewness$\downarrow$	$ADC_{min}\uparrow$, $D_{min}\uparrow$, DSD, $D^*_{max}\downarrow$, D^* skewness$\downarrow$, D^* kurtosis$\downarrow$, f skewness$\downarrow$

See subtypes — f skewness$\downarrow$

ER+ HER2− > other subtypes (D^* average); ER+ HER2− < other subtypes (D^* skewness, D^* kurtosis); ER+ HER2+ < other subtypes (ADC kurtosis); ER+ HER2+ > other subtypes (D skewness, D^* kurtosis); triple negative > other subtypes (D_{max})

↑, statistically higher; ↓, statistically lower; –, no statistical significance; n/a, not applicable.
α, Anomalous exponent; ADC, apparent diffusion coefficient; D, true diffusion (or slow) coefficient; D^*, pseudodiffusion (or fast) coefficient; DDC, distributed diffusion coefficient; ER, estrogen receptor; f, perfusion fraction; IVIM, intravoxel incoherent motion; max, maximum; MD, mean diffusivity; min, minimum; PR, progesterone receptor; sADC, synthetic ADC; DSD, D standard deviation.

excellent sensitivity and variable specificity.[34,35] Multiparametric approaches combined with IVIM can add more functional and quantitative parameters to DCE MRI and overcome the limitations of specificity.[36,37]

Wang and colleagues showed a high AUC of 0.99 in differentiating malignant from benign breast lesions using combined D value and time intensity curve (TIC) from DCE MRI among 31 malignant and 23 benign mass breast lesions.[38] Ma and colleagues found improved sensitivity and accuracy when combining IVIM with DCE MRI (85.11% and 87.50%, respectively) over those of DCE MRI alone (70.21% and 82.81%, respectively) in discriminating 81 malignant from 37 benign breast lesions.[39] Dijkstra and colleagues found that among BI-RADS 3 or 4 breast lesions, combined IVIM and DCE MRI achieved significantly higher specificity than DCE MRI alone (56.5% and 30.4%, respectively; $P = .016$) and concluded that adding IVIM could be a problem solver for BI-RADS 3 and 4 lesions.[40] Li and colleagues found that the combination of IVIM derived D, D^*, and f values with DCE MRI–derived perfusion parameters (volume transfer constant, K_{trans}; reverse volume transfer constant, K_{ep}; extravascular extracellular space volume per unit volume of tissue, V_e; and water efflux rate constant, K_{io}) resulted in the improved diagnostic accuracy with AUCs of 0.92–0.93 and specificity of 86% to 93% over DCE MRI markers alone (AUC of 0.88 and specificity of 71%) among 14 malignant and 14 benign lesions.[41] Jiang and colleagues found the combination of f and D^* to have equal discriminating power between malignant and benign breast lesions to the combination of perfusion parameters derived from DCE MRI including K_{trans}, K_{ep}, and V_e among 31 malignant and 35 benign breast lesions (AUCs of 0.834 and 0.904, respectively), but the combined IVIM + DCE MRI AUC was 0.930, which was not significantly different from perfusion parameters alone.[42] Tao and colleagues found that in terms of discriminating ductal carcinoma in situ (DCIS) from benign breast lesions, incorporation of D value improved the diagnostic efficacy of perfusion parameters from DCE MRI and yielded an AUC of 0.976 among 25 DCIS and 22 benign breast lesions.[43]

The multiparametric approach also allows combination of IVIM to other DWI-related parameters, which could be the alternative to DCE MRI in patients who have contraindications for contrast agents. Vidić and colleagues showed improved diagnostic performance for discriminating malignant from benign breast lesions of multiparametric methods, including IVIM over ADC alone with a support vector machine.[28] A multiparametric approach combining IVIM and non-Gaussian DWI is reported to have a comparable diagnostic performance to BI-RADS assessment using DCE MRI.[18] In this study, the sensitivity and specificity of the multiparametric approach using combined threshold or Bayesian analysis ranged between 92.1% and 96.1% and between 66.7% and 88.3%, respectively, comparable to those for BI-RADS (100% sensitivity and 79.2% specificity).

Several studies have investigated the correlation between IVIM and DCE MRI parameters. Some correlation between perfusion measures from the two techniques is intuitively expected, most directly between IVIM perfusion fraction f and DCE-based blood volume v_p (if included in the DCE model employed). Less directly, DCE-based transfer constant K_{trans} includes effects of total blood flow (analogous to the product fD^*) but also to vascular permeability, which is not included in the intravascular IVIM flow picture. Liu and colleagues found that IVIM-derived f value has a moderate correlation with blood volume fraction (V_p; $r = 0.692$) and K_{trans} ($r = 0.456$) in 36 malignant and 23 benign breast lesions.[44] Song and colleagues found a weak but positive correlation between f value and the proportion of delayed persistent enhancement ($r = 0.227$) in 85 invasive breast cancers.[45] On the other hand, some found no correlation between IVIM and DCE MRI parameters.[41,42] Correlations between IVIM parameters and histological microvessel density have been reported in abdominal organs of mice,[46] colorectal cancer, gastric cancer, hepatocellular carcinoma of mouse models,[47–49] brain tumors in rat models,[50] and human pancreatic tumors,[51] rectal cancer,[52] and meningioma,[53] though no correlation was found in a chemically induced rat model of mammary carcinoma.[54]

Multimodality use of IVIM in 18-fluorodeoxyglucose positron-emission tomography/MRI (FDG-PET/MRI) has also been investigated. Ostenson and colleagues found that the correlation coefficient of the standardized uptake value (SUV) and D differs between pre- and postchemotherapy status of breast cancer and correlated positively with ER and HER2/neu expression levels. The correlation coefficient of SUV and f value correlated positively with lesion size.[55] Comprehensive physiological characterization of breast tumors by acquisition of IVIM in FDG-PET/MRI may be valuable in classifying breast cancer or assessing treatment response without the use of contrast agents.

Predicting Breast Cancer Treatment Response With IVIM

Neoadjuvant chemotherapy (NAC) is becoming the standard treatment for locally advanced breast cancer. How to optimize the therapeutic effects of NAC for individual patients is under discussion, where MRI is expected to play a key role in monitoring or predicting treatment response. IVIM is considered as a promising alternative to contrast-enhanced MRI in measuring tumor vascularity and also to measure changes in tumor cellularity with treatment. The investigation of IVIM as a predictive marker of treatment response, however, is limited to studies with relatively small sample sizes, different outcome measures, and partially conflicting results.[56–58] The initial study by Che and colleagues[56] evaluated the value of IVIM-derived parameters in predicting the pathological complete response (pCR) of 36 patients (including 26 luminal B subtypes). The f value obtained from MRI before treatment was significantly higher for the pCR group versus the non-pCR group. Based on MRI after the second cycle of NAC, the D value was significantly higher and the f value was significantly lower for the pCR group than the non-pCR group. When pre- and early treatment data were compared, the change in D demonstrated the best predictive performance (AUC 0.924) for pCR. No significant difference in D^* was observed. On the other hand, another study by Cho et.al. predicting response evaluation criteria in solid tumors (RECIST) response based on pretreatment MRI of 32 lesions (including 20 luminal subtypes) showed that skewness and kurtosis of D^* (pseudodiffusion) were significantly lower among responders, and average of D^* was significantly lower among responders compared with nonresponders.[57] They found no significant difference in tissue diffusivity D. A more recent study by Kim and colleagues examined the diagnostic performance of IVIM in predicting response to NAC

(good responders defined as Miller-Payne grading system 4 and 5) among 46 patients staged as II or III, using MRI before and after two cycles of NAC.[58] Their study employed histogram analysis to capture the whole tumor. On pretreatment, MRI, mean, 50th percentile, and 75th percentile values of D were significantly higher for good responders compared with minor responders. After two cycles of NAC, mean, 25th, 50th, and 75th percentiles of D, as well as mean and 50th percentile of ADC, were significantly higher for good responders compared with minor responders. In addition, skewness of ADC and D became lower among good responders. Shift of whole-tumor D value distribution from left-sided (lower D values) to right-sided (higher D values) seemed to be the indicator of good response. These preliminary results indicate the potential of IVIM-derived parameters, yet more evidence is needed to clarify which parameters (f, D, or D^*) are useful to identify good responders.

IVIM-derived parameters can also be applied to help treatment in metastatic breast cancer. In patients undergoing radiation therapy for bone metastases, one study investigated DWI, IVIM, and DCE MRI parameters as potential valuable imaging markers of metastatic tumor response.[59] In this study, both diffusion metrics (ADC, D, D^*) and semiquantitative perfusion metrics showed significant variation over the pre- and posttreatment examinations but did not show significantly different response between metastases (such as responders vs. nonresponders). In breast cancer patients with liver metastases who underwent radioembolization, the IVIM-derived f value from posttreatment MRI was useful in response assessment and associated with overall survival.[60,61]

IVIM in Lactation

Evaluation of lactating patients with breast cancer is often challenging because of the diffuse and marked background parenchymal enhancement. MRI may have a role in managing these patients, although investigation of DWI for lactating patients remains limited. IVIM is still in the research realm; however, it might also play a role in this context.

Milk production from each breast is variable according to the period of lactation, and the DWI and IVIM parameters might be sensitive to those physiological changes. It is reported that breastfeeding has considerable effect on the IVIM and non-Gaussian diffusion parameters in lactating women. f values in FGT significantly increased after breastfeeding (1.97 vs. 2.97%, $P < .01$)[62] (Fig. 8.7). As breastfeeding itself stimulates the milk production, this IVIM change might reflect increased milk flow in dilated ducts. At the group level, D (ADC_0) and synthetic ADC ($sADC$; see later) significantly decreased, and kurtosis K increased postbreastfeeding compared with prebreastfeeding. The mechanisms of these changes are still under investigation. The observations of parameter changes together with their spatial patterns in the breast suggests a strong role of milk composition (e.g., fat, water, protein), but concomitant changes in the ductal microstructure cannot be ruled out.

Non-Gaussian DWI Biomarkers for Malignancy Determination

Differentiation of malignant and benign tumors on non-Gaussian DWI has been also increasingly investigated. Examples of typical IVIM and non-Gaussian DWI maps for malignant and benign breast tumors are shown in Fig. 8.8.

A recent meta-analysis, by Li and colleagues reviewed 13 studies using diffusion kurtosis imaging for differentiation of malignant versus benign breast tumors and considered the added benefit of the additional parameters over a simple two b value ADC when reported in the same study.[63] The considered studies varied to some degree but all contained a DWI

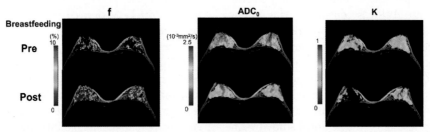

Fig. 8.7 Increase in f and K (kurtosis), and decrease in ADC_0 (diffusivity from kurtosis model) values can be observed post- compared with pre-breastfeeding. *ADC*, Apparent diffusion coefficient. (Reprinted with permission from Iima M, Kataoka M, Sakaguchi R, et al. Intravoxel incoherent motion [IVIM] and non-Gaussian diffusion MRI of the lactating breast. *Eur J Radiol Open.* 2018;5:24–30.)

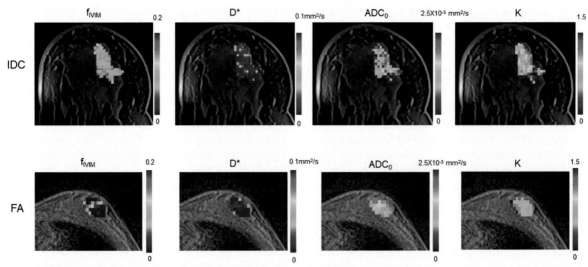

Fig. 8.8 f, D*, ADC_0, and K (kurtosis) maps of an invasive ductal carcinoma *(upper row)* and benign fibroadenoma *(lower row)*. The invasive ductal carcinoma exhibits relatively high f, low D and high K, whereas a low f/high D/low K combination is shown in the fibroadenoma.

acquisition with multiple b values (median 6; range 3–13) over an extended range (median b_{max} 2500; range 1300–3000 s/mm^2). The overall pooled result showed higher sensitivity, specificity, and receiver operating characteristic (ROC) AUC for both kurtosis fitting parameters mean kurtosis MK (0.90, 0.88, 0.90) and mean diffusivity MD (0.86, 0.88, 0.93) than for ADC (0.85, 0.83, 0.89). MK is increased in malignant lesions, whereas MD and ADC are decreased. Nevertheless, the analysis concluded that kurtosis parameters are "not overwhelmingly superior" to the more conventional DWI metric ADC. It should be noted, though, that several of the studies within the meta-analysis[64–67] and elsewhere[33,68] reported MK as the best-performing metric, which suggests that there is additional value coming explicitly from the collection of b values above 1000 s/mm^2. Additionally, Liu showed that stretched exponential DDC performed marginally better than ADC for differentiation (AUC 0.931 vs. 0.893), with α also performing reasonably well.[69] This latter approach used histogram analysis rather than simple summary statistics, and this is a general alternative approach that has also shown promise generally for lesion analysis in DWI[65,66,70] and that can be applied retrospectively.

Time-Dependent Diffusion in Breast Cancer

The effect of diffusion time has been demonstrated for breast FGT,[71] breast tumors,[71,72] and breast cancer xenografts.[20] At long diffusion times with stimulated echo sequences, time-dependent diffusion tensor imaging (DTI) DTI revealed sensitivity to large-scale structures in FGT consistent with lactiferous ducts.[71] Conversely, at short diffusion times (several ms) using oscillating gradient spin echo (OGSE) sequences,[20,72] cancerous lesions displayed significant time-dependent diffusion consistent with the microscopic scale of cellularity. These pilot studies suggest that diffusion time variation will be an increasingly used source of contrast in breast tissue and breast lesions in the future.

Ancillary Clinical Benefits of Advanced DWI in the Breast

Much of the research using DWI in breast cancer, as described here, focuses on differentiation of the lesions in terms of malignancy and, where possible, subtype[73,74,31] and expression of molecular markers (e.g., HER2, ER, and PR) and Ki-67.[70,28] In general, the choice of disease management depends most heavily on results from needle biopsy of the lesion and histological characterization, and it is here that extended diffusion measurements and associated non-Gaussian modeling are most likely to add benefit. Conventionally, the lesion is identified and defined using contrast-enhanced MRI, but there is also a possibility to use DWI to define the lesion directly[15] or to give tailored contrast for better lesion visualization.[75,76] This would reduce or remove the need for administration of gadolinium-based contrast agents, which would avoid complications from allergy, contraindications regarding impaired kidney function, and cumulative deposition, as well as additional cost for large-scale deployment. Successful and meaningful noninvasive characterization of the tumor at presentation, or from referral after conventional screening, has strong potential to considerably reduce the need for biopsy; a study by Rahbar and colleagues showed that reclassification of suspicious MR findings using ADC can avoid approximately 20% of biopsies.[77]

Image Acquisition Schemes for Breast DWI

Clinical DWI is currently performed using MRI scanners with 1.5 T or 3 T field strength. Typically, body coils are used to transmit radiofrequency (RF) pulses, and 8-channel or 16-channel dedicated breast RF coils receive the resulting emitted signal. Breast IVIM acquisition is not yet standardized, and thus a variety of b values and DWI techniques at different field strengths have been reported (some examples in Table 8.2; see also meta-analyses by Baxter[78] and Liang[25]). In terms of field strength, the majority of breast IVIM studies have been performed at 3 T versus 1.5 T. Although evidence is still accruing, studies including breast phantom data,[79] individual clinical DWI studies,[80,81] or breast DWI meta-analyses[78] have generally found minimal impact of field strength on diagnostic performance of breast DWI. Breast IVIM at 7 T may have a role in future clinical applications; however, MRI scanners with 7 T field strength are not yet widely available for clinical use.

TABLE 8.2   Intravoxel Incoherent Motion (IVIM) Acquisition Parameters

Paper	Year	Technique	Field Strength (Vendor)	Breast Coil	b values (s/mm²)	Slice Thickness (mm)	Sequence Time (min)	IVIM Analysis
Bokacheva et al.[27]	2014	Single-shot dual spin-echo EPI	3.0T (GE)	8-/16-channel	0, 30, 60, 90, 120, 400, 600, 800, 1000	5	5–6	Whole-lesion ROI
Chen et al.[82]	2017	EPI based	3.0T (Siemens)	16-channel	0, 50, 100, 150, 200, 300, 400, 800, 1000	6.5	5–6	Whole-lesion ROI/pixel-by-pixel maps
Cho et al.[26]	2016	Twice-refocused bipolar gradient single-shot TSE	3.0T (Siemens)	7-element	0, 30, 70, 100, 150, 200, 300, 400, 500, 800	4	8	Whole-lesion ROI/pixel-by-pixel maps/histogram analysis
Jiang et al.[42]	2018	Single-shot spin-echo EPI	3.0T (GE)	8-channel	0, 10, 30, 50, 70, 100, 150, 200, 400, 600, 1000, 1500	3	7–8	Whole-lesion ROI
Iima et al.[18]	2018	Single-shot EPI	3.0T (Siemens)	16-channel	5, 10, 20, 30, 50, 70, 100, 200, 400, 600, 800, 1000, 1500, 2000, 2500	3	4	Whole-lesion ROI/pixel-by-pixel maps
Lin et al.[83]	2017	Single-shot spin-echo EPI	3.0T (Philips)	4-channel	0, 50, 100, 150, 200, 500, 800	4	3:22	Whole-lesion ROI/pixel-by-pixel maps
Liu et al.[44]	2016	Single-shot spin-echo EPI	1.5T (Philips)	4-channel	0, 10, 20, 30, 50, 70, 100, 150, 200, 400, 600, 1000	5	~4	Whole-lesion ROI/pixel-by-pixel maps
Ma et al.[39]	2017	Single-shot spin-echo EPI	3.0T (Siemens)	4-channel	0, 50, 100, 150, 200, 250, 300, 400, 600, 800, 1000, 1200	5	NS	Whole-lesion ROI
Wang et al.[38]	2016	Single-shot spin-echo EPI	3.0T (GE)	8-channel	0, 10, 20, 50, 100, 200, 300, 400, 600, 800	6	~4	Whole-lesion ROI/pixel-by-pixel maps
Zhao et al.[33]	2018	Single-shot dual spin-echo EPI	3.0T (GE)	8-channel	0, 50, 100, 150, 200, 400, 500, 1000, 1500	NS	NS	Whole-lesion ROI/pixel-by-pixel maps
Kim et al.[31]	2016	Single-shot spin-echo EPI	3.0T (Philips)	Surface coil	0, 30, 70, 100, 150, 200, 300, 400, 500, 800	3	~4	Whole-lesion ROI
Lee et al.[29]	2017	Single shot spin-echo EPI	3.0T (Siemens)	Surface coil	0, 25, 50, 75, 100, 150, 200, 300, 500, 800	4	4	Whole-lesion histo-gram maps
Dijkstra et al.[84]	2016	Single-shot spin-echo EPI	1.5T (Siemens)	Circularly polarized phased-array coil	0, 50, 200, 500, 800, 1000	4	2.5	Whole-lesion ROI/pixel-by-pixel maps
Meng et al.[85]	2020	Single-shot spin-echo EPI	3T (GE)		0, 50, 75, 100, 150, 200, 400, 800, 1000	4	2–3	Whole-lesion ROI/pixel-by-pixel maps

EPI, Echo-planar imaging; *IVIM*, intravoxel incoherent motion; *NS*, not specified; *ROI*, region of interest.

Typically, DWI is performed without contrast, using single-shot diffusion weighted imaging (ss-DWI) and echo-planar imaging (EPI) readout, which is available on scanners from all major vendors; after DWI, routine DCE MRI is performed. Although meta-analyses[86] have indicated a minimal impact of contrast administration on breast DWI diagnostic performance, the IVIM technique is sensitized toward the vascular compartment and thus would be dramatically affected by the high relaxivity blood pool agent.

The EPI technique is used to achieve very fast image acquisition in order to minimize the effects of subject motion and to retain a high signal-to-noise ratio (SNR).[87] As EPI is a 2D imaging technique, volumes are acquired slice by slice with repetition times (TR) being set sufficiently long to both minimize T1 contrast and accommodate the whole volume of interest. Multiband approaches such as simultaneous multislice (SMS) acquisition have been used[88,89] to accelerate this dimension, as in other organs.[90–92] Because it employs EPI readout, ss-DWI lacks high spatial resolution and is sensitive to patient motion and magnetic field inhomogeneities, which leads to imaging artifacts (e.g., distortion, ghosting, aliasing), often preventing adequate delineation of small lesions. Readout-segmented EPI (rs-EPI) alters the conventional EPI trajectory by acquiring all phase encodes but restricting the readout acquisition in each shot as a means of limiting susceptibility artifacts.[93–95] Reduced field-of-view (rFOV) DWI captures a smaller subvolume to limit EPI echo train length and associated artifacts, providing high-resolution DWI in the breast.[96,97] Multishot (ms-) DWI EPI techniques offer higher spatial resolution but are susceptible to motion-induced phase errors because each individual shot may have suffered different slight coherent motions from pulsation, respiration, and so forth. Without correction, this results in ghosting artifacts, pixel misregistration, and low image resolution with poor diffusion contrast in the reconstructed images,[98] resulting in inaccurate measurements. Techniques such as interleaved-echo planar imaging[99] or periodically rotated overlapping parallel lines with enhanced reconstruction (PROPELLER)[100] have been introduced to reduce geometrical distortion in ms-DWI; however, they require prolonged scan times that limit their clinical applicability.[101] High resolution sequences using gradient double-echo steady-state (DESS) have also been proposed for breast lesion detection with fewer artifacts and reduced distortion relative to ss-DWI.[102,103] Recently, the multishot multiplexed sensitivity-encoding (MUSE) DWI has been proposed to amend motion-induced phase errors.[104] MUSE-DWI integrates a sensitivity-encoding (SENSE)[105] parallel imaging method and achieves a better SNR given its improved matrix inversion conditioning. MUSE splits the single-shot echo planar time. The MUSE k-space trajectory is generated by starting with the k-space pattern needed for an accelerated ss-DWI undersampled in the phase-encoding direction. The pattern is then successively shifted along the phase-encoding direction for subsequent shots. Reconstruction of this data is performed using phase maps that are estimated for each shot using a parallel imaging reconstruction method. Both the acquisition time and reconstruction time will increase with more shots; however, two shots appears reasonable for clinical diagnosis.[106] Multiple reconstruction methods are being proposed to accelerate multishot DWI data reconstruction including shot locally low-rank (shot-LLR)[107] and recently using deep learning.[108] (See Chapter 12 for more description of advanced DWI acquisition techniques.)

Data Analysis of IVIM and Non-Gaussian DWI

ANALYSIS OF IVIM DATA

The biexponential IVIM model is a well-known mathematical treatment of two-compartment systems[109] with broad applicability in the sciences. As IVIM applications continue to be explored, a detailed exploration of its challenges has also emerged, particularly regarding cases when one of two compartments in an IVIM model is a small fraction of the total, as in IVIM microcirculation or the perfusion fraction. In breast cancer, IVIM applications have grown rapidly,[10,110,111] and a number of efforts have also been made regarding protocol optimization, error minimization, and algorithm development. Some aspects of these efforts parallel that of multiexponential analysis that emerged prior to IVIM, whereas others are unique to analytic tools of the moment (e.g., machine learning). It is worthwhile to examine the range of optimization methods and algorithms for breast cancer IVIM, including the most common and robust trends, areas warranting improvement, and technologies with the highest potential for the future.

The multiexponential fitting problem is a notorious ill-conditioned nonlinear problem for IVIM. Many fitting algorithms have emerged that describe the data equally well, where the fitting algorithm converges on a "local minimum" in the residual function that may not be biologically meaningful. In some cases, however, this manifests as high spatial variability, poor reproducibility, and high image noise. The algorithm that is most prone to these errors is conventional, unconstrained, nonlinear least-squares fitting.

A common approach to limiting variability is to derive the biomarkers in a multistep process rather than simultaneously. In multistep or segmented fitting (also referred to as curve-stripping), a b value threshold (see later) is adopted above where the pseudodiffusion compartment signal is assumed to be negligible. The first step fits the remaining slow diffusion compartment above that b value to a single exponential form, which has less noise amplification than a fit to the full function. The decay rate is the slow diffusivity D. The intercept, along with measured full signal S_0, provides the perfusion fraction f. These values are then constrained (or at least used as first input) in a second fit to all b values to determine the pseudodiffusion coefficient D^*. This multistep approach typically leads to higher precision and less random error, particularly for D and f estimation, albeit at the possible expense of accuracy or systematic error if the b value threshold is not chosen judiciously.[82,112,113]

Other approaches employ computational tools to limit random noise in IVIM biomarkers. Some methods leverage prior knowledge of the system and of image noise. Conventionally, individual voxels within a region of interest would be fitted independently in parallel, and so the result from one voxel has no interaction with the result from any other. It is reasonable to assume, however, that voxels within the same tissue would tend to have similar values, and also to assume that neighboring voxels are more likely to be similar than different. This kind of information can be built into more sophisticated fitting algorithms, in particular Bayesian methods, leading to a set of techniques able to return parameter values and maps that appear smoother and can potentially be more powerful in application.[62,114–117] The Bayesian estimation approach[113,118–120,116] and related approaches (e.g., fusion bootstrap moves [FBM])[121,122] confront the ill-conditioned problem by estimating probability distributions rather than rather than single values of output parameters. This reduces variability in the reported biomarkers (e.g., mean, median, mode of distributions) and provides estimates of their precision (e.g., standard deviations). Furthermore, the prior parameter distributions required to initiate the fit may include spatial characteristics that guide the solver to produce more smoothly varying maps in lieu of high random variability. Spatial priors should be chosen carefully to avoid oversmoothing or masking of features, particularly if heterogeneity parameters are reported. For summary metrics of tumor imaging, spatial priors can often serve as appropriate means of reducing variability. Some examples are:

Bayesian shrinkage prior. The algorithm uses iteration through a Markov chain Monte Carlo framework to continually update the fitted parameter values across the whole region of interest using a prior expectation of a Gaussian distribution of fitted values.[119,118]

Local spatial prior. Iterated "fusion moves" update the fitted parameter values based on an expectation of local spatial similarity, which can be specified in the algorithm.[121,118]

Principal component analysis (PCA). This analysis is independent of analysis of the signal itself, and uses PCA to isolate noise into a lower-rank principal component, which can be omitted from a reconstruction to give a denoised image.[123]

Bayesian approaches have demonstrated advantages in simulation studies[113] and in in vivo breast cancer imaging studies.[118] In one study, diagnostic accuracy was highest when all IVIM parameters were included and Bayesian estimation versus least-squares or segmented fitting was performed.[118] Example images of breast lesion DWI parametric mapping with Bayesian approaches are shown in Fig. 8.9.

One challenge of IVIM fitting is the need to minimize error propagation across a wide range of parameter space, which could involve complex nonanalytic functional forms where intuitive strategies do not always apply. In this context, artificial intelligence approaches to IVIM may be helpful. In one study, autoencoder deep neural network architecture was used to

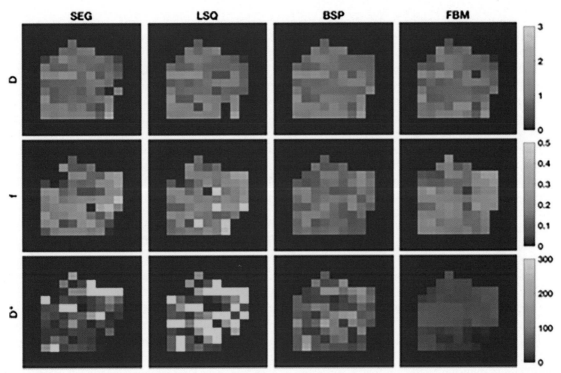

Fig. 8.9 Different fitting algorithms, including *(left to right)* segmented (SEG), least-squares (LSQ), Bayesian shrinkage prior (BSP), and fusion bootstrap moves (FBM), use the data in different ways to give more informative IVIM parameter maps, especially for pseudodiffusion parameters. Units are: diffusion coefficient *D (top)*, μm²/ms; pseudodiffusion fraction *f (middle)*, no units; pseudodiffusion coefficient *D* (bottom)*, μm²/ms. *IVIM*, Intravoxel incoherent motion. (Adapted with permission from Vidić I, Jerome NP, Bathen TF, Goa PE, While PT. Accuracy of breast cancer lesion classification using intravoxel incoherent motion diffusion-weighted imaging is improved by the inclusion of global or local prior knowledge with Bayesian methods. *J Magn Reson Imaging.* 2019;50(5):1478–1488.)

compute IVIM biomarkers from abdominal imaging.[124] In another study,[125] a combined IVIM and kurtosis model was fitted by using neural network architecture. In these and other studies, the neural network generally reduced random error and group cross-validation metrics and resulted in improved precision compared with least-squares or segmented approaches. However, the design and training of neural networks are highly dependent on the imaging protocol (*b* values) and the SNR. Artificial intelligence approaches are an active area of research and will likely be integral to breast cancer IVIM models in the future. In addition, machine learning techniques allows the use of "learned" knowledge from larger training data sets to be incorporated into decision-making (e.g., in classification or prediction of response)[126,127,28] and the fitting process.[124] In these cases, the analysis may be performed on derived metrics or directly on the images themselves without specific diffusion modeling.

Alternative parameter search algorithms including hyperspectral analysis,[128] particle swarm optimization,[129] and phasor transform[130] have been explored to meet the challenges of IVIM fitting, including in breast cancer. These algorithms hold promise but are not as far along the translational path as conventional least-squares or segmented least-squares approaches, which enjoy widespread adoption and commercial implementation.

Regardless of what fitting algorithm is chosen, the primary protocol element to ensure robust IVIM analysis is the set of diffusion weightings (*b* values). Accordingly, this has been the subject of many optimization studies, including several that are focused on breast cancer.[82,131–134] The key aspects of *b* value sampling include sufficient sampling of a low *b* value and a high *b* value to measure both microcirculation and microstructure parameters; judicious choosing of the *b* value threshold for multistep fitting; and judicious limiting of the *b* value range to be consistent with the IVIM model, in which both compartments are described by Gaussian diffusion (albeit elevated or hindered). The four IVIM parameters (S_0, f, D, D^*) imply that at least four *b* values need to be sampled, including *b* = 0. Basic numerical theory suggests that these *b* values should also include those near the inverses of the target diffusivities (1/*D* and 1/*D**), such that *b* = ~800 s/mm^2 and *b* = ~100 s/mm^2 should be present, along with an intermediate *b* value (200–300 s/mm^2). In practice, the sampling of 8 to 10 *b* values is typically done, with considerable emphasis on the low *b* value regime if *f* or *D** quantification is of particular interest. Focused sampling of key *b* values or at least nonuniform sampling has been repeatedly suggested in multiple optimization studies[41,112,131,133,134] that may lead to standardized protocols for larger-scale translation. Most breast cancer IVIM studies employing multistep fitting use threshold *b* values between 200 and 300 s/mm^2; one systematic study favored 300 s/mm^2.[82]

Finally, the upper limit of *b* values should be judiciously chosen. Although very high *b* values have a raw sensitivity to diffusion restriction that is enticing, their use should not conflict with the assumptions of the IVIM model. If non-Gaussian effects of microstructural complexity/kurtosis are sampled at high *b* values (>1000 s/mm^2), they can be accommodated in an expanded hybrid model, but otherwise they should not be confused with IVIM interpretation. To illustrate this, Fig. 8.6 shows a summary of tissue diffusivity *D* and perfusion fraction *f* across 28 clinical breast cancer studies,[18,19,24,27,29,31,39,41–45,55,83,85,118,135,26,28] including malignant and benign lesions, in order of the increasing maximum *b* value sampled. Although some consistency is observed across studies, some trends are visible; for example, lower *D* values and higher *f* values are reported for higher maximum *b* values. This is particularly evident for ultra-high *b* values (3000–4000 s/mm^2), where nonphysical perfusion fractions with reversed benign/malignant order appear, suggesting that particular caution should be taken in sampling beyond a model's range of applicability.

An encouraging aspect for the future of breast cancer IVIM is that its evidence base has been built using various platforms. Of 28 breast cancer IVIM studies from 2011 to 2020, 14 were analyzed with MRI vendor software,[14,29,31,38,42,44,45,56,83,135–138,85] three were analyzed with a commercial software package,[39,43,139] and the remaining studies were analyzed with custom code.[18,19,24,27,41,55,57,58,84,118,140–144,26,32,28] The fact that much of the footprint of breast cancer IVIM occurred with publicly available or commercial tools is a positive sign for its eventual widespread application. However, it is also evident from the variability in the literature that a concerted effort is warranted to standardize breast cancer IVIM and limit such variability if the next level of evidence is to be reached and to justify the inclusion of IVIM in larger clinical trials.

MODEL FITTING OF NON-GAUSSIAN DWI: TECHNICAL CONSIDERATIONS

The most common method for mathematical model fitting is a least-squares approach, minimizing the residual values between the recorded data and the curve described by the fitted variables. Even with simple fitting routines, there are several workflow options that need to be borne in mind.

Initialization. Where the cost function of a set of variables may have local minima, good initial values for the fitting process should result in more consistent answers. For non-Gaussian representations, this may involve initializing with a Gaussian model. Random and repeated initialization of the parameter space is much more computationally expensive but characterizes the space more fully and ensures finding any global minimum.

Covariance. A covariant relationship between two or more parameters may indicate that they are not orthogonal, meaning that the parameters are not independent and may both reflect some of the same characteristics. This does not invalidate the result but may indicate a nonoptimal representation.

Fixed values. With more variables, fixing one or more to a known or arbitrary value may make the fitting more stable, although inaccuracy in the fixed value will necessarily be accommodated by changes in the solution for the fitted variables.[145] Sequential fitting, such as the segmented fitting approach for IVIM, may be appropriate for certain representations.

Constrained values. For certain models, physiology dictates valid ranges for certain parameters, which can be imposed on the fitting process. DWI data is often noisy, particularly at a voxel level, and so it can legitimately give values outside these ranges; imposing limits without flagging that the limit has been hit has the potential to introduce bias into the estimate. Examining the occurrence of these flags, or fitting without limits and examining nonphysiological values, tells the researcher something about the quality of the data and its ability to support the model (including the suitability of the chosen model).[146]

Fitting algorithm. Different fitting algorithms operate in different ways, and this also should not be overlooked.[147,148] In addition, algorithm options that are normally hidden, such as limits on fitting iterations and stopping criteria, should be considered. If a Bayesian approach is chosen, the prior should be chosen carefully and consistently with the desired resolution.

NOISE HANDLING

One of the most significant features of acquisitions that intend to use a non-Gaussian representation, such

as described earlier, is their higher maximum b value. In these images, the signal is attenuated to the point that consideration of noise becomes a critical part of analysis. Through the reconstruction of magnitude images from complex k-space data, the noise in DWI images can be considered Rician in nature and thus has a finite, positive expectation value. The increased net dephasing at higher b values means the signal can approach this "noise floor," and thus noise can be incorrectly modeled as true signal and introduce bias to derived DWI metrics (Fig. 8.10). Correct handling of noise is challenging and requires knowledge of the noise floor value. Careful attention must therefore be paid to the SNR in the region of interest (ROI), which is also dependent on the tissue type, signal averaging, and voxel size in the acquisition. Above a suitable SNR threshold (~5–10), noise may be considered Gaussian in nature and does not need an explicit

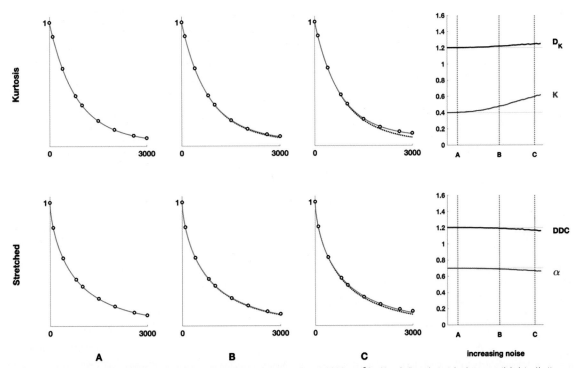

Fig. 8.10 Effect of noise on DWI-derived metrics. Synthetic DKI (*top row;* $D = 0.0012$ mm²/s, $K = 0.4$) and stretched exponential data (*bottom row;* $DDC = 0.0012$ mm²/s, $\alpha = 0.7$), with fitted curves (*colors*) and underlying true curve (*black dashed curve*). Y-axis is signal, X-axis is b value in s/mm². Increasing Rician noise contribution (subplots A–C) can affect fitted parameters from non-Gaussian representations, as shown in right-hand column (subplot locations shown by *dashed lines*, true values are *gray horizontal lines*). Scale on right-hand plots is 10^{-3} mm²/s for D and DDC, no units for K and α. Noise should be explicitly accounted for when fitting non-Gaussian representations to high-b value data. *DDC,* Distributed diffusion coefficient; *DKI,* diffusional kurtosis imaging; *DWI,* diffusion-weighted imaging.

noise correction. Several methods are available for accounting for the presence of noise, including correction[11,19,149,150] and removal[151] as well as appropriate design of acquisition protocol.

COMPARISON OF REPRESENTATION PERFORMANCE

Having acquired multiple *b* value DWI data, it is possible to perform retrospective analyses using a range of representations; comparison of the quality of fit can be indicative of suitability and therefore give insight to the microstructure of the system. Simplistically, smaller residuals from the fitted curve indicates a favored representation, although in the case of varying number of fitted parameters it is necessary to compare through an information criterion, such as the Akaike (AIC) or Bayesian (BIC). Such a comparison cannot

speak to the suitability of the model to the system, but it can indicate whether the use of that representation is supported by the information in the acquired data. In particular, high levels of noise will disfavor more complicated models (Fig. 8.11).

This complexity has been borne out in prospective clinical studies as well. Suo and colleagues[30] and Vidić and colleagues[11] compared various representations of non-Gaussian DWI in breast lesions (monoexponential, biexponential, kurtosis, and stretched exponential), with indeterminate results. Both numerical criteria (e.g., AIC/BIC) and clinical criteria (e.g., AUC for benign/malignant differentiation) were found to vary between models, lesion types, and even sublesion regions with no universally preferred model. This behavior underscores the fact that although

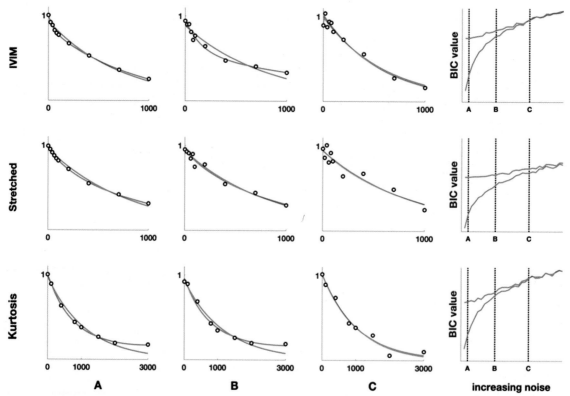

Fig. 8.11 Increasingly noisy data (increasing A–C) favors representations with fewer parameters, as indicated by lower BIC values. *(Top row)* Synthetic IVIM data ($f = 0.15$, $D = 0.0012$ mm²/s, $D^* = 0.022$ mm²/s). *(Middle row)* Synthetic stretched exponential data ($DDC = 0.0012$ mm²/s, $\alpha = 0.75$). *(Bottom row)* Synthetic DKI data ($D = 0.0012$ mm²/s, $K = 0.87$). *Blue curve* is the "correct" non-Gaussian representation, *red* is single exponential, both fitted to the synthetic data points. *(Right column)* Lower BIC values show that the non-Gaussian representation is clearly favored at low noise (A), but at increasingly higher noise (B and C) this distinction disappears, because the data no longer supports the more complex representation. *BIC*, Bayesian information criterion; *DKI*, diffusional kurtosis imaging; *IVIM*, intravoxel incoherent motion.

higher-order treatments like non-Gaussian DWI do reveal more tissue features and associated clinical specificity, the choice of "correct" representation may not be universal for all applications.

"DIRECT" (MODEL-FREE, NONFITTING) APPROACHES

There exist some approaches investigated without model or fitting in the traditional sense. Direct estimation of IVIM and NGD parameters from limited sets of b values has been introduced in Fig. 8.10. One approach includes the sADC, which is calculated using b value combinations of 200 and 1500 s/mm^2 for better diagnostic performance of distinguishing between malignant and benign tumors.[152] The other approach is the signature index, also a model-free method, which allows direct differentiation of tissue types while shortening acquisition and processing times.[152,153] This signature index is calculated from the resemblance of the diffusion MRI signal profile of a tissue in vivo to a database or library of "signature" signal profiles acquired in advance. sADC and signature index were reported to be biomarkers to differentiate molecular prognostic markers, such as PR expression.[18,153] Combination of the signature index with BI-RADS scores yielded higher specificity than BI-RADS alone (94.7% vs. 60.5%) and a high sensitivity.[153] On the other hand, there are some drawbacks, which require a sufficient database of prior examinations to establish the "library," which should be as broad in disease types and morphological characteristics. They need separate "training" for each clinical task of interest.

Relative enhanced diffusivity (RED) is also known as a nonfitting method related to IVIM using a minimal acquisition of three b values; it was found to be correlated with signal enhancement ratio from DCE MRI and linearly proportional to the IVIM parameter f.[154]

Balancing Biophysical Complexity and Practical Clinical Benefit

In this chapter, we have reviewed many examples of the clinical potential of IVIM and non-Gaussian DWI approaches for such clinical tasks as diagnosing malignancy, prognostic factor classification, and treatment response prediction. In many cases, these applications benefit from a more complete description of the signal behavior and its biophysical origins (microstructure, cellularity, vascularity). As supported by the meta-analyses reviewed here, this potential goes beyond exploratory single site studies and suggests these biomarkers can be deployed broadly and with high impact. However, to achieve this goal, attention must be paid to practical issues of translation (added diagnostic value, scan time optimization and reproducibility) that ensure reliable use.

Conventional DWI and the simple ADC model— despite its oversimplicity in representing the tissue— perform well in many tasks, with a meta-analysis by Surov and colleagues[155] of 123 studies showing a robust and clear separation of malignant and benign lesions (and giving a proposed threshold of $<1.00 \times 10^{-3}$ mm^2/s as an indicator of malignancy). The number of pooled analyses available for IVIM and non-Gaussian DWI is not as high, making comparisons nonideal. At the global level, the analyses of Liang and colleagues for IVIM[25] and Li and colleagues for DKI[63] show clear benefits of advanced diffusion MRI over ADC for some clinical tasks, but more complexities exist at a more granular level. Some studies looking at DKI either fail to outperform ADC[62,30,156] or are similar enough that the extension of the scanning protocol is not clearly justified.[63] Some similar reports have shown the same for the fractional order calculus, statistical, and stretched exponential approaches,[11,69,157] or in a number of IVIM studies, where D (essentially a perfusion-insensitive ADC) is sometimes the best-performing parameter.[1] Given the current state of evidence, the 2020 consensus and mission statement from the EUSOBI International Breast Diffusion-Weighted Imaging working group concludes that currently "there is no reliable evidence regarding the clinical value superiority of advanced DWI techniques over standard *ADC* assessment."[158]

In addition to sensitivity and specificity, the repeatability of potential biomarkers is crucial when considering clinical adoption. ADC is known to be remarkably robust despite representing complex combinations of diffusion phenomena in a single value,[159] and this remains to be shown at the same level for advanced diffusion metrics. A brief review of repeatability in IVIM metrics in the selected studies where it was evaluated[1] showed that pseudodiffusion parameters (f and D^*) were much less repeatable than D, and this has also been shown specifically for one cohort of benign breast lesions,[146] with stretched exponential parameters performing better for a b value range below 1000 s/mm². Studies by Iima and colleagues[160] and Kuai and colleagues[161] show that DKI and stretched exponential parameters have acceptable variability and repeatability, which is encouraging and reasonable when considering parameters reflecting signal changes over wider diffusion-weighting ranges. The importance of repeatability has been recognized as crucial to wide scale translation and clinical adoption of MRI biomarkers by multiple international consortia (e.g., Quantitative Imaging Network [QIN], Quantitative Imaging Biomarkers Alliance [QIBA]), and the aforementioned studies thus provide key input into this process (see also Chapter 14). Despite demonstrated single-site diagnostic/prognostic potential, it may be that wider-scale deployment of non-Gaussian methods cannot rely solely on conventional analysis methods without context-driven constraints or noise-conscious heterogeneity mapping (e.g., Bayesian fitting). Continuing efforts should take this current state of evidence into maximal account, and multisite studies should continue to emphasize practical translation of non-Gaussian DWI biomarkers.

Although the additional scientific insight from IVIM and non-Gaussian DWI seems to be agreed upon in the context of research, the future role of such acquisitions in clinical breast cancer management is not yet resolved. The accumulated evidence needs to be verified with larger patient cohorts and multicenter studies. Although there remain many divergent approaches in terms of acquisition and analysis choices, generalizability of acquisitions to future, pooled, and retrospective analyses will benefit. This suggests the inclusion of a detailed recording and reporting of all acquisition parameters, including those that may not be routine, such as diffusion time and duration (Δ and δ). The power of strategies such as machine learning that use the richness of large data sets and are not confined to individual representations[162,163,28] may be able to overcome much of interstudy and intersite protocol variation. In any case, the DWI community should recognize the responsibility and opportunity to move toward standardized and fully reported protocols, including

finding consensus on the role and benefits of extended acquisitions for acquisition and interrogation of IVIM and non-Gaussian diffusion in the breast.

In summary, evidence has continued to accrue on the diagnostic utility of IVIM biomarkers in breast lesions, their dependence (or lack thereof) on acquisition parameters, and their translation amid different processing tools. A variety of imaging readouts have also been brought to bear for breast DWI that may amplify the performance of breast IVIM even further. Guided by successes in large scale translation of breast DWI, IVIM biomarkers have great potential to amplify clinical management of breast lesions both in the diagnostic and prognostic settings.

REFERENCES

1. Orton MR, Jerome NP, Rata M, Koh D-M. IVIM in the body: a general overview. In: Le Bihan D, Iima M, Federau C, et al, eds. *Intravoxel Incoherent Motion (IVIM) MRI: Principles and Applications*. Pan Stanford Publishing; 2018:145–174.
2. Koh D-M, Collins DJ, Orton MR. Intravoxel incoherent motion in body diffusion-weighted MRI: reality and challenges. *Am J Roentgenol*. 2011;196(6):1351–1361.
3. Maki JH, Macfall JR, Johnson GA. The use of gradient flow compensation to separate diffusion and microcirculatory flow in MRI. *Magn Reson Med*. 1991;17(1):95–107.
4. Ahlgren A, Knutsson L, Wirestam R, et al. Quantification of microcirculatory parameters by joint analysis of flow-compensated and non-flow-compensated intravoxel incoherent motion (IVIM) data. *NMR Biomed*. 2016;29(5):640–649.
5. Wetscherek A, Stieltjes B, Laun FB. Flow-compensated intravoxel incoherent motion diffusion imaging. *Magn Reson Med*. 2015;74(2):410–419.
6. Moulin K, Aliotta E, Ennis DB. Effect of flow-encoding strength on intravoxel incoherent motion in the liver. *Magn Reson Med*. 2019;81(3):1521–1533.
7. Jensen JH, Helpern JA, Ramani A, Lu H, Kaczynski K. Diffusional kurtosis imaging: the quantification of non-Gaussian water diffusion by means of magnetic resonance imaging. *Magn Reson Med*. 2005;53(6):1432–1440.
8. Rosenkrantz AB, Padhani AR, Chenevert TL, et al. Body diffusion kurtosis imaging: basic principles, applications, and considerations for clinical practice. *J Magn Reson Imaging*. 2015;42(5):1190–1202.
9. Jensen JH, Helpern JA. MRI quantification of non-Gaussian water diffusion by kurtosis analysis. *NMR Biomed*. 2010;23(7):698–710.
10. Egnell L, Vidić I, Jerome NP, Bofin AM, Bathen TF, Goa PE. Stromal collagen content in breast tumors correlates with in vivo diffusion-weighted imaging: a comparison of multi b value DWI with histologic specimen from benign and malignant breast lesions. *J Magn Reson Imaging*. 2020;51:1868–1878.
11. Vidić I, Egnell L, Jerome NP, et al. Modeling the diffusion-weighted imaging signal for breast lesions in the b = 200 to 3000 s/mm² range: quality of fit and classification accuracy for different representations. *Magn Reson Med*. 2020;84(2):1011–1023.

12. Pfeuffer J, Provencher SW, Gruetter R. Water diffusion in rat brain in vivo as detected at very large b values is multicompartmental. *MAGMA*. 1999;8(2):98–108.

13. Chevallier O, Wang YXJ, Guillen K, Pellegrinelli J, Cercueil J-P, Loffroy R. Evidence of tri-exponential decay for liver intravoxel incoherent motion MRI: a review of published results and limitations. *Diagnostics*. 2021;11:379.

14. Chevallier O, Zhou N, Cercueil JP, He J, Loffroy R, Wáng YXJ. Comparison of tri-exponential decay versus bi-exponential decay and full fitting versus segmented fitting for modeling liver intravoxel incoherent motion diffusion MRI. *NMR Biomed*. 2019;32(11):e4155.

15. Andreassen MMS, Rodríguez-Soto AE, Conlin CC, et al. Discrimination of breast cancer from healthy breast tissue using a three-component diffusion-weighted MRI model. *Clin Cancer Res*. 2021;27(4):1094–1105.

16. Baalen SV, Leemans A, Dik P, Lilien MR, Haken BT, Froeling M. Intravoxel incoherent motion modeling in the kidneys: comparison of mono-, bi-, and triexponential fit. *J Magn Reson Imaging*. 2017;46(1):228–239.

17. Bennett KM, Schmainda KM, Bennett RT, Rowe DB, Lu H, Hyde JS. Characterization of continuously distributed cortical water diffusion rates with a stretched-exponential model. *Magn Reson Med*. 2003;50(4):727–734.

18. Iima M, Kataoka M, Kanao S, et al. Intravoxel incoherent motion and quantitative non-gaussian diffusion MR imaging: evaluation of the diagnostic and prognostic value of several markers of malignant and benign breast lesions. *Radiology*. 2018;287(2):432–441.

19. Iima M, Yano K, Kataoka M, et al. Quantitative non-Gaussian diffusion and intravoxel incoherent motion magnetic resonance imaging: differentiation of malignant and benign breast lesions. *Invest Radiol*. 2015;50(4):205–211.

20. Iima M, Nobashi T, Imai H, et al. Effects of diffusion time on non-Gaussian diffusion and intravoxel incoherent motion (IVIM) MRI parameters in breast cancer and hepatocellular carcinoma xenograft models. *Acta Radiol Open*. 2018;7(1):1–8.

21. Rodríguez-Soto AE, Andreassen MMS, Conlin CC, et al. Characterization of the Diffusion Signal of Breast Tissues using Multi-exponential Models. *Magn Reson Med*. 2022;87(4):1938–1951.

22. Panagiotaki E, Chan RW, Dikaios N, et al. Microstructural characterization of normal and malignant human prostate tissue with vascular, extracellular, and restricted diffusion for cytometry in tumours magnetic resonance imaging. *Invest Radiol*. 2015;50(4):218–227.

23. Folkman J. Tumor angiogenesis: therapeutic implications. *N Engl J Med*. 1971;285(21):1182–1186.

24. Sigmund EE, Cho GY, Kim S, et al. Intravoxel incoherent motion imaging of tumor microenvironment in locally advanced breast cancer. *Magn Reson Med*. 2011;65(5):1437–1447.

25. Liang J, Zeng S, Li Z, et al. Intravoxel incoherent motion diffusion-weighted imaging for quantitative differentiation of breast tumors: a meta-analysis. *Front Oncol*. 2020;10:585486.

26. Cho GY, Moy L, Kim SG, et al. Evaluation of breast cancer using intravoxel incoherent motion (IVIM) histogram analysis: comparison with malignant status, histological subtype, and molecular prognostic factors. *Eur Radiol*. 2016;26(8):2547–2558.

27. Bokacheva L, Kaplan JB, Giri DD, et al. Intravoxel incoherent motion diffusion-weighted MRI at 3.0 T differentiates malignant breast lesions from benign lesions and breast parenchyma. *J Magn Reson Imaging*. 2014;40(4):813–823.

28. Vidić I, Egnell L, Jerome NP, et al. Support vector machine for breast cancer classification using diffusion-weighted MRI histogram features: preliminary study. *J Magn Reson Imaging*. 2018;47(5):1205–1216.

29. Lee YJ, Kim SH, Kang BJ, et al. Intravoxel incoherent motion (IVIM)–derived parameters in diffusion-weighted MRI: associations with prognostic factors in invasive ductal carcinoma. *J Magn Reson Imaging*. 2017;45(5):1394–1406.

30. Suo S, Cheng F, Cao M, et al. Multiparametric diffusion-weighted imaging in breast lesions: association with pathologic diagnosis and prognostic factors. *J Magn Reson Imaging*. 2017;46(3):740–750.

31. Kim Y, Ko K, Kim D, et al. Intravoxel incoherent motion diffusion-weighted MR imaging of breast cancer: association with histopathological features and subtypes. *Br J Radiol*. 2016;89(1063):20160140.

32. Kawashima H, Miyati T, Ohno N, et al. Differentiation between luminal-A and luminal-B breast cancer using intravoxel incoherent motion and dynamic contrast-enhanced magnetic resonance imaging. *Acad Radiol*. 2017;24(12):1575–1581.

33. Zhao M, Fu K, Zhang L, et al. Intravoxel incoherent motion magnetic resonance imaging for breast cancer: a comparison with benign lesions and evaluation of heterogeneity in different tumor regions with prognostic factors and molecular classification. *Oncol Lett*. 2018;16(4):5100–5112.

34. Leithner D, Wengert GJ, Helbich TH, et al. Clinical role of breast MRI now and going forward. *Clin Radiol*. 2018;73(8):700–714.

35. Morrow M, Waters J, Morris E. MRI for breast cancer screening, diagnosis, and treatment. *Lancet*. 2011;378(9805):1804–1811.

36. Pinker K, Helbich TH, Morris EA. The potential of multiparametric MRI of the breast. *Br J Radiol*. 2016;90(1069):20160715.

37. Marino MA, Helbich T, Baltzer P, Pinker-Domenig K, Multiparametric MRI of the breast: a review. *J Magn Reson Imaging*. 2018;47(2):301–315.

38. Wang Q, Guo Y, Zhang J, Wang Z, Huang M, Zhang Y. Contribution of IVIM to conventional dynamic contrast-enhanced and diffusion-weighted MRI in differentiating benign from malignant breast masses. *Breast Care (Basel)*. 2016;11(4):254–258.

39. Ma D, Lu F, Zou X, et al. Intravoxel incoherent motion diffusion-weighted imaging as an adjunct to dynamic contrast-enhanced MRI to improve accuracy of the differential diagnosis of benign and malignant breast lesions. *Magn Reson Imaging*. 2017;36:175–179.

40. Dijkstra H, Dorrius MD, Wielema M, Pijnappel RM, Oudkerk M, Sijens PE. Quantitative DWI implemented after DCE-MRI yields increased specificity for BI-RADS 3 and 4 breast lesions. *J Magn Reson Imaging*. 2016;44(6):1642–1649.

41. Li K, Machireddy A, Tudorica A, et al. Discrimination of malignant and benign breast lesions using quantitative multiparametric MRI: a preliminary study. *Tomography*. 2020;6(2):148–159.

42. Jiang L, Lu X, Hua B, Gao J, Zheng D, Zhou Y. Intravoxel incoherent motion diffusion-weighted imaging versus dynamic contrast-enhanced magnetic resonance imaging: comparison of the diagnostic performance of perfusion-related parameters in breast. *J Comput Assist Tomogr*. 2018;42(1):6–11.

43. Tao WJ, Zhang HX, Zhang LM, et al. Combined application of pharmacokinetic DCE-MRI and IVIM-DWI could improve detection efficiency in early diagnosis of ductal carcinoma in situ. *J Appl Clin Med Phys*. 2019;20(7):142–150.

44. Liu C, Wang K, Chan Q, et al. Intravoxel incoherent motion MR imaging for breast lesions: comparison and correlation with pharmacokinetic evaluation from dynamic contrast-enhanced MR imaging. *Eur Radiol.* 2016;26(11):3888–3898.

45. Song SE, Cho KR, Seo BK, et al. Intravoxel incoherent motion diffusion-weighted MRI of invasive breast cancer: correlation with prognostic factors and kinetic features acquired with computer-aided diagnosis. *J Magn Reson Imaging.* 2019;49(1):118–130.

46. Eberhardt C, Wurnig MC, Wirsching A, et al. Intravoxel incoherent motion analysis of abdominal organs: computation of reference parameters in a large cohort of C57Bl/6 mice and correlation to microvessel density. *MAGMA.* 2016;29(5):751–763.

47. Lee HJ, Rha SY, Chung YE, et al. Tumor perfusion-related parameter of diffusion-weighted magnetic resonance imaging: correlation with histological microvessel density. *Magn Reson Med.* 2014;71(4):1554–1558.

48. Song XL, Kang HK, Jeong GW, et al. Intravoxel incoherent motion diffusion-weighted imaging for monitoring chemotherapeutic efficacy in gastric cancer. *World J Gastroenterol.* 2016;22(24):5520–5531.

49. Lee Y, Lee SS, Cheong H, et al. Intravoxel incoherent motion MRI for monitoring the therapeutic response of hepatocellular carcinoma to sorafenib treatment in mouse xenograft tumor models. *Acta Radiol.* 2017;58(9):1045–1053.

50. Iima M, Reynaud O, Tsurugizawa T, et al. Characterization of glioma microcirculation and tissue features using intravoxel incoherent motion magnetic resonance imaging in a rat brain model. *Invest Radiol.* 2014;49(7):485–490.

51. Klau M, Mayer P, Bergmann F, et al. Correlation of histological vessel characteristics and diffusion-weighted imaging intravoxel incoherent motion-derived parameters in pancreatic ductal adenocarcinomas and pancreatic neuroendocrine tumors. *Invest Radiol.* 2015;50(11):792–797.

52. Surov A, Meyer HJ, Hohn AK, et al. Correlations between intravoxel incoherent motion (IVIM) parameters and histological findings in rectal cancer: preliminary results. *Oncotarget.* 2017;8(13):21974–21983.

53. Togao O, Hiwatashi A, Yamashita K, et al. Measurement of the perfusion fraction in brain tumors with intravoxel incoherent motion MR imaging: validation with histopathological vascular density in meningiomas. *Br J Radiol.* 2018;91(1085):20170912.

54. Jerome NP, Boult JK, Orton MR, et al. Characterisation of fibrosis in chemically-induced rat mammary carcinomas using multi-modal endogenous contrast MRI on a 1.5 T clinical platform. *Eur Radiol.* 2018;28(4):1642–1653.

55. Ostenson J, Pujara AC, Mikheev A, et al. Voxelwise analysis of simultaneously acquired and spatially correlated (18) F-fluorodeoxyglucose (FDG)-PET and intravoxel incoherent motion metrics in breast cancer. *Magn Reson Med.* 2017;78(3):1147–1156.

56. Che S, Zhao X, Ou Y, et al. Role of the intravoxel incoherent motion diffusion weighted imaging in the pre-treatment prediction and early response monitoring to neoadjuvant chemotherapy in locally advanced breast cancer. *Medicine (Baltimore).* 2016;95(4):e2420.

57. Cho GY, Gennaro L, Sutton EJ, et al. Intravoxel incoherent motion (IVIM) histogram biomarkers for prediction of neoadjuvant treatment response in breast cancer patients. *Eur J Radiol Open.* 2017;4:101–107.

58. Kim Y, Kim SH, Lee HW, et al. Intravoxel incoherent motion diffusion-weighted MRI for predicting response to

59. Gaeta M, Benedetto C, Minutoli F, et al. Use of diffusion-weighted, intravoxel incoherent motion, and dynamic contrast-enhanced MR imaging in the assessment of response to radiotherapy of lytic bone metastases from breast cancer. *Acad Radiol.* 2014;21(10):1286–1293.

60. Pieper CC, Meyer C, Sprinkart AM, et al. The value of intravoxel incoherent motion model-based diffusion-weighted imaging for outcome prediction in resin-based radioembolization of breast cancer liver metastases. *Onco Targets Ther.* 2016;9:4089.

61. Pieper CC, Sprinkart AM, Meyer C, et al. Evaluation of a simplified intravoxel incoherent motion (IVIM) analysis of diffusion-weighted imaging for prediction of tumor size changes and imaging response in breast cancer liver metastases undergoing radioembolization: a retrospective single center analysis. *Medicine (Baltimore).* 2016;95(14).

62. Iima M, Kataoka M, Sakaguchi R, et al. Intravoxel incoherent motion (IVIM) and non-Gaussian diffusion MRI of the lactating breast. *Eur J Radiol Open.* 2018;5:24–30.

63. Li Z, Li X, Peng C, et al. The diagnostic performance of diffusion kurtosis imaging in the characterization of breast tumors: a meta-analysis. *Front Oncol.* 2020;10(October):1–14.

64. Sun K, Chen X, Chai W, et al. Breast cancer: diffusion kurtosis MR imaging-diagnostic accuracy and correlation with clinical-pathologic factors. *Radiology.* 2015;277(1):46–55.

65. Liu W, Wei C, Bai J, Gao X, Zhou L. Histogram analysis of diffusion kurtosis imaging in the differentiation of malignant from benign breast lesions. *Eur J Radiol.* 2019;117(June):156–163.

66. Li T, Hong Y, Kong D, Li K. Histogram analysis of diffusion kurtosis imaging based on whole-volume images of breast lesions. *J Magn Reson Imaging.* 2020;51(2):627–634.

67. Huang Y, Lin Y, Hu W, et al. Diffusion kurtosis at 3.0T as an in vivo imaging marker for breast cancer characterization: correlation with prognostic factors. *J Magn Reson Imaging.* 2019;49(3):845–856.

68. Meng N, Wang X, Sun J, et al. A comparative study of the value of amide proton transfer-weighted imaging and diffusion kurtosis imaging in the diagnosis and evaluation of breast cancer. *Eur Radiol.* 2021;31(3):1707–1717.

69. Liu C, Wang K, Li X, et al. Breast lesion characterization using whole-lesion histogram analysis with stretched-exponential diffusion model. *J Magn Reson Imaging.* 2018;47(6):1701–1710.

70. You C, Li J, Zhi W, et al. The volumetric-tumour histogram-based analysis of intravoxel incoherent motion and non-Gaussian diffusion MRI: association with prognostic factors in HER2-positive breast cancer. *J Transl Med.* 2019;17(1)182.

71. Teruel JR, Cho GY, Moccaldi Rt M, et al. Stimulated echo diffusion tensor imaging (STEAM-DTI) with varying diffusion times as a probe of breast tissue. *J Magn Reson Imaging.* 2017;45(1):84–93.

72. Iima M, Honda M, Sigmund EE, Ohno Kishimoto A, Kataoka M, Togashi K. Diffusion MRI of the breast: current status and future directions. *J Magn Reson Imaging.* 2020;52(1):70–90.

73. Horvat VJ, Bernard-Davila B, Helbich TH, et al. Diffusion-weighted imaging (DWI) with apparent diffusion coefficient (ADC) mapping as a quantitative imaging biomarker for prediction of immunohistochemical receptor status, proliferation rate, and molecular subtypes of breast cancer. *J Magn Reson Imaging.* 2019;50(3):836–846.

74. Xie T, Zhao Q, Fu C, et al. Differentiation of triple-negative breast cancer from other subtypes through whole-tumor

histogram analysis on multiparametric MR imaging. *Eur Radiol.* 2019;29(5):2535–2544.

75. Blackledge MD, Leach MO, Collins DJ, Koh D-M. Computed diffusion-weighted MR imaging may improve tumor detection. *Radiology.* 2011;261(2):573–581.

76. Cheng L, Blackledge MD, Collins DJ, et al. T2-adjusted computed diffusion-weighted imaging: a novel method to enhance tumour visualisation. *Comput Biol Med.* 2016;79(August):92–98.

77. Rahbar H, Zhang Z, Chenevert TL, et al. Utility of diffusion weighted imaging to decrease unnecessary biopsies prompted by breast MRI: a trial of the ECOG-ACRIN Cancer Research Group (A6702). *Clin Cancer Res.* 2019;25(6):1756–1765.

78. Baxter GC, Graves MJ, Gilbert FJ, Patterson AJ. A meta-analysis of the diagnostic performance of diffusion MRI for breast lesion characterization. *Radiology.* 2019;291(3):632–641.

79. Keenan KE, Peskin AP, Wilmes LJ, et al. Variability and bias assessment in breast ADC measurement across multiple systems. *J Magn Reson Imaging.* 2016;44(4):846–855.

80. Eghtedari M, Ma J, Fox P, Guvenc I, Yang WT, Dogan BE. Effects of magnetic field strength and b value on the sensitivity and specificity of quantitative breast diffusion-weighted MRI. *Quant Imaging Med Surg.* 2016;6(4):374–380.

81. Newitt DC, Zhang Z, Gibbs JE, et al. Test-retest repeatability and reproducibility of ADC measures by breast DWI: results from the ACRIN 6698 trial. *J Magn Reson Imaging.* 2019;49(6):1617–1628.

82. Chen W, Zhang J, Long D, Wang Z, Zhu JM. Optimization of intra-voxel incoherent motion measurement in diffusion-weighted imaging of breast cancer. *J Appl Clin Med Phys.* 2017;18(3):191–199.

83. Lin N, Chen JY, Hua J, Zhao JH, Zhao J, Lu JS. Intravoxel incoherent motion MR imaging in breast cancer: quantitative analysis for characterizing lesions. *Int J Clin Exp Med.* 2017;10(1):1705–1714.

84. Dijkstra H, Dorrius MD, Wielema M, et al. Semi-automated quantitative intravoxel incoherent motion analysis and its implementation in breast diffusion-weighted imaging. *J Magn Reson Imaging.* 2016;43(5):1122–1131.

85. Meng N, Wang XJ, Sun J, et al. Comparative study of amide proton transfer-weighted imaging and intravoxel incoherent motion imaging in breast cancer diagnosis and evaluation. *J Magn Reson Imaging.* 2020;52(4):1175–1186.

86. Dorrius MD, Dijkstra H, Oudkerk M, Sijens PE. Effect of b value and pre-admission of contrast on diagnostic accuracy of 1.5-T breast DWI: a systematic review and meta-analysis. *Eur Radiol.* 2014;24(11):2835–2847.

87. Partridge SC, Nissan N, Rahbar H, Kitsch AE, Sigmund EE. Diffusion-weighted breast MRI: clinical applications and emerging techniques. *J Magn Reson Imaging.* 2017;45(2):337–355.

88. Song SE, Woo OH, Cho KR, et al. Simultaneous multislice readout-segmented echo planar imaging for diffusion-weighted MRI in patients with invasive breast cancers. *J Magn Reson Imaging.* 2021;53(4):1108–1115.

89. Filli L, Ghafoor S, Kenkel D, et al. Simultaneous multi-slice readout-segmented echo planar imaging for accelerated diffusion-weighted imaging of the breast. *Eur J Radiol.* 2016;85(1):274–278.

90. Blaimer M, Choli M, Jakob PM, Griswold MA, Breuer FA. Multiband phase-constrained parallel MRI. *Magn Reson Med.* 2013;69(4):974–980.

91. Duan F, Zhao T, He Y, Shu N. Test-retest reliability of diffusion measures in cerebral white matter: a multiband diffusion MRI study. *J Magn Reson Imaging.* 2015;42(4):1106–1116.

92. Schmitter S, Adriany G, Waks M, et al. Bilateral multiband 4D flow MRI of the carotid arteries at 7T. *Magn Reson Med.* 2020;84(4):1947–1960.

93. Bogner W, Pinker-Domenig K, Bickel H, et al. Readout-segmented echo-planar imaging improves the diagnostic performance of diffusion-weighted MR breast examinations at 3.0 T. *Radiology.* 2012;263(1):64–76.

94. McKay JA, Church AL, Rubin N, et al. A comparison of methods for high-spatial-resolution diffusion-weighted imaging in breast MRI. *Radiology.* 2020;297(2):304–312.

95. Kishimoto AO, Kataoka M, Iima M, et al. Evaluation of malignant breast lesions using high-resolution readout-segmented diffusion-weighted echo-planar imaging: comparison with pathology. *Magn Reson Med Sci.* 2021;20(2):204–215.

96. Singer L, Wilmes LJ, Saritas EU, et al. High-resolution diffusion-weighted magnetic resonance imaging in patients with locally advanced breast cancer. *Acad Radiol.* 2012;19(5):526–534.

97. McLaughlin RL, Newitt DC, Wilmes LJ, et al. High resolution in vivo characterization of apparent diffusion coefficient at the tumor-stromal boundary of breast carcinomas: a pilot study to assess treatment response using proximity-dependent diffusion-weighted imaging. *J Magn Reson Imaging.* 2014;39(5):1308–1313.

98. Wu W, Miller KL. Image formation in diffusion MRI: a review of recent technical developments. *J Magn Reson Imaging.* 2017;46(3):646–662.

99. Madore B, Chiou JY, Chu R, Chao TC, Maier SE. Accelerated multi-shot diffusion imaging. *Magn Reson Med.* 2014;72(2):324–336.

100. Wang FN, Huang TY, Lin FH, et al. PROPELLER EPI: an MRI technique suitable for diffusion tensor imaging at high field strength with reduced geometric distortions. *Magn Reson Med.* 2005;54(5):1232–1240.

101. Li Z, Pipe JG, Lee CY, Debbins JP, Karis JP, Huo D. X-PROP: a fast and robust diffusion-weighted propeller technique. *Magn Reson Med.* 2011;66(2):341–347.

102. Daniel BL, Granlund KL, Moran CJ, et al. Breast MRI without gadolinium: utility of 3D DESS, a new 3D diffusion weighted gradient-echo sequence. *Eur J Radiol.* 2012;81(suppl 1):S24–26.

103. Granlund KL, Staroswiecki E, Alley MT, Daniel BL, Hargreaves BA. High-resolution, three-dimensional diffusion-weighted breast imaging using DESS. *Magn Reson Imaging.* 2014;32(4):330–341.

104. Chen NK, Guidon A, Chang HC, Song AW. A robust multi-shot scan strategy for high-resolution diffusion weighted MRI enabled by multiplexed sensitivity-encoding (MUSE). *Neuroimage.* 2013;72:41–47.

105. Pruessmann KP, Weiger M, Scheidegger MB, Boesiger P. SENSE: sensitivity encoding for fast MRI. *Magn Reson Med.* 1999;42(5):952–962.

106. Daimiel Naranjo I, Lo Gullo R, Morris EA, et al. High-spatial-resolution multishot multiplexed sensitivity-encoding diffusion-weighted imaging for improved quality of breast images and differentiation of breast lesions: a feasibility study. *Radiology: Imaging Cancer.* 2020;2(3):e190076.

107. Hu Y, Ikeda DM, Pittman SM, et al. Multishot diffusion-weighted MRI of the breast with multiplexed sensitivity encoding (MUSE) and shot locally low-rank (shot-LLR) reconstructions. *J Magn Reson Imaging.* 2021;53(3):807–817.

108. Hu Y, Xu Y, Tian Q, et al. RUN-UP: accelerated multishot diffusion-weighted MRI reconstruction using an unrolled network with U-Net as priors. *Magn Reson Med.* 2020;85(2):709–720.

109. Istratov AA, Vyvenko OF. Exponential analysis in physical phenomena. *Rev Sci Instrum.* 1999;70(2):1233–1257.

110. Bailey C, Siow B, Panagiotaki E, et al. Microstructural models for diffusion MRI in breast cancer and surrounding stroma: an ex vivo study. *NMR Biomed.* 2017;30(2):1–13.

111. Ma W, Mao J, Wang T, et al. Distinguishing between benign and malignant breast lesions using diffusion weighted imaging and intravoxel incoherent motion: A systematic review and meta-analysis. *Eur. J. Radiol.* 2021;141:109809.

112. Jalnefjord O, Montelius M, Starck G, Ljungberg M. Optimization of b value schemes for estimation of the diffusion coefficient and the perfusion fraction with segmented intravoxel incoherent motion model fitting. *Magn Reson Med.* 2019;82(4):1541–1552.

113. While PT. A comparative simulation study of bayesian fitting approaches to intravoxel incoherent motion modeling in diffusion-weighted MRI. *Magn Reson Med.* 2017; 78(6):2373–2387.

114. Jalnefjord O, Andersson M, Montelius M, et al. Comparison of methods for estimation of the intravoxel incoherent motion (IVIM) diffusion coefficient (D) and perfusion fraction (f). *MAGMA.* 2018;31(6):715–723.

115. Lanzarone E, Mastropietro A, Scalco E, Vidiri A, Rizzo G. A novel Bayesian approach with conditional autoregressive specification for intravoxel incoherent motion diffusion-weighted MRI. *NMR Biomed.* 2020;33(3):1–17.

116. Gustafsson O, Montelius M, Starck G, Ljungberg M. Impact of prior distributions and central tendency measures on Bayesian intravoxel incoherent motion model fitting. *Magn Reson Med.* 2018;79(3):1674–1683.

117. Gurney-Champion OJ, Klaassen R, Froeling M, et al. Comparison of six fit algorithms for the intravoxel incoherent motion model of diffusion weighted magnetic resonance imaging data of pancreatic cancer patients. *PLoS One.* 2018;13(4):1–18.

118. Vidić I, Jerome NP, Bathen TF, Goa PE, While PT. Accuracy of breast cancer lesion classification using intravoxel incoherent motion diffusion-weighted imaging is improved by the inclusion of global or local prior knowledge with Bayesian methods. *J Magn Reson Imaging.* 2019;50(5):1478–1488.

119. Orton MR, Collins DJ, Koh DM, Leach MO. Improved intravoxel incoherent motion analysis of diffusion weighted imaging by data driven Bayesian modeling. *Magn Reson Med.* 2014;71(1):411–420.

120. Neil JJ, Bretthorst GL. On the use of Bayesian probability theory for analysis of exponential decay data: an example taken from intravoxel incoherent motion experiments. *Magn Reson Med.* 1993;29(5):642–647.

121. Freiman M, Perez-Rossello JM, Callahan MJ, et al. Reliable estimation of incoherent motion parametric maps from diffusion-weighted MRI using fusion bootstrap moves. *Med Image Anal.* 2013;17(3):325–336.

122. Taimouri V, Afacan O, Perez-Rossello JM, et al. Spatially constrained incoherent motion method improves diffusion-weighted MRI signal decay analysis in the liver and spleen. *Med Phys.* 2015;42(4):1895–1903.

123. Gurney-Champion OJ, Collins DJ, Wetscherek A, et al. Principal component analysis for fast and model-free denoising of multi b value diffusion-weighted MR images. *Phys Med Biol.* 2019;64(10):105015.

124. Barbieri S, Gurney-Champion OJ, Klaassen R, Thoeny HC. Deep learning how to fit an intravoxel incoherent motion model to diffusion-weighted MRI. *Magn Reson Med.* 2020;83(1):312–321.

125. Bertleff M, Domsch S, Weingartner S, et al. Diffusion parameter mapping with the combined intravoxel incoherent motion and kurtosis model using artificial neural networks at 3 T. *NMR Biomed.* 2017;30(12).

126. Sutton EJ, Dashevsky BZ, Oh JH, et al. Breast cancer molecular subtype classifier that incorporates MRI features. *J Magn Reson Imaging.* 2016;44(1):122–129.

127. Nindrea RD, Aryandono T, Lazuardi L, Dwiprahasto I. Diagnostic accuracy of different machine learning algorithms for breast cancer risk calculation: a meta-analysis. *Asian Pac J Cancer Prev.* 2018;19(7):1747–1752.

128. Chan SW, Chang YC, Huang PW, et al. Breast tumor detection and classification using intravoxel incoherent motion hyperspectral imaging techniques. *Biomed Res Int.* 2019; 2019:3843295.

129. Ertas G. Fitting intravoxel incoherent motion model to diffusion MR signals of the human breast tissue using particle swarm optimization. *IJOCTA.* 2019;9(2):105–112.

130. van Rijssel MJ, Froeling M, van Lier A, Verhoeff JJC, Pluim JPW. Untangling the diffusion signal using the phasor transform. *NMR Biomed.* 2020;33(12):e4372.

131. Cho GY, Moy L, Zhang JL, et al. Comparison of fitting methods and b value sampling strategies for intravoxel incoherent motion in breast cancer. *Magn Reson Med.* 2015;74(4):1077–1085.

132. While PT, Teruel JR, Vidić I, Bathen TF, Goa PE. Relative enhanced diffusivity: noise sensitivity, protocol optimization, and the relation to intravoxel incoherent motion. *MAGMA.* 2018;31(3):425–438.

133. Zhang JL, Sigmund EE, Rusinek H, et al. Optimization of b value sampling for diffusion-weighted imaging of the kidney. *Magn Reson Med.* 2012;67(1):89–97.

134. Lemke A, Stieltjes B, Schad LR, Laun FB. Toward an optimal distribution of b values for intravoxel incoherent motion imaging. *Magn Reson Imaging.* 2011;29(6):766–776.

135. Jin YN, Zhang Y, Cheng JL, Zheng DD, Hu Y. mono-exponential, Biexponential, and stretched-exponential models using diffusion-weighted imaging: A quantitative differentiation of breast lesions at 3.0T. *J Magn Reson Imaging.* 2019;50(5):1461–1467.

136. Doudou NR, Liu Y, Kampo S, Zhang K, Dai Y, Wang S. Optimization of intravoxel incoherent motion (IVIM): variability of parameters measurements using a reduced distribution of b values for breast tumors analysis. *MAGMA.* 2020;33(2):273–281.

137. Chen BY, Xie Z, Nie P, et al. Multiple b value diffusion-weighted imaging in differentiating benign from malignant breast lesions: comparison of conventional mono-, bi- and stretched exponential models. *Clin Radiol.* 2020;75(8): 642.e1–642.e8.

138. Liu C, Liang C, Liu Z, Zhang S, Huang B. Intravoxel incoherent motion (IVIM) in evaluation of breast lesions: comparison with conventional DWI. *Eur J Radiol.* 2013;82(12):e782–e789.

139. Mao X, Zou X, Yu N, Jiang X, Du J. Quantitative evaluation of intravoxel incoherent motion diffusion-weighted imaging (IVIM) for differential diagnosis and grading prediction of benign and malignant breast lesions. *Medicine (Baltimore).* 2018;97(26):e11109.

140. Suo S, Lin N, Wang H, et al. Intravoxel incoherent motion diffusion-weighted MR imaging of breast cancer at 3.0 Tesla: comparison of different curve-fitting methods. *J Magn Reson Imaging.* 2015;42(2):362–370.

141. Yuan J, Wong OL, Lo GG, Chan HH, Wong TT, Cheung PS. Statistical assessment of bi-exponential diffusion weighted

imaging signal characteristics induced by intravoxel incoherent motion in malignant breast tumors. *Quant Imaging Med Surg.* 2016;6(4):418–429.

142. Panek R, Borri M, Orton M, et al. Evaluation of diffusion models in breast cancer. *Med Phys.* 2015;42(8):4833–4839.

143. Bedair R, Priest AN, Patterson AJ, et al. Assessment of early treatment response to neoadjuvant chemotherapy in breast cancer using non-mono-exponential diffusion models: a feasibility study comparing the baseline and mid-treatment MRI examinations. *Eur Radiol.* 2017;27(7):2726–2736.

144. Chen F, Chen P, Hamid Muhammed H, Zhang J. Intravoxel incoherent motion diffusion for identification of breast malignant and benign tumors using chemometrics. *Biomed Res Int.* 2017;2017:3845409.

145. Meeus EM, Novak J, Withey SB, Zarinabad N, Dehghani H, Peet AC. Evaluation of intravoxel incoherent motion fitting methods in low-perfused tissue. *J Magn Reson Imaging.* 2017;45(5):1325–1334.

146. Jerome NP, Vidić I, Egnell L, et al. Understanding diffusion-weighted MRI analysis: repeatability and performance of diffusion models in a benign breast lesion cohort. *NMR Biomed.* 2021;34(7):e4508.

147. Barbieri S, Donati OF, Froehlich JM, Thoeny HC. Impact of the calculation algorithm on biexponential fitting of diffusion-weighted MRI in upper abdominal organs. *Magn Reson Med.* 2016;75(5):2175–2184.

148. Jones DK, Cercignani M. Twenty-five pitfalls in the analysis of diffusion MRI data. *NMR Biomed.* 2010;23(7):803–820.

149. Karunamuni RA, Kuperman J, Seibert TM, et al. Relationship between kurtosis and bi-exponential characterization of high *b* value diffusion-weighted imaging: application to prostate cancer. *Acta Radiol.* 2018;59(12):1523–1529.

150. Koay CG, Basser PJ. Analytically exact correction scheme for signal extraction from noisy magnitude MR signals. *J Magn Reson.* 2006;179(2):317–322.

151. Glenn GR, Tabesh A, Jensen JH. A simple noise correction scheme for diffusional kurtosis imaging. *Magn Reson Imaging.* 2015;33(1):124–133.

152. Iima M, Le Bihan D. Clinical intravoxel incoherent motion and diffusion MR imaging: past, present, and future. *Radiology.* 2016;278(1):13–32.

153. Goto M, Le Bihan D, Yoshida M, Sakai K, Yamada K. Adding a model-free diffusion MRI marker to BI-RADS assessment improves specificity for diagnosing breast lesions. *Radiology.* 2019;292(1):84–93.

154. Teruel JR, Goa PE, Sjøbakk TE, Østlie A, Fjøsne HE, Bathen TF. A simplified approach to measure the effect of the microvasculature in diffusion-weighted MR imaging applied to breast tumors: preliminary results. *Radiology.* 2016;281(2):373–381.

155. Surov A, Meyer HJ, Wienke A. Can apparent diffusion coefficient (ADC) distinguish breast cancer from benign breast findings? A meta-analysis based on 13,847 lesions. *BMC Cancer.* 2019;19(1):1–14.

156. Palm T, Wenkel E, Ohlmeyer S, et al. Diffusion kurtosis imaging does not improve differentiation performance of breast lesions in a short clinical protocol. *Magn Reson Imaging.* 2019;63(May):205–216.

157. Bickelhaupt S, Steudle F, Paech D, et al. On a fractional order calculus model in diffusion weighted breast imaging to differentiate between malignant and benign breast lesions detected on x-ray screening mammography. *PLoS One.* 2017;12(4):1–14.

158. Baltzer P, Mann RM, Iima M, et al. Diffusion-weighted imaging of the breast—a consensus and mission statement from the EUSOBI International Breast Diffusion-Weighted Imaging working group. *Eur Radiol.* 2020;30(3):1436–1450.

159. Winfield JM, Tunariu N, Rata M, et al. Extracranial soft-tissue tumors: repeatability of apparent diffusion coefficient estimates from diffusion-weighted MR imaging. *Radiology.* 2017;284(1):88–99.

160. Iima M, Kataoka M, Kanao S, et al. Variability of non-Gaussian diffusion MRI and intravoxel incoherent motion (IVIM) measurements in the breast. *PLoS One.* 2018;13(3):e0193444.

161. Kuai ZX, Sang XQ, Yao YF, Chu CY, Zhu YM. Evaluation of non-monoexponential diffusion models for hepatocellular carcinoma using *b* values up to 2000 s/mm²: A short-term repeatability study. *J Magn Reson Imaging.* 2019;50(1):297–304.

Chapter 9

Diffusion Tensor Imaging (DTI) of the Breast

Eric E. Sigmund, PhD, Edna Furman-Haran, PhD, Pascal A. T. Baltzer, MD, and
Savannah C. Partridge, PhD

Diffusion tensor imaging (DTI) is a widely applied quantitative magnetic resonance imaging (MRI) approach to characterize tissue microstructure throughout the body. In addition to quantifying the amount of water diffusion hindrance by tissue, DTI also captures the orientational bias (anisotropy) caused by a microstructural environment with a preferred direction. Although the initial application of DTI largely occurred in the axonal nerve bundles of the brain, a growing literature of studies have performed DTI of the breast, applied most often to study breast cancer. This has led to extensive DTI research of both breast cancer lesions themselves and the surrounding fibroglandular tissue (FGT) to identify DTI properties distinguishing the two that can aid in diagnosis. Lesions tend to be dense, cellular, and disorganized, whereas FGT comprises more freely diffusing fluid-filled ducts and collagen oriented within the ductal tree. Thus both degree of restriction and its orientation may be diagnostic breast MR biomarkers. DTI metrics have shown promise to facilitate biological stratification of breast lesions (related to presence of malignancy, prognostic factors, and subtypes) and to aid in prediction of response to therapy. Finally, the Gaussian anisotropic model behind DTI is only one of a variety of models to capture tissue microstructure, and other models are also under exploration for the case of the breast. This chapter will summarize DTI in the breast in these areas, including technical issues, interpretive frameworks, and clinical potential. As with each organ of the body, the application of DTI to the breast is unique in both challenges and benefits.

DTI in the Breast: Basics, Metrics, and Pitfalls

In recent years, diffusion-weighted imaging (DWI) and DTI have been explored as complementary tools in breast MRI to improve lesion characterization, and enhance specificity.[1-4] Both DWI and DTI allow the quantification of an average diffusion coefficient (i.e., apparent diffusion coefficient [ADC] or mean diffusivity [MD]) that is sensitive to variations in the water diffusion caused by the differences in tissue complexity, such as cell density, cell size, membrane permeability, and extracellular tortuosity. By also capturing diffusion anisotropy, DTI can give a more complete tissue description of both healthy and pathological tissues and potentially provide higher value clinical tools. This includes extraction of additional information reflecting glandular microstructure: the ductal lumens, the epithelial cells, and the surrounding supporting stromal tissue. Specifically, the mammary ductal network comprises a "tree" pattern that facilitates lactation, such that locally (i.e., within an MRI voxel) the orientation of lactiferous ducts and adjacent collagen fibers displays a common direction. Water molecules whose transport is hindered by the ductal wall or collagen fibers will show anisotropic diffusion (i.e., displace further along the duct than across it, on average). Malignant transformation may in turn cause blockage of the ducts by proliferating neoplastic cells and loss of structured organization, potentially resulting in a concomitant reduction of anisotropy measures. Future sections will delve into this literature, sources of contrast, and comparison with pathological lesions in detail. Here we will review the metrics of

DTI and the technical requirements to ensure confidence in their deployment, as reviewed recently[5] and in Chapter 1.

DTI extends the average diffusivity derived by DWI by applying diffusion gradients in multiple directions and allowing characterization of water diffusion directionality or anisotropy. Mathematically, at least six noncollinear directions are required given the need to calculate six independent elements of the symmetrical 3×3 diffusion tensor D_{ij}.[6] The tensor is then typically transformed to its principal frame where its diagonal elements (eigenvalues) (λ_1, λ_2, and λ_3) are the principal diffusivities, their average is the MD, and their corresponding eigenvectors (v_1, v_2, and v_3) define the principal diffusion directions. Anisotropy indices are different combinations of the directional diffusion coefficients, such as the normalized variance called fractional anisotropy (FA), which indirectly describe structural elements such as fibers or ducts that partially restrict water diffusion (Fig. 9.1). Although the ADC and MD are in principle equivalent markers of diffusion, the sampling scheme and tensor analysis of DTI add robustness to MD in comparison with ADC measurements by single direction or average of three orthogonal directions in terms of signal-to-noise ratio

(SNR) and sensitivity to gradient hardware directional differences. In other organs such as the brain or skeletal muscle, optimization studies have been conducted to determine b value and number of directions choices to minimize noise-induced bias or uncertainty[7,8]; a minimum 20 or 30 directions are typically recommended, but it is advised to apply diffusion-weighted images in many directions as allowed by scan time limitation.[8,9] Analogous efforts have been performed for breast DTI for the application of tractography.[10] In most breast DTI studies, FA has been the common anisotropy index applied both for characterization of the FGT and for cancer diagnosis. It has been shown that water diffusion anisotropy in the healthy breast can be similarly mapped by other normalized anisotropy indices, such as relative anisotropy (RA), and 1-volume ratio (1-VR), as well as by the nonnormalized absolute maximal anisotropy index ($\lambda_1 - \lambda_3$).[11] However, there is no consensus regarding which is the optimal parameter to best describe anisotropy for breast cancer diagnosis.[11]

As will be reviewed in later sections, a consensus of studies have shown that MD, similarly to standard ADC, strongly discriminates malignant lesions from benign lesions and from FGT, because malignant

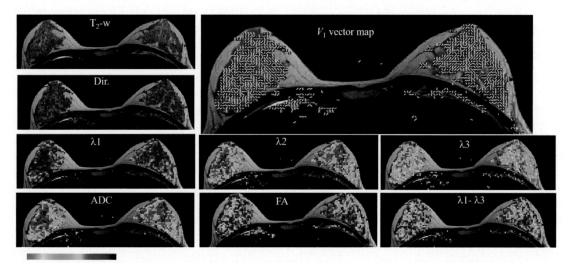

Fig. 9.1 Example for output of parametric DTI maps of a central slice in the breasts of a 32-year-old healthy volunteer overlaid on anatomical T_2-weighted images of the same slice. Dir: direction map with red indicating left to right, green indicating anterior to posterior, and blue indicating head to feet. All diffusion coefficients are in units of 10^{-3} mm²/s. FA is unitless. The scale bar from left to right is 0.8–2.3 × 10^{-3} mm²/s for λ_1, λ_2, λ_3 and ADC, 0.2–1.2 × 10^{-3} mm²/s for $\lambda_1 - \lambda_3$ and 0.05–0.3 for FA. DTI acquisition parameters: bipolar EPI acquisition, 30 directions; $b = 0, 700$ s/mm²; TE = 120 ms; resolution 1.9 × 1.9 × 2.5 mm³. Images were analyzed with the DDE MRI software (DDE MRI Solutions Ltd., Tel Aviv, Israel). *ADC,* Apparent diffusion coefficient; *DTI,* diffusion tensor imaging; *EPI,* echo-planar imaging; *FA,* fractional anisotropy; *TE,* echo time.

invasive ductal carcinoma lesions tend to feature dense cellularity. Furthermore, measures of anisotropy conceptually should help discriminate between healthy structured FGT and the more typically disordered cancerous or precancerous lesions. This is indeed borne out in some DTI studies comparing FGT to lesions,[12,13] but not all.[11,14–16] Similarly, some studies find FA distinguishes benign from malignant lesions,[13,14,17] whereas others do not.[12,15,16] This clinical diagnostic performance will be reviewed later in this chapter.

Part of those discrepancies might relate to the influence of SNR on the output DTI metrics.[5] Because anisotropy reflects directional variance of diffusion captured in the diffusion eigenvalues, it can be distorted or amplified by random signal variance introduced by signal noise. This effect is sometimes termed "eigenvalue repulsion,"[18] because the eigenvalue spread is artificially enhanced by noise due to the nonlinear diagonalization process; primary eigenvalue λ_1 increases and tertiary eigenvalue λ_3 decreases. FA values, eigenvalue difference $\lambda_1 - \lambda_3$ eigenvalue ratio λ_1/λ_3, and RA all increase in the process. In some cases, this may have the effect of increasing sensitivity to disease, but this nonbiological "boost" in utility should be considered cautiously.

Fibroglandular Tissue (FGT) DTI

DTI PARAMETERS OF NORMAL FIBROGLANDULAR TISSUE

DTI measurements of the normal breast have allowed characterization of the breast ductal/glandular structure.[14,16,19–21] Table 9.1 shows the broad range of reported diffusion parameters that were measured in normal breast tissue of healthy volunteers. Because of the lack of standardization, different DTI protocols were applied in the various studies, making comparison between different scan protocols difficult and resulting in reported mean MD and FA values that span a large range (1.69–2.05 $\times 10^{-3}$ mm²/s and 0.11–0.32, respectively). Water diffusion is independent of field strength, whereas differences in the DTI protocols (b values, diffusion time, echo time [TE], number of sensitizing diffusion directions, spatial resolution) affect the intensity in the diffusion-weighted images and thus the calculated

parameters. For example, selection of the b value affects the derived diffusion coefficients: higher b values lead to a reduction in the SNR and a reduction in the derived MD (or ADC in DWI studies) but not necessarily in FA.[5,10,19,22] In addition to SNR-based artificial decreases, this decrease in MD/ADC can also be explained by the presence of several different diffusion compartments, or equivalently the presence of microstructural complexity gives rise to non-Gaussian diffusion kurtosis effects. Additional differences in the derived values emerge from the size and placement of the regions of interest (ROIs) for the analysis, from partial volume effects due to unsuppressed fat, or from biological effects due to age and/or hormonal status.

Additionally, selection of the diffusion time (which in spin-echo echo-planar imaging [SE-EPI] is about TE/2) is a compromise between SNR and sensitivity to restriction. Water diffusion in a complex microenvironment will depend on the time allotted (i.e., diffusion time), because at longer diffusion times, more water molecules encounter barriers to their transport. This reduces the average displacement per time of the ensemble and therefore the measured diffusion coefficient. Not only does this decrease of diffusivity increase the measured contrast in the tissue of interest, but with biophysical modeling it can provide quantitative microstructural estimates. Teruel and colleagues,[23] using a stimulated-echo approach with variable diffusion times (69–903 ms), showed that the MD in healthy FGT decreased with increasing diffusion time. This decrease was attributed mainly to a decrease in the radial diffusivity (corresponding to diffusion in the direction perpendicular to the ductal walls), whereas the axial diffusivity (corresponding to free diffusion parallel to the ducts) remained at a similar value in the various diffusion times (Fig. 9.2). Consequently, an increase of FA with the diffusion time was observed.[23] A first-order modeling of the decline of radial diffusion using the Mitra theory to estimate surface-to-volume ratio provided size estimates of the order of magnitude (hundreds of microns) represented by duct diameters, consistent with histological quantification of human breast specimens.[24] Similar results were obtained in a study that used bipolar SE-EPI and compared the derived anisotropy indices obtained with a TE of 90 ms versus 120 ms (corresponding to diffusion times

TABLE 9.1   Reported Diffusion Tensor Imaging Parameters of the Normal Fibroglandular Breast in Healthy Volunteers

Publication	Age (Years), Number of Participants (n)	TE (t0) (ms)	Field, Protocol #Directions/ b Value	Resolution (mm)	Parameter (Average ± SD) (10^{-3} mm²/s)					
					MD	λ_1	λ_2	λ_3	$\lambda_1 - \lambda_3$	FA
Partridge et al.[19]	25–72, $n = 12$	71.5 (35) 71.5 (35)	1.5 T, SE-EPI 6/600 s/mm² 6/1000 s/mm²	1.9 × 1.9 × 4–5	1.95 ± 0.24 1.77 ± 0.29	2.51 ± 0.28	1.89 ± 0.25	1.39 ± 0.26	n/a	0.29 ± 0.05 0.30 ± 0.05
Tagliafico et al.[20]	28–85, $n = 60$	minimum	3 T, SE-EPI 32/1000 s/mm²	2.7 × 2 × 2	1.92 ± 0.30	n/a	n/a	n/a	n/a	0.32 ± 0.09
Plaza et al.[77]	50 ± 10, 35 breasts in 21 patients. Fatty FGT, $n = 15$ Heterogeneous FGT, $n = 20$	80–120	3 T, Bipolar SE-EPI 6/600 s/mm² Observer1, Observer2 Observer1 Observer2	2.2–2.7 × 2.2–2.7 × 4	1.97 ± 0.24 2.05 ± 0.24 1.99 ± 0.30 1.94 ± 0.37	2.33 ± 0.18 2.43 ± 0.19 2.33 ± 0.34 2.33 ± 0.42	1.94 ± 0.23 2.03 ± 0.25 1.97 ± 0.31 1.94 ± 0.36	1.63 ± 0.34 1.66 ± 0.38 1.66 ± 0.34 1.60 ± 0.39	0.70 ± 0.23 0.77 ± 0.30 0.67 ± 0.26 0.73 ± 0.30	0.19 ± 0.08 0.19 ± 0.07 0.18 ± 0.07 0.19 ± 0.08
Wang et al.[10]	25–65, $n = 7$ Another group, $n = 7$	minimum	1.5 T, SE-EPI 6/600 s/mm² 15/600 s/mm² 31/600 s/mm² 6/400, 600, 800 or 1000 s/mm²	2.8 × 2.8 × 3	n/a	n/a	n/a	n/a	n/a	0.16 ± 0.10 0.12 ± 0.05 0.11 ± 0.06 0.28–0.29 ± 0.1
Nissan et al.[21]	22–34, $n = 15$	120 (47)	3 T, Bipolar SE-EPI 30/700 s/mm²	1.9 × 1.9 × 2.5	1.95 ± 0.18	2.44 ± 0.16	1.91 ± 0.19	1.49 ± 0.21	0.95 ± 0.13	0.25 ± 0.04
Teruel et al.[23]	25–34, $n = 6$	45 (68.5) 45 (902.5)	3 T, STEAM-DTI 6/500 s/mm²	2.1 × 2.1 × 5	1.97 ± 0.26 1.77 ± 0.25	2.21 ± 0.27 2.17 ± 0.24		$(\lambda_2 + \lambda_3)/2$: 1.85 ± 0.26 1.57 ± 0.26	n/a n/a	0.13 ± 0.03 0.23 ± 0.06
Eyal et al.[16]	29–66, $n = 21$	120 (47)	3 T, Bipolar SE-EPI 30/700 s/mm²	1.9 × 1.9 × 1.9 – 2.5	1.76	2.17	1.76	1.36	0.77	0.23
Scaranelo et al.[78]	37–69, $n = 6$	86 (~43)	3 T, SE-EPI 30/700 s/mm²	1.9 × 1.9 × 4	1.69	2.20	1.64	1.10	0.99	n/a
Furman-Haran et al.[11]	23–68, $n = 6$	90 (33) 120 (47)	3 T, Bipolar SE-EPI 30/700 s/mm²	1.9 × 1.9 × 1.9 – 2.5	n/a	n/a	n/a	n/a	0.87 ± 0.08 1.14 ± 0.13	0.24 ± 0.02 0.31 ± 0.03

DTI, Diffusion tensor imaging; *FA*, fractional anisotropy; *FGT*, fibroglandular tissue; *MD*, mean diffusivity; *n/a*, not applicable; *SD*, standard deviation; *SE-EPI*, spin-echo echo-planar imaging; *STEAM*, stimulated echo diffusion tensor imaging; *TE*, echo time.

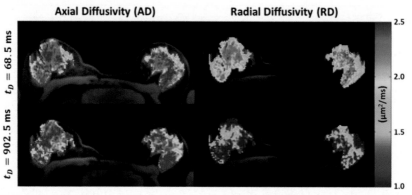

Fig. 9.2 **Axial and radial diffusivity parametric maps of fibroglandular tissue in a 28-year-old volunteer.** *(Upper row)* Diffusion time, $t_D = 68.5$ ms. *(Lower row)* Images acquired with $t_D = 902.5$ ms. Parametric maps are shown by direct overlay on corresponding slices of T1-weighted anatomical images. (Adapted with permission from Teruel JR, Cho GY, Moccaldi Rt M, et al. Stimulated echo diffusion tensor imaging (STEAM-DTI) with varying diffusion times as a probe of breast tissue. *J Magn Reson Imaging.* 2017;45(1):84–93.)

of 33 ms and 47 ms, respectively),[11] whereas all tested anisotropy indices (FA, RA, 1-VR, and $\lambda_1 - \lambda_3$) showed an increase in the derived values following an increase in the diffusion time. These findings are consistent with the higher sensitivity to microstructural features with the increased diffusion time, as more water molecules approach the structural barriers (see Fig. 9.2). According to the Einstein equation[25] (in one dimension, $x^2 = 2Dt_D$, where x is the mean displacement of water molecules, D is the diffusion coefficient, and t_D is the diffusion time; see also Chapter 1), for diffusion times in the range 30 to 50 ms (typical for most clinical DTI protocols), the mean displacement is about 7 to 10 µm (assuming D of free water at 37 degrees of ~3.0 × 10^{-3} mm²/s).[26] Because the mean diameter of most normal ducts is considerably larger (average of 90 µm, ranging from 40 µm to 314 reported in a post-mortem specimens study[24]), only a fraction of molecules—those close to the ductal walls—experience restriction and to a different extent across the various clinical DTI protocols. Additionally, partial volume effects due to voxel sizes being significantly larger than the ductal diameters contribute to reduction in sensitivity to restricted water diffusion.

Several studies have investigated the distribution of the DTI parameters in the various regions of the normal breast tissue.[19,20,27] In a study by Partridge and colleagues,[19] image analysis comparing ROIs (~130 mm² in size) subjectively placed in anterior, central, and posterior regions in 12 healthy

volunteers revealed that MD and FA are affected by location in the breast, with higher MD values in the central breast regions and higher FA in outer posterior regions.[19] In contrast, in the study of Tagliafico and colleagues,[20] small ROIs (30 mm² in size) placed in anterior, central, and posterior breast regions were compared, and no significant regional differences were observed in breast MD and FA. A possible explanation for this controversy is the use of minimal possible TE by Tagliafico and colleagues that reduced the sensitivity to restriction. Another explanation may be the small size of the ROIs and their subjective placement.

Weiderer and colleagues,[27] in an attempt to avoid dependence on ROI positioning, applied 2D histogram analysis and mapped the diffusion parameters in a cohort of seven healthy premenopausal volunteers. In this study, in agreement with the work of Partridge and colleagues,[19] the highest MD values were found in the central areas of the breast parenchyma, which are directed toward the breast papilla, whereas toward the periphery of the breast a decline was seen. The higher MD values in central areas may be due to larger areas of FGT in this region, resulting in less partial volume averaging with adipose tissue. Pixel-by-pixel statistical analysis further revealed that the central areas of high MD corresponded to areas of low FA, whereas the peripheral areas of low MD showed relatively high FA.[27] Higher anisotropy in outer and posterior regions was also demonstrated by mapping the various anisotropy indices in a cohort of six healthy volunteers.[11] The higher restriction in outer and posterior regions is presumably due to a higher concentration of small peripheral ducts and terminal ductal lobular units with low diameter in these regions and hence higher restriction of water diffusion in the directions orthogonal to the ductal walls. On the other hand, regions with low anisotropy values in the healthy FGT indicate the absence of water-restricting structures, presumably regions that are predominantly composed of fibrous connective tissue or regions with ducts near the nipple that—despite their directionality toward the nipple, the combination of their large diameter,[28,29] and the relatively short diffusion time—reduced the sensitivity to restriction. An example for the spatial distribution of the DTI parameters is shown in Fig. 9.1.

A similar but more pronounced distribution of the DTI parameters was reported by Nissan and colleagues in the lactating breast,[30] wherein the distribution of all diffusion coefficients (λ_1, λ_2, λ_3 and MD) indicated faster diffusion in the anterior regions close to the nipple compared with posterior regions. The distribution of the anisotropy indices λ_1 –λ_3 and FA revealed low anisotropy in anterior regions close to the nipple that increased toward the posterior regions (Fig. 9.3). The low anisotropy in regions close to the nipple can be explained by the presence of ducts with large diameter similar to the spatial resolution of the DTI protocol (about 2 mm). Indeed, in vivo ultrasound of the lactating breast showed that the mean diameter of the ducts in the base of the nipple was 2.0 ± 0.8 mm (range 1.1–4.4 mm).[31] In these large ducts, only a small fraction of the molecules (those close to the walls) are restricted, and therefore the average anisotropy is relatively low.

HORMONAL REGULATION OF BREAST DTI PARAMETERS DURING THE MENSTRUAL CYCLE

Because of the increased interest in clinical usage of diffusion-weighted MRI, hormonal-induced changes on the diffusion MR imaging parameters were investigated. Nissan and colleagues[21] have investigated the

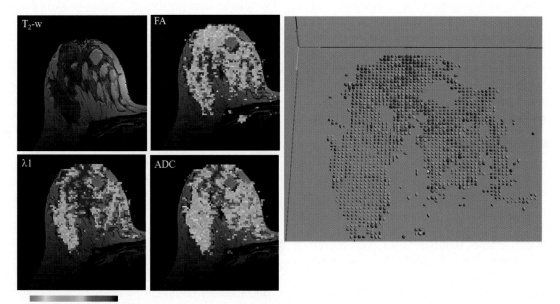

Fig. 9.3 **Ellipsoids and parametric DTI maps of a central slice in the breast of a 33-year-old lactating healthy volunteer overlaid on T₂-weighted images of the same slice.** The colors of the ellipsoids refer to the main direction of *v*1 with green indicating posterior-anterior, red indicating right-left, and blue indicating head-feet. Note the low restriction and high diffusivity near the nipple and the high anisotropy in the lobular-posterior regions. The scale bar from left to right is (0.8–2.3) × 10⁻³ mm²/s for λ_1 and ADC, and 0 to 0.3 for FA. DTI acquisition parameters: bipolar EPI acquisition, 64 directions; b = 0, 700 s/mm²; TE = 120 ms; resolution 1.9 × 1.9 × 2.5 mm³. Images were analyzed with the DDE MRI software (DDE MRI Solutions Ltd., Tel Aviv, Israel). *ADC,* Apparent diffusion coefficient; *DTI,* diffusion tensor imaging; *EPI,* echo-planar imaging; *TE,* echo time.

parameters obtained with DTI of the breast in premenopausal healthy volunteers throughout the menstrual cycle phases ($n = 15$). It was shown that the diffusion coefficients (λ_1, λ_2, λ_3 and ADC) and the anisotropy indexes (FA and $\lambda_1 - \lambda_3$) were almost constant throughout the menstrual cycle, with a very small within-subject coefficient of variance of 1% to 2% for the diffusion coefficients and 5% to 6% for the anisotropy parameters. Additionally, comparing between a group of premenopausal nonlactating volunteers who used oral contraceptive (OC; $n = 7$) to OC-free volunteers ($n = 8$) did not show significant differences for all DTI parameters. Wiederer and colleagues[27] likewise reported no statistical significant changes in MD and FA derived from a breast DTI study of premenopausal OC free volunteers with regular menstrual cycle that were examined in four consecutive weeks ($n = 7$).

These results are in general agreement with studies that investigated menstrual cycle effects on ADC derived from DWI studies of the breast,[32–36] as described in Chapter 7. Furthermore, even reported menstrual changes in diffusion metrics[36] are relatively small in comparison to more than 30% reduction in ADC in breast tumors in comparison to ADC of normal tissue.[4,37] Thus the diagnostic accuracy of DWI/DTI parameters of the normal breast FGT is likely minimally affected by the histological changes of the epithelial and stromal components and vascular changes that occur during the menstrual cycle,[38,39] and thus the timing for performing breast DWI/DTI is not restricted throughout the menstrual cycle.

DTI OF THE POSTMENOPAUSAL BREAST

It has been suggested that falling serum estradiol and progesterone in postmenopausal women can cause a reduction in the water-containing glandular epithelium, collagenization of the interlobular stroma, and thickening of the lobular basement membranes, all of which reduce water diffusion[32] (see also Chapter 7). Indeed, comparing breast ADC values of premenopausal to postmenopausal women who did not use hormonal replacement therapy (HRT) revealed that the diffusion coefficients (λ_1, λ_2, λ_3 and ADC) were significantly higher by 9% to 14% in premenopausal women, but there were no differences in anisotropy indices.[21] Reduced average ADC of normal FGT in postmenopausal women without HRT versus premenopausal

women was also observed in DWI studies of healthy volunteers[32] and in the normal contralateral FGT of breast cancer patients[33,34] (Table 9.2).

In accord with the expected hormonal effect of HRT,[40] there were no significant differences in DTI parameters between premenopausal volunteers and the postmenopausal volunteers who used HRT.[21] Additionally, a significantly higher value of λ_1, λ_2, λ_3 and ADC by 6% to 12% in volunteers who used HRT ($n = 8$) in comparison to volunteers that did not use HRT ($n = 11$) was found. However, there were no significant differences in anisotropy (FA and $\lambda_1 - \lambda_3$) between the two groups.[21] Higher ADC values in postmenopausal women who were taking HRT compared with women who were not were also observed in DWI studies,[32,33] although they did not reach statistical significance because of the small number of participants in these studies (see Table 9.2). Further studies with larger cohorts are required to validate these findings.

DTI OF THE LACTATING BREAST

DTI was also applied to follow and characterize microstructural changes in the mammary gland of healthy volunteers from the time of lactation to 3 to 11 months postweaning ($n = 10$).[30] The lactating and postweaning FGT were characterized by similar mean value of the prime diffusion coefficient λ_1 ((2.11 ± 0.13) $\times$ 10^{-3} mm²/s for both), which was statistically significantly lower ($P = .01$) than in an age-matched control group ((2.29 ± 0.13) $\times 10^{-3}$ mm²/s, $n = 10$). Because milk is a colloid of fat globules within a water-based fluid that contains dissolved carbohydrates and protein aggregates with minerals, the viscosity of milk is higher than that of the normal water fluid in the ducts, and thus the water diffusion coefficients of lactating breasts are lower than those of nonlactating premenopausal women. The fact that λ_1 remained similar during lactation and postweaning and did not return to the range of normal values suggests that the fluid in the ductal/glandular tissue during the first year postweaning may still contain ingredients that increase the ductal fluid viscosity.

The mean value of the two radial diffusion coefficients λ_2 and λ_3 decreased significantly (from (1.65 ± 0.10) $\times 10^{-3}$ mm²/s to (1.55 ± 0.14) $\times 10^{-3}$ mm²/s, $P = .016$ for λ_2 and from (1.28 ± 0.12) $\times 10^{-3}$ mm²/s to (1.09 ± 0.15) $\times 10^{-3}$ mm²/s, $P = .0008$ for λ_3),

TABLE 9.2 Reported Comparison of Breast Diffusion Tensor Imaging Parameters of Premenopausal and Postmenopausal Volunteers With and Without Hormonal Replacement Therapy Usage

Publication	ADC (Mean ± SD) (x10⁻³ mm²/s)			Statistical Significance (P)		
	Premenopausal	Postmenopausal With HRT	Postmenopausal Without HRT	Premenopausal vs. Postmenopausal With HRT	Premenopausal vs. Postmenopausal Without HRT	Postmenopausal With vs. Without HRT
Nissan et al.[21]	1.95 ± 0.18, $n = 15$	1.90 ± 0.07, $n = 8$	1.73 ± 0.13, $n = 11$	.35	.001	.003
Cakir et al.[15]	1.66 ± 0.07, $n = 32$	1.50 ± 0.09, $n = 14$			.08	–
O'Flynn et al.[32]	1.84 ± 0.26, $n = 13$	1.53 ± 0.5, $n = 4$	1.43 ± 0.24, $n = 14$	–	–	.46
		1.46 ± 0.3, $n = 18$			<.001	
Shin et al.[34]	1.64, $n = 73$	–	1.38, $n = 51$	–	<.001	–
Kim et al.[33]	1.75 ± 0.27, $n = 29$	1.66 ± 0.35, $n = 5$	1.58 ± 0.29, $n = 23$	–	.035	.684
		1.60 ± 0.30, $n = 28$			.030	

Diffusion protocols with different *b* values were applied in the various studies.
ADC, Apparent diffusion coefficient; *DTI*, diffusion tensor imaging; *HRT*, hormonal replacement therapy; *SD*, standard deviation.

leading to reduced MD postweaning (from $(1.68 \pm 0.11) \times 10^{-3}$ mm²/s to $(1.58 \pm 0.14) \times 10^{-3}$ mm²/s, $P = .022$).[30] In parallel, the mean anisotropy significantly increased from lactating to postweaning by $32.1\% \pm 20.2\%$ for FA and by $26.1\% \pm 17.9\%$ for $\lambda_1 - \lambda_3$. The reduced radial diffusivity and increased anisotropy emerge from restriction by the ductal walls and are related to the reduction in the radial size of the ductal/glandular system reflecting the ductal involution postweaning.[31,41]

BREAST DTI IN PREGNANCY

Breast MRI during pregnancy is limited due to both the inconvenience involved in lying prone during the scan and safety concerns related to the usage of gadolinium-based contrast agents that are an essential part of the diagnostic breast MRI workup. DTI parameters of the healthy pregnant breast were so far described only in a pilot study of pregnancy-associated breast cancer patients.[42] Images were acquired on a 1.5 T scanner with monopolar SE-EPI acquisition

with $b = 0$ and 700 s/mm², applied in 32 directions, TE of 91 ms, and resolution of $1.9 \times 2.6 \times 2.5$ mm³. Analysis included ROI delineation of the entire FGT in the healthy contralateral breast ($n = 9$) in a single slice at the level of the nipple. The derived mean DTI parameters were similar to previously reported measurements in young premenopausal women acquired with a similar scanning protocol.[21]

RECONSTRUCTION OF THE DUCTAL TREE

Our knowledge of the structure of the mammary gland is based on several detailed anatomical studies of breast autopsies and mastectomy specimens.[43–46] In studies by Sir Astley Cooper using colored wax injection to lactating breast cadavers, it was shown that the human mammary gland comprises several separate lobes that vary in size and shape, and each lobe presents a ductal tree with a central duct and its peripheral branches (Fig. 9.4). Attempts to image the ductal system ("ductography"), which involved injecting a contrast into the duct orifice at the nipple and

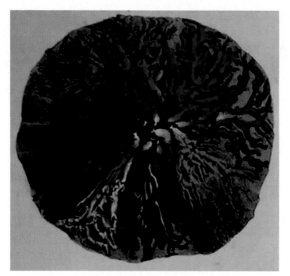

Fig. 9.4 An artistic drawing of the mammary ducts injected with colored wax. (Adapted with permission from Cooper AP. *Anatomy of the Breast.* London; 1840.)

subsequent x-ray[47] or MR[48] imaging, were able to illustrate a portion of the ductal system. Preliminary ultrasound studies of the lactating breast were also applied and allowed in vivo quantifying and measuring of the main glandular ducts[31] and reconstructing sections of the 3D ductal system.[49] However, these measurements were limited by the ductal diameters, and none of these approaches has so far succeeded in imaging the entire ductal system. This is also owing to the fact that only single pathologically dilated ducts (e.g., involving nipple discharge) can be probed by ductography equipment.

DTI analysis allows modeling of water diffusion in each voxel as an ellipsoid wherein the direction of water diffusion in three orthogonal directions (v_1, v_2, v_3) and the magnitude of the directional water diffusion coefficients (λ_1, λ_2, λ_3) are defined. Because water diffusion in the mammary gland is anisotropic, with free water movement in the direction of the ducts and restricted diffusion in the direction perpendicular to the ducts, the dominant direction of the ellipsoids of $v1$ allows the tracking of the main ductal orientation in the mammary gland.[14,50] Indeed, in a high-resolution DTI study ($1.5 \times 1.5 \times 1.5$ mm^3 resolution), Baltzer and colleagues reported that the unaffected FGT showed on color-coded directional maps a dominant anterior-posterior

diffusion direction—the direction of the majority of glandular ducts toward the nipple—in a large fraction of patients (66.1%; 39 of 59 patients).[14] In the example shown in Fig. 9.3, each pixel in the FGT is modeled as an ellipsoid, and the color coding reflects the direction of the prime eigenvector v_1, demonstrating the dominant anterior-posterior direction and the potential of v_1 vector maps/ellipsoid model to track the 3D structure of the mammary tree.

DTI-based tracking was originally developed for white matter tracking in the brain.[51] However, the size, shape, and structure of the ductal tree and the origin of water restriction are remarkably different in the mammary gland from those in the brain white matter fibers. Additionally, the anisotropy in the mammary gland is relatively low (FA 0–0.3) in comparison to white matter tracks (FA in the brain is most commonly >0.5), and the diffusion coefficients are higher than those in the brain. Hence the optimization of the acquisition protocols and the development of new dedicated tools for tracking the ductal tree are required.

An initial attempt for in vivo 3D tracking of the entire ductal system was applied in a study by Reisert and colleagues.[52] In this study, DTI data were acquired in a sagittal orientation, with b = 0 and b = 700 s/mm^2, 64 diffusion sensitizing gradient directions, and $1.9 \times 1.9 \times 2.5$ mm^3 resolution. The tracking approach was based on an algorithm that was developed for brain white matter tractography[53] and included probabilistic tracking and accumulating the directions of the tracts, using the nipple as a seed followed by streamline tracking from the nipple and applying clustering of the streamlines tracts to obtain the ductal tree structure. Fig. 9.5 shows an example for 3D tracking of the ductal tree obtained using this algorithm,[52] demonstrating its capability to reveal detailed anatomical information of the ductal tree and its directional architecture toward the nipple.

Wang and colleagues[10] investigated the effect of the selected *b* value (400, 600, 800, and 1000 s/mm^2), voxel size ($2.8 \times 2.8 \times 3$ mm^3, $1.9 \times 1.9 \times 5$ mm^3, and $1.4 \times 1.4 \times 5$ mm^3), and the number of applied diffusion directions (6, 15, and 31) on DTI acquired for tractography. In this study, the quality of the protocol was assessed by comparing the SNR and by calculating the mean length and mean number of reconstructed tracks. DTI tractography was applied to an ROI of fixed

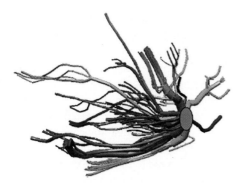 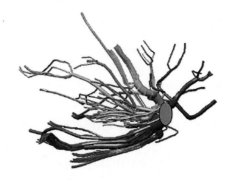

Fig. 9.5 The ductal tree. A view of 3D tracking of the ductal tree in a healthy volunteer that was obtained using the algorithm developed by Reisert and colleagues. *(Left)* The ductal tree based on 10 initial ducts. *(Right)* The ductal tree based on six initial ducts. (Adapted with permission from Reisert M, Weigel M, Eyal E, Grobgeld D, Degani H, Hennig J. Diffusion tensor based reconstruction of the ductal tree. Paper presented at: Annual Meeting of the International Society of Magnetic Resonance in Medicine (ISMRM); May 7–13, 2011; Montreal, Canada.)

size located in the central portion at the largest slice of the breast tissue using a continuous tracking algorithm that was developed for brain DTI (Diffusion Toolkit software) and applying default thresholds of minimum FA = 0.05 and a maximum turning angle of 50 degrees. The results suggested using a b value of 600 s/mm^2 and spatial resolution of 2.8 × 2.8 × 3 mm^3 that allowed isotropic voxels, and applying a 31-direction scan for the optimal fiber tracking. Although the tractography in this study could not be validated by histology, the results demonstrated the presence of anisotropy, the dominant anterior-posterior directions of the tracts, and the feasibility of breast DTI tractography.

Although additional validation is warranted, these preliminary results are encouraging and suggest that tracking of the ductal system by DTI with advanced algorithms and optimized acquisition parameters is feasible. In the future, detailed 3D information of the mammary ductal architecture could be obtained in order to follow individual differences.

Clinical Application of Breast DTI

DIFFERENTIAL DIAGNOSIS: BENIGN VERSUS MALIGNANT LESIONS

DTI is a valuable tool to differentiate breast cancer from benign lesions with high sensitivity and specificity. In a meta-analysis by Wang and colleagues[54] of 16 studies including 1636 patients, DTI metrics (λ_1, λ_2, λ_3, MD, and FA) were investigated for this purpose.

In this analysis, λ_1 showed the highest diagnostic performance characteristics (AUC 0.97, sensitivity 93%, specificity 92%), followed by MD (AUC 0.92, sensitivity 87%, specificity 83%). MD is significantly higher in benign (range of reported mean MD values (1.41 – 1.91) × 10^{-3} mm^2/s, one outlier 1.08 × 10^{-3} mm^2/s)[15,55,56] compared with malignant breast lesions (range of reported mean MD values (0.71 – 1.25) × 10^{-3} mm^2/s, one outlier of 1.62 × 10^{-3} mm^2/s)[13,15,56] with a standardized mean difference (a normalized metric allowing pooling of variable parameters across studies) of −2.1 (95% CI; −2.58 to −1.63). λ_1 was reported lower in malignant compared with benign lesions, with a standardized mean difference of −2.75 (95% CI; −3.69 to −1.82). FA was significantly higher in malignant (0.15–0.55) than benign (0.1–0.38) lesions, with a standardized mean difference of 0.55 (95% CI; 0.19–0.92), but provided only a moderate diagnostic value, with the lowest AUC of 0.76 among the parameters. There are still controversies in the usage of FA for the differentiation between breast cancer and benign lesions, and caution should be paid for its usage.[5] Although all these findings were associated with significant heterogeneity between studies, suggesting several potential technical and biological/study design biases, the findings for λ_1 further demonstrated significant publication bias. More generally, it should also be noted that the studies surveyed by Wang and colleagues[54] were carried out with a range of TEs, b values, direction sets, and spatial resolution that undoubtedly contributed heterogeneity to the group results and to controversies regarding parameter performance. This underscores the need for harmonization of protocols across studies when large evidence level accrual is the goal, as suggested by recent consortia.[4]

DIAGNOSIS OF BREAST CANCER INVASIVENESS OR SUBTYPE

DTI metrics have been investigated regarding their ability to distinguish invasive from noninvasive (ductal carcinoma in situ [DCIS]) breast cancer lesions. Investigated metrics were MD and FA. Table 9.3 shows details from several studies testing diagnostic accuracy of invasive from DCIS lesions. MD[12,57,58] was found significantly lower in invasive breast cancer compared with DCIS (significant standardized mean difference of 0.76; 95% CI; −1.4 to −0.12 reported by Wang and colleagues[54]), whereas the FA metric did not differ between both malignant subtypes. Although the results must be considered preliminary as these studies comprised 163 (MD) and 414 (FA) malignant lesions only, it can be concluded that the general FA metric is not a promising biomarker for this diagnostic task, whereas the findings for MD are well in line with those reported for the ADC metric reported in standard DWI.[59] As shown in selected studies, lesion subgrouping impacts the diagnostic performance of DTI metrics. For example, Luo and colleagues[56] demonstrated better diagnostic performance in mass lesions than nonmass lesions for both MD (AUC 0.84 vs. 0.63) and FA (AUC 0.69 vs. 0.50).

HISTOLOGICAL PROPERTIES AND DTI METRICS

A number of researchers have associated DTI metrics with prognostic factors in breast cancer. Results are contradictory, and their comparison is hampered by different statistical methods used (e.g., correlation analysis vs. comparison of mean/median values). In a study of 80 histologically verified breast lesions, 58 of them malignant, Yamaguchi and colleagues[60] reported no association of ADC/MD values with prognostic factors (ER, PR, HER2, grade, subtype, lymph node (LN) status), whereas FA values were found higher in lesions with more favorable prognostic factors such as positive estrogen receptor

status, lower nuclear grade and intrinsic subtype. The reported *P*-values were borderline significant, even not considering alpha error accumulation that was not addressed statistically.[60] Kim and coworkers[58] reported on 251 patients with breast cancer lesions, 230 of them invasive. In line with Yamaguchi and colleagues,[60] they reported lower FA values in lesions with higher histological grade but also a negative correlation with lesion size. No significant FA differences were found between lesions with positive versus negative estrogen or progesterone receptor or lymph node status. The authors also investigated Ki-67 and p53 status and found a nonsignificant tendency toward lower FA values if both were high or positive. On the other hand, they reported significant associations of MD with grade (higher discriminatory power than FA), lymphovascular invasion, and lymph node status as well as Ki-67 status.[58] Two clinical examples from one of our institutions are seemingly well in line with the findings of Yamaguchi and colleagues and Kim and colleagues, showing lower MD values in a triple negative lesion (Fig. 9.6) than in an HR+/HER2+ lesion (Fig. 9.7). Ozal and colleagues[55] investigated the DTI metrics MD, FA, RA and volume ratio (VR) in a study comprising 63 women with breast cancer. They reported significantly lower MD values in grade 3 breast cancers but no difference of FA, RA, and VR between histological grades. Although FA, RA, and VR showed higher values in lesions with higher grade, only RA and VR showed statistical significance, and no alpha error correction was applied. The authors further reported higher MD and lower FA, RA, and VR values in hormonal receptor positive cancers; only MD proved statistically significant, whereas FA was borderline significant regarding progesterone receptor status.[55] These contradictory results point out a controversial role of the investigated DTI metrics to predict surrogate markers of breast cancer aggressiveness.

In addition to ductal microarchitecture, other features have been considered for their contribution to observed diffusion anisotropy within and around cancerous lesions. Kakkad and colleagues[61] performed a study on breast cancer specimens on an 11.7 T scanner with high resolution (62.5 × 62.5 × 62.5 μm^3) and b = 2100 s/mm^2; a correlation between observed anisotropy and collagen content was shown, though

TABLE 9.3 Reported Diffusion Tensor Imaging Parameters and Their Ability to Distinguish Invasive Breast Cancer From Ductal Carcinoma in Situ

Publication	TE (ms)	Field, Protocol #Directions/b Value	Resolution (mm)	MD (Average ± SD) (x10⁻³ mm²/s), #lesion			FA (Average ± SD)		
				IBC	DCIS	P	IBC	DCIS	P
Partridge et al.[12]	71.5	1.5 T, SE-EPI 6/600 s/mm²	1.9 × 1.9 × 5	1.14 ± 0.29, n = 62	1.43 ± 0.21, n = 14	<.001	0.24 ± 0.07	0.22 ± 0.07	0.17
Wang et al.[76]	minimum	1.5 T, SE-EPI 6/600 s/mm²	2.65 × 2.65 × 3	1.03 ± 0.22, n = 53	1.28 ± 0.20, n = 11	.001	0.16 ± 0.09	0.13 ± 0.04	0.288
Jiang et al.[75]	90	1.5 T, SE-EPI 6/1000 s/mm²	2.6 × 1.5 × 5	0.94 ± 0.33, n = 23	0.96 ± 0.21, n = 11	>.05	0.20 ± 0.06	0.17 ± 0.06	>0.05
Kim et al.[58]	74	3 T, Bipolar SE-EPI 20/1000 s/mm²	2.1 × 2.1 × 3	1.01 ± 0.25, n = 230	1.27 ± 0.14, n = 21	<.001	0.29 ± 0.09	0.30 ± 0.04	0.226
Jiang et al.[57]	90	1.5 T, SE-EPI 6/1000 s/mm²	2.6 × 1.5 × 5	Grade I–II: 1.00 ± 0.33, n = 15 Grade III: 0.85 ± 0.14, n = 30	1.04 ± 0.31, n = 14	.022	Grade I–II: 0.20 ± 0.05 Grade III: 0.20 ± 0.05	0.18 ± 0.03	0.417
Luo et al.[56]	61	3 T, SE-EPI 6/100, 800 s/mm²	1.5 × 1.5 × 5	n/a n = 73	n/a n = 17		0.30	0.22	0.026

DCIS, Ductal carcinoma in situ; FA, fractional anisotropy; IBC, invasive breast cancer; MD, mean diffusivity; n/a, not applicable; SD, standard deviation; SE-EPI, spin-echo echo-planar imaging; TE, echo time.

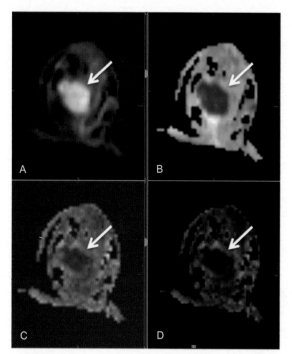

Fig. 9.6 Perimenopausal woman with a newly diagnosed, nonpalpable mammographic mass. The trace diffusion-weighted image (A, b = 800 s/mm²) shows a hyperintense mass. MD (B) was quantified as 0.76 × 10⁻³ mm²/s. FA (C) was measured as 0.15 and the FA map with color-coded main tensor direction overlay (D) revealed a disruption of the predominant green (anterior-posterior) diffusion direction as well as a marked hypointensity due to the low FA. Subsequent ultrasound-guided biopsy revealed a triple negative invasive breast cancer G3 not otherwise specified; the Ki-67 count was 90%. DTI acquisition parameters: EPI acquisition, 20 directions; b = 0, 800 s/mm²; TE = 87 ms; resolution 1.8 × 1.8 × 4 mm³. Images were analyzed with Siemens Syngo software. *DTI*, Diffusion tensor imaging; *EPI*, echo-planar imaging; *FA*, fractional anisotropy; *MD*, mean diffusivity.

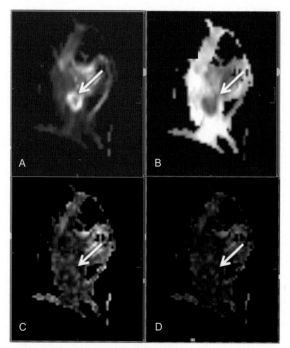

Fig. 9.7 Perimenopausal woman with a newly diagnosed, nonpalpable mammographic mass. The trace diffusion-weighted image (A, b = 800 s/mm²) shows a mass with circular hyperintensity. MD (B) was quantified as 0.82 × 10⁻³ mm²/s. Note the low MD values also in the area corresponding to the hypointense signal on (A). Fractional anisotropy (C) was measured as 0.42 and the FA map with color-coded main tensor direction overlay (D) revealed a disruption of the predominant green (anterior-posterior) diffusion direction but no hypointensity due to the FA that was similar to healthy breast tissue. Subsequent ultrasound-guided biopsy revealed a hormonal receptor positive, HER2-negative invasive breast cancer G2 not otherwise specified; the Ki-67 count was 10% (luminal A type). DTI acquisition parameters: EPI acquisition, 20 directions; b = 0, 800 s/mm²; TE = 87 ms; resolution 1.8 × 1.8 × 4 mm³. Images were analyzed with Siemens Syngo software. *DTI*, Diffusion tensor imaging; *EPI*, echo-planar imaging; *FA*, fractional anisotropy; *MD*, mean diffusivity.

the non-Gaussian *b* value regime should be noted. Bailey and colleagues,[62] using a 9.4 T scanner and a high-resolution (250 × 250 μm²) DTI protocol with *b* values up to 1500 s/mm², found analogous correlations of fibrous stroma and diffusion directionality zones in human breast tissue specimens containing invasive breast cancers. Thus although ducts are likely the dominant source of diffusion anisotropy in the breast, accompanying stromal features may also play a role, depending on the image resolution, applied *b* value, and SNR; on a related note, stromal collagen has been recently found to contribute to diffusion properties in breast lesions.[63]

PREDICTION AND MONITORING OF RESPONSE TO TREATMENT

Only limited data on 54 patients exist regarding the value of DTI metrics in the assessment of response to neoadjuvant breast cancer treatment.[64,65] Wilmes and colleagues[64] investigated DTI metrics ADC, FA, and principal eigenvalues before and after three cycles of taxane-based therapy in 34 patients. They reported somewhat lower ADC values in the pCR group ($n = 9$) compared with the non-pCR group ($n = 25$) before treatment; also λ_2 was slightly lower in the pCR group.

Upon early response, none of the DTI metrics differed between both pCR and non-pCR groups. Most pronounced differences were found investigating the change of DTI metrics over time, with all eigenvalues and ADC showing a higher and statistically significant increase after treatment in the pCR group. The highest AUC values were found for ADC (83%) and λ_1 (82%). FA was not significantly associated with pCR and showed a moderate negative correlation with tumor volume. However, the change in eigenvalue difference ($\lambda_1 - \lambda_3$) trended toward significant association with pCR ($P = .07$). Furman-Haran and colleagues[65] reported on 20 breast cancer patients before and after neoadjuvant treatment. They included residual disease in their responder definition and reported significantly higher changes of eigenvalue metrics and MD in responders ($n = 12$) compared with nonresponders ($n = 8$), reporting AUC values for distinguishing responders from nonresponders of up to 0.84 for λ_1 and 0.83 for MD. Significant differences were reported for all eigenvalues, MD, and ($\lambda_1 - \lambda_3$), but not FA. Neither group reported benchmarking results against standard of care metrics, including clinical and conventional assessment, although both showed correlation to tumor volume from dynamic contrast-enhanced (DCE) MRI. Neither explicitly compared the performance of DTI-specific metrics over conventional ADC.[64,65] The added value of DTI over DWI in monitoring therapeutic response in breast cancer requires further investigation.

CLINICAL DECISION-MAKING

Though there is accumulating evidence that DTI metrics provide additional and independent insights into breast pathology compared with the ADC/MD, there is still a lack of conclusive evidence that DTI-derived metrics are superior to standard DWI metrics for all diagnostic pathways, and sparse and even contradicting evidence exists regarding prognostic/predictive applications. From a clinical perspective, DTI is still a research tool and currently not indicated to base clinical decisions upon its results. Larger phase III and multicenter diagnostic studies[66] are required to estimate the potential of DTI in the multimodal imaging-based diagnosis and treatment of breast cancer.

As indicated throughout this review, heterogeneity among studies in acquisition (b values, TEs,

directions, resolution) and analysis (anisotropy metrics, ROI definition) may contribute to the inconsistency of some findings (e.g., prognostic factor correlations, anisotropy metric diagnostic/prognostic value). Now that sufficient evidence has been collected demonstrating potential of DTI metrics beyond single site trials, efforts are warranted to harmonize protocols and analysis strategies when multisite data is to be compared or pooled for enhanced impact. A blueprint for this harmonization has been laid out recently for breast DWI that should guide future study design.[4]

Breast DTI: Advances and Extensions

Diffusion MRI has proven a very versatile probe of tissue microstructure and microcirculation throughout the body. The combination of expanded diffusion encoding patterns and associated theoretical signal models allows quantification of increasingly complex features that provide markers of tissue function and pathology. Breast FGT and breast lesions have also been studied with such advanced approaches.

One example encoding parameter is the diffusion time, as described earlier, for the longer diffusion time regime (~1 s) than the conventional one (~40 ms). In the other extreme, very small diffusion times (9.6 ms and 27.6 ms) and a range of b values (0–4000 s/mm^2) were employed by Iima and colleagues, allowing diffusion lengths on the order of cancer cell dimensions to be probed, with an oscillating gradient spin echo (OGSE) pulse sequence in both preclinical cancer models.[67] In a human breast cancer lesion study by Iima and colleagues,[68] malignant lesions showed a more significant change (with diffusion time from 4.7 to 97 ms) than did benign lesions. Although the diagnostic accuracy of this ΔADC parameter (reflecting the rate of change in ADC values with diffusion time) was similar to that of the two ADC values individually, correlations with prognostic factors (in particular Ki-67 expression) were much stronger using ΔADC. This implies improved utility in differentiating variants in cellular architecture when protocols go beyond single ADC values.

As mentioned, a general research effort of diffusion imaging throughout the body is aimed to reach a more detailed and multiparametric encoding scheme that, combined with biophysical modeling, may yield more specific biological biomarkers. One example of such an approach is restriction spectrum imaging (RSI). RSI combines measurement of a broad range of diffusion contrast (b value, direction, diffusion time) with a linear mixture model of prototypical components (e.g., hindered anisotropic compartment, isotropic restricted compartment) representing features like dense cellularity or directional fibers/ducts. As originally applied to brain tumors,[69] "the RSI framework is designed to strike a balance between model complexity and interpretability by minimizing a priori assumptions on microstructure while preserving biophysical interpretability of the resulting estimates." The application of RSI to brain cancer has involved eight such components, whose component weights comprise a "restriction spectrum"; weighted averages of this spectrum are computed to represent such features as cell density. The RSI approach has recently been extended to breast lesions[70] to probe the appropriate spectrum of compartments for that tissue type and its clinical questions (tumor conspicuity, benign/malignant classification, and lesion subtyping). Initial results favor a three-compartment triexponential diffusion model wherein the diffusion signal across all acquired b values, $S(b)$, is defined as $S(b) = N[C_1e^{-bADC_1} + C_2e^{-bADC_3} + C_3e^{-bADC_3}]$. Here,

C_i denotes the signal contribution from each component nominally representing perfusion, hindered, and restricted diffusion (Fig. 9.8),[70] with new metrics derived from combinations of their weights (e.g., the product $C_1 \times C_2$). Though this treatment has not yet involved anisotropic diffusion in the breast, future implementations in the breast may introduce this aspect as in prior RSI studies.

Diffusion tensor distribution (DTD) imaging similarly involves measurement of multiple diffusion directions and b values in a model of distributed diffusion tensors in both magnitude and direction. DTD belongs to a family of approaches[71] that apply "tensor-valued" diffusion encoding waveforms (linear, planar, spherical encoding) to disentangle tissue components based on the sizes, shapes, and orientations of their diffusion tensor. Again, this formalism allows more detailed characterization and separation of both lesions and surrounding FGT, because both carry properties of restriction and anisotropy to a different degree.[72] However, this pilot demonstration requires continued development before clinical deployment.

Finally, recent work by Tan and colleagues,[73] guided by analogous work in the brain,[74] applied a multicompartment analysis to highly sampled multiple b value, multiple diffusion direction data in breast

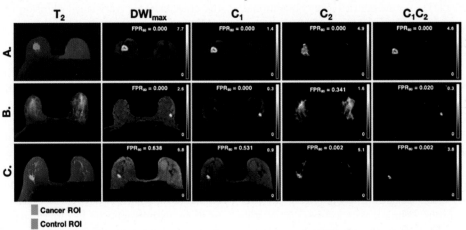

Cancer ROI
Control ROI

Fig. 9.8 Example RSI analysis for breast lesions. Parameter maps for DWImax, C_1, C_2, and C_1C_2 with FPR80, T_2-weighted images with cancer *(red)* and control *(green)* ROI overlay for three representative cases. FPR80 vary depending on healthy tissue composition in relation to the magnitude of C_1 and C_2 in cancer tissue. (A) Mixed tissue composition with cancer high on both dimensions. (B) Abundant fibroglandular tissue and high C_1-magnitude of cancer. (C) Abundant fat tissue and high C_2-magnitude of cancer. DWImax and C_1 performance is poorest in (B), C_2 in (C), whereas C_1C_2 has perfect performance across cases. Gray level windows for all images are scaled to the maximum and minimum signal intensity of each case and given in arbitrary units. *Au,* Arbitrary unit; *C,* signal contribution; *DWImax,* image acquired at maximum b value; *FPR80,* false positive rate given sensitivity 80%; *ROI,* region of interest; *RSI,* restriction spectrum imaging. (Adapted with permission from Andreassen MMS, Rodriguez-Soto AE, Conlin CC, et al. Discrimination of breast cancer from healthy breast tissue using a three-component diffusion-weighted MRI model. *Clin Cancer Res.* 2021;27(4):1094–1104.)

tissue. A model-based denoising method was applied that included a total of 20 isotropic compartments for tumor, vascular, and fat fractions and a composite of 40 anisotropic compartments of varying orientation that constitute normal FGT. From this high-dimensional model-based denoising, fractions of canonical compartments are distilled (restricted, hindered, and free). This denoising strategy also decreased coefficient of variation of many derived breast DWI metrics, importantly for this chapter including FA. Qualitative image quality and differentiation of normal from tumorous regions were improved by this denoising processing. Thus a more complete signal description while applying a denoising approach allowed an improved view of metrics of diffusion anisotropy in the breast, though scan time (10 minutes) remains moderately high.

Viewing this literature together, it is apparent that a new stage of research is emerging beyond characterization of one feature at a time to instead incorporate many signal features in comprehensive models. If the history of diffusion imaging is any indication, these trends will continue to refine both diagnostic and prognostic tools for management of breast cancer patients.

Overview/Outlook

DTI has been demonstrated to provide compelling biomarkers of both FGT and benign/malignant lesions in the human breast. Diffusion anisotropy, most commonly quantified by FA, is a common feature observed in FGT and provides impetus for continued research to depict ductal architecture via diffusion tractography. Of the DTI metrics, MD shows high diagnostic value for lesion malignancy, aggressiveness, and treatment response prediction, whereas anisotropy measures show some complementary utility with less consistency across studies. Applying acquisition schemes with multiple diffusion times and a wide range of b values have potential to amplify both diagnostic utility and biophysical modeling. Multicompartment modeling approaches (RSI, DTD, model-based denoising) including anisotropic elements shows promise for a more complete and ultimately useful tissue description for breast DWI.

Finally, as alluded to throughout this discussion, the clinical potential of DTI reviewed in this volume may only be truly realized at a large scale when combined with efforts of standardization and harmonization for data intended for large-scale pooling and evidence amplification, as recently suggested for breast DWI generally.[4] Such effort does not oppose ongoing innovation of DTI as described here; rather it is a necessary parallel process for the breast imaging community to achieve clinical impact with DTI.

REFERENCES

1. Ei Khouli RH, Jacobs MA, Mezban SD, et al. Diffusion-weighted imaging improves the diagnostic accuracy of conventional 3.0-T breast MR imaging. *Radiology*. 2010;256(1):64–73.
2. Shapiro-Feinberg M, Weisenberg N, Zehavi T, et al. Clinical results of DTI. *Eur J Radiol*. 2012;81(suppl 1):S151–S152.
3. Partridge SC, McDonald ES. Diffusion weighted magnetic resonance imaging of the breast: protocol optimization, interpretation, and clinical applications. *Magn Reson Imaging Clin N Am*. 2013;21(3):601–624.
4. Baltzer P, Mann RM, Iima M, et al. Diffusion-weighted imaging of the breast—a consensus and mission statement from the EUSOBI International Breast Diffusion-Weighted Imaging working group. *Eur Radiol*. 2020;30(3):1436–1450.
5. Iima M, Partridge SC, LE Bihan D. Six DWI questions you always wanted to know but were afraid to ask: clinical relevance for breast diffusion MRI. *Eur Radiol*. 2020;30(5):2561–2570.
6. Le Bihan D, Mangin JF, Poupon C, et al. Diffusion tensor imaging: concepts and applications. *J Magn Reson Imaging*. 2001;13(4):534–546.
7. Froeling M, Nederveen AJ, Nicolay K, Strijkers GJ. DTI of human skeletal muscle: the effects of diffusion encoding parameters, signal-to-noise ratio and T2 on tensor indices and fiber tracts. *NMR Biomed*. 2013;26(11):1339–1352.
8. Jones DK. The effect of gradient sampling schemes on measures derived from diffusion tensor MRI: a Monte Carlo study. *Magn Reson Med*. 2004;51(4):807–815.
9. Jones DK, Horsfield MA, Simmons A. Optimal strategies for measuring diffusion in anisotropic systems by magnetic resonance imaging. *Magn Reson Med*. 1999;42(3):515–525.
10. Wang Y, Zhang XP, Li YL, et al. Optimization of the parameters for diffusion tensor magnetic resonance imaging data acquisition for breast fiber tractography at 1.5 T. *Clin Breast Cancer*. 2014;14(1):61–67.
11. Furman-Haran E, Grobgeld D, Nissan N, Shapiro-Feinberg M, Degani H. Can diffusion tensor anisotropy indices assist in breast cancer detection? *J Magn Reson Imaging*. 2016; 44(6):1624–1632.
12. Partridge SC, Ziadloo A, Murthy R, et al. Diffusion tensor MRI: preliminary anisotropy measures and mapping of breast tumors. *J Magn Reson Imaging*. 2010;31(2):339–347.
13. Tsougos I, Svolos P, Kousi E, et al. The contribution of diffusion tensor imaging and magnetic resonance spectroscopy for the differentiation of breast lesions at 3T. *Acta Radiol*. 2014;55(1):14–23.
14. Baltzer PA, Schafer A, Dietzel M, et al. Diffusion tensor magnetic resonance imaging of the breast: a pilot study. *Eur Radiol*. 2011;21(1):1–10.
15. Cakir O, Arslan A, Inan N, et al. Comparison of the diagnostic performances of diffusion parameters in diffusion weighted

imaging and diffusion tensor imaging of breast lesions. *Eur J Radiol*. 2013;82(12):e801–e806.

16. Eyal E, Shapiro-Feinberg M, Furman-Haran E, et al. Parametric diffusion tensor imaging of the breast. *Invest Radiol*. 2012;47(5):284–291.

17. Teruel JR, Goa PE, Sjobakk TE, Ostlie A, Fjosne HE, Bathen TF. Diffusion weighted imaging for the differentiation of breast tumors: from apparent diffusion coefficient to high order diffusion tensor imaging. *J Magn Reson Imaging*. 2016;43(5):1111–1121.

18. Mehta ML. *Random Matrices*. 2nd ed. Academic Press; 1991.

19. Partridge SC, Murthy RS, Ziadloo A, White SW, Allison KH, Lehman CD. Diffusion tensor magnetic resonance imaging of the normal breast. *Magn Reson Imaging*. 2010;28(3):320–328.

20. Tagliafico A, Rescinito G, Monetti F, et al. Diffusion tensor magnetic resonance imaging of the normal breast: reproducibility of DTI-derived fractional anisotropy and apparent diffusion coefficient at 3.0 T. *Radiol Med*. 2012;117(6):992–1003.

21. Nissan N, Furman-Haran E, Shapiro-Feinberg M, Grobgeld D, Degani H. Diffusion-tensor MR imaging of the breast: hormonal regulation. *Radiology*. 2014;271(3):672–680.

22. Bogner W, Gruber S, Pinker K, et al. Diffusion-weighted MR for differentiation of breast lesions at 3.0 T: how does selection of diffusion protocols affect diagnosis? *Radiology*. 2009;253(2):341–351.

23. Teruel JR, Cho GY, Moccaldi Rt M, et al. Stimulated echo diffusion tensor imaging (STEAM-DTI) with varying diffusion times as a probe of breast tissue. *J Magn Reson Imaging*. 2017;45(1):84–93.

24. Mayr NA, Staples JJ, Robinson RA, Vanmetre JE, Hussey DH. Morphometric studies in intraductal breast carcinoma using computerized image analysis. *Cancer*. 1991;67(11):2805–2812.

25. Einstein A. *Investigations on the Theory of the Brownian Movement*. Dover Publications, Inc; 1956.

26. Simpson J, Carr H. Diffusion and nuclear spin relaxation in water. *Phys Rev*. 1958;111(5):1201–1202.

27. Wiederer J, Pazahr S, Leo C, Nanz D, Boss A. Quantitative breast MRI: 2D histogram analysis of diffusion tensor parameters in normal tissue. *MAGMA*. 2014;27(2):185–193.

28. Taneri F, Kurukahvecioglu O, Akyurek N, et al. Microanatomy of milk ducts in the nipple. *Eur Surg Res*. 2006;38(6):545–549.

29. Rusby JE, Brachtel EF, Michaelson JS, Koerner FC, Smith BL. Breast duct anatomy in the human nipple: three-dimensional patterns and clinical implications. *Breast Cancer Res Treat*. 2007;106(2):171–179.

30. Nissan N, Furman-Haran E, Shapiro-Feinberg M, Grobgeld D, Degani H. Monitoring in-vivo the mammary gland microstructure during morphogenesis from lactating to post-weaning using diffusion tensor MRI. *J Mammary Gland Biol Neoplasia*. 2017;22(3):193–202.

31. Ramsay DT, Kent JC, Hartmann PE. Anatomy of the lactating human breast redefined with ultrasound imaging. *J Anat*. 2005;206(6):525–534.

32. O'Flynn EAM, Morgan VA, Giles SL, deSouza NM. Diffusion weighted imaging of the normal breast: reproducibility of apparent diffusion coefficient measurements and variation with menstrual cycle and menopausal status. *Eur Radiol*. 2012;22(7):1512–1518.

33. Kim JU, Suh HB, KAng HJ, et al. Apparent diffusion coefficient of breast cancer and normal fibroglandular tissue in diffusion-weighted imaging: the effects of menstrual cycle and menopausal status. *Breast Cancer Res Treat*. 2016;157(1):31–40.

34. Shin S, Ko ES, Kim RB, et al. Effect of menstrual cycle and menopausal status on apparent diffusion coefficient values and detectability of invasive ductal carcinoma on diffusion-weighted MRI. *Breast Cancer Res Treat*. 2015;149:751–759.

35. Partridge SC, McKinnon GC, Henry RG, Hylton NM. Menstrual cycle variation of apparent diffusion coefficients measured in the normal breast using MRI. *J Magn Reson Imaging*. 2001;14(4):433–438.

36. Clendenen TV, Kim S, Moy L, et al. Magnetic resonance imaging (MRI) of hormone-induced breast changes in young premenopausal women. *Magn Reson Imaging*. 2013;31(1):1–9.

37. Shi R, Yao Q, Wu L, Xu J. Breast lesions: diagnosis using diffusion weighted imaging at 1.5T and 3.0T—systematic review and meta-analysis. *Clin Breast Cancer*. 2018;18(3):e305–e320.

38. Vogel PM, Feorgiade NG, Fetter BF, Vogel SF, McCarty KS. The correlation of histologic changes in the human breast with the menstrual cycle. *Am J Pathol*. 1981;104(1):23–34.

39. Weinstein SP, Conant EF, Sehgal CM, Woo IP, Patton JA. Hormonal variations in the vascularity of breast tissue. *J Ultrasound Med*. 2005;24(1):67–72.

40. Söderqvist G. Effects of sex steroids on proliferation in normal mammary tissue. *Ann Med*. 1998;30(6):511–524.

41. Geddes DT. Inside the lactating breast: the latest anatomy research. *J Midwifery Womens Health*. 2007;52(6):556–563.

42. Nissan N, Furman-Haran E, Allweis T, et al. Noncontrast breast MRI during pregnancy using diffusion tensor imaging: a feasibility study. *J Magn Reson Imaging*. 2019;49(2):508–517.

43. Cooper AP. *Anatomy of the Breast*. London; 1840.

44. Ohtake T, Kimijima I, Fukushima T, et al. Computer-assisted complete three-dimensional reconstruction of the mammary ductal/lobular systems: implications of ductal anastomoses for breast-conserving surgery. *Cancer*. 2001;91(12):2263–2272.

45. Love SM, Barsky SH. Anatomy of the nipple and breast ducts revisited. *Cancer*. 2004;101(9):1947–1957.

46. Going JJ, Moffat DF. Escaping from Flatland: clinical and biological aspects of human mammary duct anatomy in three dimensions. *J Pathol*. 2004;203(1):538–544.

47. Cardenosa G, Doudna C, Eklund GW. Ductography of the breast: technique and findings. *AJR Am J Roentgenol*. 1994;162(5):1081–1087.

48. Kanemaki Y, Kurihara Y, Itoh D, et al. MR mammary ductography using microscopy coil for assessment of intraductal lesions. *Am J Roentgenol*. 2004;182(5):1340–1342.

49. Gooding MJ, Mellor M, Shipley JA, Broadbent KA, Goddard DA. Automatic mammary duct detection in 3D ultrasound. *Med Image Comput Comput Assist Interv*. 2005;8(pt 1):434–441.

50. Nissan N, Furman-Haran E, Feinberg-Shapiro M, et al. Tracking the mammary architectural features and detecting breast cancer with magnetic resonance diffusion tensor imaging. *J Vis Exp*. 2014;94:52048.

51. Basser PJ, Mattiello M, LeBijan D. MR diffusion tensor spectroscopy and imaging. *Biophys J*. 1994;66(1):259–267.

52. Reisert M, Weigel M, Eyal E, Grobgeld D, Degani H, Hennig J. Diffusion tensor based reconstruction of the ductal tree. Paper presented at: Annual Meeting of the International Society of Magnetic Resonance in Medicine (ISMRM). May 7–13, Montreal, Canada; 2011.

53. Kerher BW, Schnell S, Mader I, et al. Connecting and merging fibers: pathway extraction by combining probability maps. *Neuroimage*. 2008;43(1):81–89.

54. Wang K, Li Z, Wu Z, et al. Diagnostic performance of diffusion tensor imaging for characterizing breast tumors: a comprehensive meta-analysis. *Front Oncol*. 2019;9:1229.

55. Ozal ST, Inci E, Gemici AA, Turgut H, Cikot M, Karabulut M. Can 3.0 tesla diffusion tensor imaging parameters be prognostic indicators in breast cancer? *Clin Imaging*. 2018;51:240–247.

56. Luo J, Hippe DS, Rahbar H, Parsian S, Rendi MH, Partridge SC. Diffusion tensor imaging for characterizing tumor microstructure and improving diagnostic performance on breast MRI: a prospective observational study. *Breast Cancer Res*. 2019;21(1):102.

57. Jiang R, Ma Z, Dong H, Sun S, Zeng X, Li X. Diffusion tensor imaging of breast lesions: evaluation of apparent diffusion coefficient and fractional anisotropy and tissue cellularity. *Br J Radiol*. 2016;89(1064): 20160076.

58. Kim JY, Kim JJ, Kim S, et al. Diffusion tensor magnetic resonance imaging of breast cancer: associations between diffusion metrics and histological prognostic factors. *Eur Radiol*. 2018;28(8):3185–3193.

59. Bickel H, Pinker-Domenig K, Bogner W, et al. Quantitative apparent diffusion coefficient as a noninvasive imaging biomarker for the differentiation of invasive breast cancer and ductal carcinoma in situ. *Invest Radiol*. 2015;50(2):95–100.

60. Yamaguchi K, Nakazono T, Egashira R, et al. Diagnostic performance of diffusion tensor imaging with readout-segmented echo-planar imaging for invasive breast cancer: correlation of ADC and FA with pathological prognostic markers. *Magn Reson Med Sci*. 2017;16(3):245–252.

61. Kakkad S, Zhang J, Akhbardeh A, et al. Collagen fibers mediate MRI-detected water diffusion and anisotropy in breast cancers. *Neoplasia*. 2016;18(10):585–593.

62. Bailey C, Siow B, Panagiotaki E, et al. Microstructural models for diffusion MRI in breast cancer and surrounding stroma: an ex vivo study. *NMR Biomed*. 2017;30(2):e3679.

63. Egnell L, Vidic I, Jerome NP, Bofin AM, Bathen TF, Goa PE. Stromal collagen content in breast tumors correlates with in vivo diffusion-weighted imaging: a comparison of multi b value DWI with histologic specimen from benign and malignant breast lesions. *J Magn Reson Imaging*. 2020;51(6):1868–1878.

64. Wilmes LJ, Li W, Shin HJ, et al. Diffusion tensor imaging for assessment of response to neoadjuvant chemotherapy in patients with breast cancer. *Tomography*. 2016;2(4):438–447.

65. Furman-Haran E, Nissan N, Ricart-Selma V, Martinez-Rubio C, Degani H, Camps-Herrero J. Quantitative evaluation of breast cancer response to neoadjuvant chemotherapy by diffusion tensor imaging: initial results. *J Magn Reson Imaging*. 2018;47(4):1080–1090.

66. Gluud C, Gluud LL. Evidence based diagnostics. *BMJ*. 2005;330(7493):724–726.

67. Iima M, Nobashi T, Imai H, et al. Effects of diffusion time on non-Gaussian diffusion and intravoxel incoherent motion (IVIM) MRI parameters in breast cancer and hepatocellular carcinoma xenograft models. *Acta Radiol Open*. 2018;7(1): 2058460117751565.

68. Iima M, Kataoka M, Honda M, et al. The rate of apparent diffusion coefficient change with diffusion time on breast diffusion-weighted imaging depends on breast tumor types and molecular prognostic biomarker expression. *Invest Radiol*. 2021;56(8):501–508.

69. White NS, McDonald C, Farid N, et al. Diffusion-weighted imaging in cancer: physical foundations and applications of restriction spectrum imaging. *Cancer Res*. 2014;74(17): 4638–4652.

70. Andreassen MMS, Rodriguez-Soto AE, Conlin CC, et al. Discrimination of breast cancer from healthy breast tissue using a three-component diffusion-weighted MRI model. *Clin Cancer Res*. 2021;27(4):1094–1104.

71. Reymbaut A, Zheng Y, Li S, et al. Clinical research with advanced diffusion encoding methods in MRI. In: Topgaard D, ed. *Advanced Diffusion Encoding Methods in MRI*. Royal Society of Chemistry; 2020.

72. Naranjo ID, Reymbaut A, Brynolfsson P, Lo Gullo R, Bryskhe K, Topgaard D, Giri DD, Reiner JS, Thakur SB, Pinker-Domenig K. Multidimensional diffusion magnetic resonance imaging for characterization of tissue microstructure in breast cancer patients: a prospective pilot study. *Cancers (Basel)* 2021;13(7): 1606.

73. Tan ET, Wilmes LJ, Joe BN, et al. Denoising and multiple tissue compartment visualization of multi-*b*-valued breast diffusion MRI. *J Magn Reson Imaging*. 2021;53(1):271–282.

74. Sperl JI, Sprenger T, Tan ET, Menzel MI, Hardy CJ, Marinelli L. Model-based denoising in diffusion-weighted imaging using generalized spherical deconvolution. *Magn Reson Med*. 2017;78(6):2428–2438.

75. Jiang R, Zeng X, Sun S, Ma Z, Wang X. Assessing detection, discrimination, and risk of breast cancer according to anisotropy parameters of diffusion tensor imaging. *Med Sci Monit*. 2016;22:1318–1328.

76. Wang Y, Zhang X, Cao K, Li Y, Li X, Qi L, Tang L, Wang Z, Gao S. Diffusion-tensor imaging as an adjunct to dynamic contrast-enhanced MRI for improved accuracy of differential diagnosis between breast ductal carcinoma in situ and invasive breast carcinoma. *Chin J Cancer Res* 2015;27(2):209–217. doi: 10.3978/j.issn.1000–9604.2015.03.04

77. Plaza MJ, Morris EA, Thakur SB. Diffusion tensor imaging in the normal breast: influences of fibroglandular tissue composition and background parenchymal enhancement. *Clinical Imaging* 2016;40(3):506–511.

78. Scaranelo AM, Degani H, Grobgeld D, Talbot N, Bodolai K, Furman-Haran E. Effect of IV Administration of a Gadolinium-Based Contrast Agent on Breast Diffusion-Tensor Imaging. *American Journal of Roentgenology* 2020;215(4):1030–1036.

Artificial Intelligence—Enhanced Breast MRI and DWI: Current Status and Future Applications

Katja Pinker, MD, PhD, Roberto Lo Gullo, MD, Sarah Eskreis-Winkler, MD, PhD, Almir Bitencourt, MD, Peter Gibbs, PhD, and Sunitha B. Thakur, MSc, PhD

Background

Personalized medicine is yielding increasingly precise treatment and prevention strategies for groups of individuals based on their genetic makeup, environment, and lifestyle, as enabled by approaches including genomics, transcriptomics, proteomics, metabolomics, and so forth. In oncology, the goal of using such approaches is to increasingly harness individual-level information versus population-level or traditional clinical information (e.g., tumor stage, age, gender) to select the most successful cancer treatment regimen for each patient.[1]

Molecular tumor characterization can be performed using genomic and proteomic approaches, but this requires tissue sampling from invasive surgery or biopsy.[2] Currently, large-scale genome cancer characterization that would include genetic testing for every individual is not feasible because of the high costs, considerable time burden, and technically complex data analysis and interpretation.[3] Moreover, even when molecular characterization is performed using tissue sampling, samples may not accurately represent the entire lesion as they are often obtained from a small portion of a heterogeneous lesion with inherent selection bias during biopsy.[3]

By contrast, imaging can provide a more comprehensive view of the tumor in its entirety via radiomics and radiogenomics. Radiomics is an approach pertaining to the extraction and correlation of multiple imaging parameters with different variables of interest (patient characteristics as well as histopathologic, genomic, molecular, or outcome data) to create decision support models. Such models can be used for multiple purposes, such as treatment planning, risk assessment, and outcome prediction. When imaging data is correlated with genetic data in particular, this approach is referred to as radiogenomics.[1–3] Coupling with artificial intelligence (AI) techniques allows us to more fully harness the power of radiomics/genomics. Because of the noninvasive nature of medical imaging and its ubiquitous use in clinical practice, the field of AI-enhanced imaging is rapidly evolving.[4–7]

With continuous advances in radiomics analysis and machine learning (ML), such as deep learning (DL), we are now on the cusp of providing more effective, more efficient, and even more patient-centric breast cancer care than ever before. In this chapter, we will begin with the basic concepts of radiomics, radiogenomics, and AI methodology in breast magnetic resonance imaging (MRI). The rest of the chapter will be devoted to reviewing AI-enhanced MRI and AI-enhanced diffusion-weighted imaging (DWI), whereby we will present the current knowledge and future applications of AI-enhanced MRI and DWI in clinical practice and address their challenges and limitations.

Basic Concepts of Radiomics and AI Methodology

Radiomics analysis can be divided into two arms based on how imaging information is transformed into mineable data: handcrafted and AI based (Fig. 10.1). Handcrafted radiomics extracts features that are used to fingerprint phenotypical characteristics in images, whereas AI uses a complex network to create its own features.

Handcrafted radiomics methodology usually follows this workflow: image acquisition (2D, 3D, 4D); normalization to pixel intensities evenly across a data set and within a standardized range; image annotation and segmentation (manual, semiautomatic, or fully automatic; Fig. 10.2) and for definition of region of interest (ROI) and feature extraction; radiomics analysis (feature selection and reduction); and classification and modeling. Handcrafted radiomics analysis includes first-order features based on the distribution of pixel intensities (histogram based) and higher-order features based on how pixels are positioned in relation to each other (e.g., co-occurrence matrices, run length matrices, size zone matrices, neighborhood gray-level dependence matrices, Minkowski functionals, local binary patterns, wavelet analysis). Because a large quantity of imaging features are extracted, which are not necessarily all relevant to the task proposed to the model, feature selection and reduction is an essential step, followed by classification and modeling to answer the specific question we are proposing. Handcrafted radiomics studies typically use AI methods (e.g., decision trees, support vector machines, random forests, neural networks) to select features and construct models. Ideally, the model's performance should be validated in external data sets to avoid overfitting, which refers to spurious correlations in the data that do not allow generalization to other similar data sets. If no external validation data set is available, cross-validation techniques can be applied to split the data into different subsets (training and validation sets). To be able to expand the interoperability of models to all hardware, acquisition, and reconstruction parameters in general clinical practice, rigorous standardization is necessary but is hard to achieve. Standardized data collection, evaluation criteria, and reporting guidelines will be required for radiomics to mature as a discipline. To gauge the quality of published radiomics studies, a radiomics quality score has been proposed (Fig. 10.3),[4] and to address the issue of radiomic feature reproducibility, some harmonization methods such as Combine Batches (ComBat) have been investigated in the literature.[5]

DL is a new class of ML that uses neural networks with multiple layers of processing inspired by human brain architecture. In contrast to traditional radiomics-based ML approaches, where humans engage in handcrafted feature extraction, DL networks learn both the

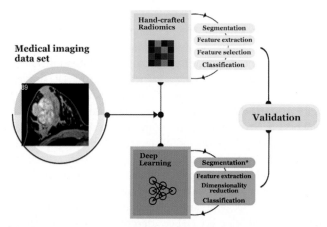

Fig. 10.1 Development of imaging biomarkers using quantitative image analysis. *Segmentation is not a necessity in the automated radiomics pipeline. (Modified and reprinted with permission from Ibrahim A, Primakov S, Beuque M, et al. Radiomics for precision medicine: current challenges, future prospects, and the proposal of a new framework. *Methods.* 2021;188:20–29.)

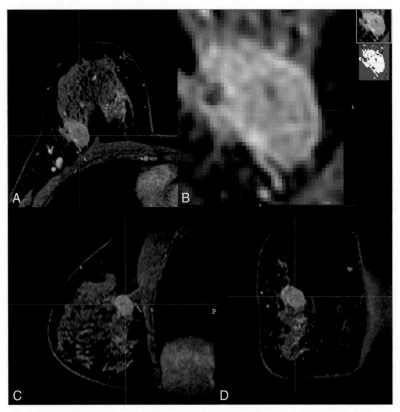

Fig. 10.2 Example of manual semiautomated tumor segmentation using edge-based snakes. Dynamic contrast-enhanced MRI and segmented region indicated in red: (A) axial, (B) axial detail, (C) sagittal, and (D) coronal—for radiomics analysis in a 43-year-old woman with a biopsy-proven, poorly differentiated triple negative (TN) breast cancer in the 10 o'clock axis of the left breast.

feature extraction and classification steps in tandem and are able to extract very high-level features from imaging data. These recent advances in software and also hardware (to support higher computational power requirements) have given DL models the potential to surpass human performance in some image analyses tasks.

To date, most DL applications in medical imaging use convolutional neural networks (CNNs), which are particularly well suited to visual tasks. CNNs can be used for both image classification and image segmentation. In supervised learning approaches, which constitute almost all the DL in medical imaging literature to date, it is necessary to supply the CNN with large numbers of labeled imaging data. To develop a CNN model, imaging data sets must be divided into three independent groups: training, validation, and testing

data sets. First the DL model is trained on the training set images and learns to predict the label. This process is repeated many times with different model hyperparameters, with intermittent evaluation of performance using the validation data set to prevent overfitting. Then, once the DL model parameters and hyperparameters have been finalized, the held-out test set is used to evaluate final CNN performance and results are reported with a standard set of relevant statistical metrics (e.g., area under the curve [AUC], precision recall, sensitivity, specificity). DL studies must pass through rigorous validation steps, which includes definition of the image sets (training, validation, and test sets) and ground truth reference standard; detailed description of the model, training approach, and metrics of model performance; and validation or testing on external data.[11,12]

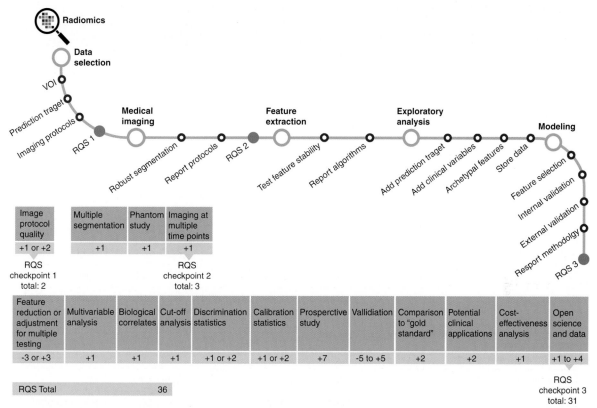

Fig. 10.3 Flowchart depicting the workflow of radiomics and the application of the RQS. The workflow includes the necessary steps in a radiomic analysis. The RQS both rewards and penalizes the methodology and analyses of a study, consequently encouraging the best scientific practice. *RQS*, Radiomics quality score; *VOI*, volume of interest. (Reprinted with permission from Lambin P, Leijenaar RTH, Deist TM, et al. Radiomics: the bridge between medical imaging and personalized medicine. *Nat Rev Clin Oncol.* 2017;14(12):749–762.)

Further reviews of the process of radiomics/genomics analysis coupled with AI (image acquisition, volume of interest selection, segmentation, feature extraction and quantification, database building, classifier modeling, and data sharing) are described in detail elsewhere.[4,6–14]

AI-Enhanced Breast MRI

Breast MRI is the most sensitive modality for breast cancer detection, with a pooled sensitivity of 93% and pooled specificity of 71%.[15] Dynamic contrast-enhanced MRI (DCE MRI) is the primary sequence of the breast MRI examination, which relies on intravenous injection of a gadolinium-based contrast agent and provides excellent morphological information and functional information about abnormal vascularization as a tumor-specific feature. DCE MRI is regarded as the most sensitive imaging technique for breast cancer detection. However, it has been criticized for its variable specificity.

To overcome limitations in DCE MRI specificity and to obtain more valuable functional data, additional MRI sequences have been combined with DCE MRI; this approach is known as multiparametric MRI (mpMRI). In the multiparametric context, DWI with apparent diffusion coefficient (ADC) mapping or more advanced markers (see Chapter 8) has emerged as the most robust and valuable additional parameter, with a reported sensitivity of up to 96% for breast cancer detection and a specificity of up to 100% for breast tumor characterization; it is therefore increasingly implemented in clinical routine.[16–19]

Compared with other imaging modalities, breast MRI is the most sensitive for detection and

TABLE 10.1   Current Studies and Their Use Cases for Artificial Intelligence (AI)-Enhanced Breast Diffusion-Weighted Imaging (DWI)

Use Case	Field Strength (T)	b-Values	Segmentation	Input	AI Approach
Detection					
Bickelhaupt et al.[26]	1.5	0, 1500	3D, manual	DWI, DWIBS, ADC	Radiomics/ML
Dalmis et al.[21]	3	50, 800	2D, marker placement	DCE, T2, ADC	DL
Lo Gullo et al.[29]	1.5/3	0, 800	2D, semiautomated	DCE, ADC	Radiomics/ML
Molecular Subtyping					
Leithner et al.[49]	3	0, 1000	2D, manual	DCE, ADC	Radiomics/ML
Leithner et al.[50]	3	0, 1000	2D, manual	ADC	Radiomics/ML
Sun et al.[52]	1.5/3	0, 1000	2D, manual	DCE, DWI	Radiomics/ML
Xie et al.[53]	3	0, 400, 800	3D, semiautomated	DCE, ADC	Radiomics/ML
Zhang et al.[54]	3	50,800	3D, semiautomated	ADC	Radiomics/ML
Treatment Response Prediction and Assessment					
Amornsiripanitch et al.[69]	3	0, 800	2D, manual	DWI, ADC	ML
Liu et al.[60]	3	0, 1000	3D, manual	DCE, T2, DWI, ADC	Radiomics/ML
Tahmassebi et al.[59]	3	50,850	n/a	DCE, T2, ADC	ML
Thakur et al.[68]	3	0, 600, 800	2D, manual	DWI, ADC	n/a

ADC, Apparent diffusion coefficient; *DCE*, dynamic contrast enhanced; *DL*, deep learning; *DWIBS*, DWI with background suppression; *ML*, machine learning.

additionally offers quantitative biomarkers with value for breast cancer diagnosis. As a result, it is well suited to AI-based research, and AI-enhanced breast MRI is increasingly studied for a variety of applications, particularly for lesion detection and classification.[20] Table 10.1 summarizes the current studies and its use cases for AI-enhanced breast DWI.

Use Cases

DETECTION

Fully automated detection of breast cancer on screening MRI using CNN has shown to be possible, not only for systematic diagnostic interpretation[21] but also to identify tumor-containing slices stored on picture archiving and communication systems.[22] The latter can be particularly useful for nonsystematic image review, such as for research purposes or interdisciplinary tumor board meetings. The growing use of breast MRI for both screening and conventional imaging problem-solving purposes has posed significant challenges in clinical practice due to the high number of incidental MR-detected lesions. In this context, different approaches have been tested to help classify breast lesions identified on MRI as benign or malignant.[21,23–25] For example, Truhn and colleagues[23] compared the diagnostic performance of radiomics with ML and CNN to radiologists for the classification of DCE MRI–enhancing lesions. They evaluated 447 patients with 1294 lesions and found that CNN (AUC = 0.88) was superior to radiomics/ML (AUC = 0.81) for lesion classification, but both approaches were inferior to radiologists' performance.

Focusing on DWI used in a biparametric contrast-agent-free MRI context, Bickelhaupt and colleagues[26] investigated radiomics with DWI in combination with T2-weighted imaging for the classification of lesions that were deemed to be suspicious on breast cancer screening with mammography as benign and malignant. In this study, 50 asymptomatic women who underwent screening mammography and who were diagnosed with a suspicious finding were examined with multiparametric MRI with DCE, T2-weighted, DWI, and DWI with background suppression (DWIBS) sequences with ADC mapping. For the purpose of this study, out of this standard multiparametric MRI protocol an unenhanced, abbreviated DWI (ueMRI) including T2-weighted, DWI, and DWIBS sequences and corresponding DC maps was extracted and used for radiomics analysis. Three-dimensional segmentations of the MR index lesions were generated manually and performed separately on T2TSE images, and DWIBS *b*-1500 images and radiomics features were extracted. Segmentations of the background parenchyma on DWIBS *b*-1500 images and normal-appearing fat on the T2-weighted image, which were used to normalize the MR intensities of the corresponding images in terms of lesion-to-background ratio, were performed. In addition to radiomics analysis, an expert radiologist assessed this unenhanced abbreviated protocol for lesion classification as well as a full multiparametric protocol, including DCE MRI. From the ueMRI with DWI, DWIBS, and T2-weighted imaging, three Lasso-supervised ML classifiers were constructed (i.e., univariate mean ADC model, unconstrained radiomic model, and constrained radiomic model with mandatory inclusion of mean ADC) and compared with the clinical performance of a highly experienced radiologist. The radiomic classifiers allowed a differentiation of malignant from benign lesions with a AUC of 84.2% for the unconstrained and 85.1% for the constrained, respectively, compared with 77.4% for mean ADC and 95.9% for the ueMRI protocol and 95.9% for the full multiparametric protocol of the experienced radiologist. The results of this study indicate that DWI

radiomics classifiers can perform well in breast cancer diagnosis and achieve higher performance than the mean ADC parameter alone. Diagnostic performance was lower than that of an experienced breast radiologist, but results indicate the potential of AI-enhanced DWI to provide a diagnostic decision tool to benefit less-experienced readers to achieve near expert reader performance.

Dalmis and colleagues[21] also applied AI for classification of breast lesions using a multiparametric MRI protocol with ultrafast DCE MRI, T2-weighted imaging, and DWI. A final AI system combining all imaging information achieved an AUC of 0.852, significantly higher than ultrafast DCE alone ($P = .002$) and with fewer false positives when operating at the same sensitivity level of radiologists. Thus, the application of AI for the interpretation of multiparametric breast MRI may improve specificity, reducing the number of unnecessary breast biopsies. In another study, a similar conclusion was reached using a DCE MRI radiomics AI 4D classifier including automatically extracting BI-RADS curve types and pharmacokinetic enhancement features, which was able to avoid up to 36.2% of unnecessary biopsies.[27]

The ability to accurately classify and reduce the number of unnecessary breast biopsies is particularly important in the setting of screening-detected, nonpalpable lesions such as subcentimeter lesions, nonmass-like lesions, and high-risk lesions. AI can improve the diagnosis of these type of lesions in breast MRI.[28] For example, Lo Gullo and colleagues[29] evaluated subcentimeter enhancing lesions in *BRCA* mutation carriers and showed that radiomics/ML based on multiparametric breast MRI improved diagnostic accuracy compared with qualitative morphological assessment using BI-RADS classification and could be used as an adjunct to spare unnecessary biopsies for benign-appearing small breast masses in this population. However, DWI signal analysis did not contribute to the accuracy of assessing these lesions; the authors stated that this might be partly due to the limited spatial resolution of DWI, which makes it challenging to accurately evaluate subcentimeter masses on DWI. In another study, the same group investigated whether radiomics coupled with ML based on multiparametric MRI could help in predicting malignant upgrade in atypical ductal hyperplasia (a high-risk lesion) to avoid surgical excision.[30] Unfortunately, this approach was not able to accurately predict which biopsy-proven atypical ductal hyperplasia lesions would be upgraded to malignancy; radiomic features from DWI in particular did not add any value to the ML model.

MOLECULAR SUBTYPING

In the past decade, gene-expression profiling has revolutionized breast cancer classification and replaced traditional categorizations based on immunohistochemistry with molecular subtypes.[31,32] Four intrinsic molecular subtypes of breast cancer have been revealed from extensive profiling at the DNA, microRNA, and protein levels by the Cancer Genome Atlas (TCGA) Network[33]: luminal A, luminal B, HER2-enriched, and triple negative (TN). Molecular breast cancer subtypes are unevenly distributed within patients, occur with different tumor phenotypes, and are associated with distinct prognosis, response to treatment, preferential sites of metastasis, and recurrence or disease-free survival outcomes.[34] Since 2011, the St. Gallen International Expert Consensus panel has maintained molecular subtype–based recommendations for systemic therapies for breast cancer.[31,32]

Associations between MRI characteristics and molecular breast cancer subtypes have been investigated in several studies. In a systematic review and meta-analysis published in 2014, Elias and colleagues[35] reported that higher tumoral enhancement is associated with the luminal B subtype, whereas HER2-enriched cancers are more likely to show fast initial enhancement or washout kinetics with circumscribed margins. Elsewhere, TN cancers have been associated with high T2 signal intensity and the presence of rim enhancement.[36,37] In a more recent study by Grimm and colleagues,[38] associations between breast MRI findings using the BI-RADS lexicon descriptors and breast cancer molecular subtypes were assessed. For this purpose, qualitative BI-RADS descriptors were evaluated on DCE MRI in 278 patients with breast cancer presenting as masses or nonmass enhancement (NME); results showed significant correlations between mass shape and basal cancers, mass margin and HER2 cancers, and internal enhancement and luminal B cancers. In another study, Yamaguchi and colleagues[39] assessed the relationship between the delayed phase of enhancement of DCE

MRI and molecular subtypes, finding that ER-positive and/or PgR-positive and HER2-negative cancers demonstrated less washout. Focusing on DWI in particular, HER2-enriched tumors have been shown to have the highest ADC values, whereas luminal B/HER2-negative cancers showed the lowest values.[40–42]

More recently, radiomic features have themselves been associated with molecular breast cancer subtypes. While most of the data is available for DCE MRI, the concept of molecular subtyping can be extended to other MRI sequences including DWI.

In DCE MRI, Mazurowski and colleagues[43] showed that extracted MRI radiomics features that relate to an increased ratio of tumor-to-background parenchymal enhancement were associated with HER2-positive cancers. This difference might be due to the increased vascularization found in HER2-positive subtypes mediated by VEGF, which leads to increased vessel diameter, vascular permeability, and extracellular fluid. Grimm and colleagues[44] found correlations between extracted morphological, texture, and dynamic radiomics features from routine MRI and luminal A and B breast cancer subtypes. In a study including 143 patients, Leithner and colleagues evaluated the diagnostic performance of radiomic signatures extracted from DCE MRI for the assessment of breast cancer receptor status and molecular subtypes.[45] In the training data set, radiomic signatures yielded the following accuracies >80%: luminal B versus luminal A, 84.2% (mainly based on co-occurrence matrix [COM] features); luminal B versus TN, 83.9% (mainly based on geometry features [GEO]); luminal B versus all others, 89% (mainly based on COM features); and HER2-enriched versus all others, 81.3% (mainly based on COM features). Radiomic signatures were successfully validated in the separate validation data set for luminal A versus luminal B (79.4%) and luminal B versus TN (77.1%). The authors concluded that radiomic signatures with DCE MRI have the potential for the assessment of breast cancer receptor status and molecular subtypes with high diagnostic accuracy. Other studies reported similar findings, and the data indicates that specific molecular subtypes seem to carry radiomics signatures on DCE MRI images that can be used to accurately classify lesions with respect to receptor status and molecular subtypes.[45–48] These signatures may have the potential to provide prognostic indicators derived from the whole tumor, while biopsy

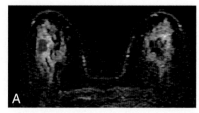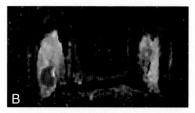

Fig. 10.4 (A) ADC map of a 49-year-old patient with a luminal A cancer in the right breast. (B) ADC map of a 67-year-old patient with a luminal B cancer in the right breast. In our patient, collective and radiomic signatures derived from DWI differentiated luminal A from luminal B cancers with an accuracy of 91.5% when tumor segmentation was performed on the ADC map (89.5% when segmented on high b-value DWI and copied to the ADC map). *ADC*, Apparent diffusion coefficient; *DWI*, diffusion-weighted imaging. (Reprinted with permission from Leithner D, Bernard-Davila B, Martinez DF, et al. Radiomic signatures derived from diffusion-weighted imaging for the assessment of breast cancer receptor status and molecular subtypes. *Mol Imaging Biol*. 2020;22(2):453–461.)

sampling, currently used for molecular subtyping, is only giving a portion of the bigger picture. This could be especially useful to monitor biological changes during treatment, which may vary throughout the tumor.

Focusing on DWI in particular, in a study by Leithner and colleagues,[49] features extracted from ADC maps achieved accuracies over 80% for breast cancer subtype differentiation. The authors found that luminal B and HER2-positive cancers seemed to carry distinct radiomic features that were different from others. Further investigation with multiparametric MRI also showed AUCs over 0.80 for noninvasive differentiation of TN and luminal A breast cancers from other subtypes.[50] Accuracy was superior for radiomics features extracted directly from the ADC map (Fig. 10.4). In another recent study, Wang and colleagues explored whether radiomic features on DWI can be used to identify TN breast cancer (TNBC) and other subtypes (non-TNBC). They showed that breast tumors exhibit differences in radiomic features with DWI, allowing a good discrimination between TNBC and non-TNBC tumors with an accuracy of 83.4% and an AUC of 0.804.[51]

To further exploit the combined benefits of breast multiparametric MRI in this context, several authors have assessed the performance of multiparametric MRI-based radiomics in conjunction with AI for the assessment of breast cancer receptor status and molecular subtypes (Leithner and colleagues; Fig. 10.5).[50,52,53] Results indicate that radiomics signatures derived from multiparametric MRI enable the determination of certain treatment-naïve molecular breast cancer subtypes with high accuracy. Although radiomics and AI are unlikely to replace invasive tissue sampling, multiparametric radiomics imaging biomarkers could

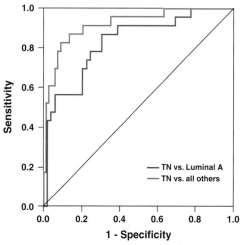

Fig. 10.5 Multilayer perceptron feed-forward artificial neural network–based separation of luminal A and triple negative cancers. The separation yielded an overall median area under the receiver operating characteristic (ROC) curve (area under the curve [AUC]) of 0.8 (0.75–0.83), with median accuracies of 74% in the training data set and 68.2% in the validation data set *(blue ROC curve)*. The separation of TN from all other cancers was even more successful, with an overall median AUC of 0.86 (0.77–0.92), with median accuracies of 85.9% in the training data set and 85.2% in the validation data set *(red ROC curve)*. *ROC*, Receiver operating characteristic; *TN*, triple negative. (Reprinted with permission from Leithner D, Mayerhoefer ME, Martinez DF, et al. Non-invasive assessment of breast cancer molecular subtypes with multiparametric magnetic resonance imaging radiomics. *J Clin Med*. 2020;9(6):1853.)

potentially serve as auxiliary parameters and provide a noninvasive method to derive prognostic and predictive information from the entire tumor before and during treatment.

In efforts to noninvasively assess breast cancer proliferation rates with DWI, Zhang and colleagues[54] developed a radiomics model for predicting the Ki-67 proliferation index in patients with invasive ductal breast cancer preoperatively. Radiomics features were extracted from ADC maps, and a good identification ability was shown for the ADC-based radiomics model, with AUCs of 0.72 in the test set for differentiation of low (Ki-67 proliferation index <14%) and high (Ki-67 proliferation index ≥ 14%) Ki-67 expression. Advanced DWI relying on intravoxel incoherent motion (IVIM) and non-Gaussian diffusion (see Chapter 8) have also shown that some markers, such as the shifted ADC and the tissue signature index, could predict ER, PgR, HER2, and Ki-67 status noninvasively.[19,55]

Recently Bismeijer and colleagues[56] linked gene expression levels from RNA sequencing to seven DCE MRI radiomics features (tumor size, shape, initial enhancement, late enhancement, smoothness of enhancement, sharpness, and sharpness variation). They found an association between enhancement and sharpness of the tumor margin and the expression of ribosomal proteins, which suggests that MRI features may be imaging biomarkers for drugs targeting the ribosome.

TREATMENT RESPONSE PREDICTION AND ASSESSMENT

AI-enhanced MRI has been used to predict response to neoadjuvant chemotherapy (NAC) at an early stage or even before the commencement of NAC.[57,58] This application of AI would be useful to avoid administering ineffective potentially toxic therapies and to expedite surgery in patients who would not benefit from neoadjuvant chemotherapy. Furthermore, there is interest to determine whether surgery can be potentially avoided in patients with pathological complete response (pCR) after NAC, which relies on accurate noninvasive determination of pCR. Tahmassebi and colleagues[59] showed that ML with multiparametric MRI allowed early prediction of pCR after only two cycles of NAC (AUC: 0.86) and survival outcomes with high accuracy. In this study, the most relevant features for the prediction of pCR were changes in lesion size, pattern of shrinkage, and mean transit time on DCE MRI; minimum apparent ADC on DWI; and peritumoral edema on T2-weighted imaging. Similar results were achieved by a radiomics multiparametric model in a multicenter study; this model included four radiomic signatures based on pre-NAC T2-weighted

imaging, DWI, and contrast-enhanced T1-weighted imaging.[60] When Ha and colleagues investigated the response of axillary nodes in particular to NAC, the developed CNN algorithm based on primary breast cancer features achieved an accuracy of 83% to predict axillary response to NAC using pretreatment breast MRI.[61]

The prediction of response to NAC in HER2-positive patients in particular has been reported with AI-enhanced DCE MRI but not yet with AI-enhanced DWI. Bitencourt and colleagues used clinical and MRI radiomic features coupled with ML to assess HER2 expression level and predict pCR in HER2 overexpressing breast cancer patients receiving NAC.[62] In this retrospective study, which included 311 patients with an overall pCR rate of 60.5%, selected radiomics parameters were advanced to ML modeling alongside clinical MRI-based parameters (lesion type, multifocality, size, and nodal status). The final model to predict HER2 heterogeneity used three MRI parameters (two clinical, one radiomic) for a sensitivity of 99.3%, specificity of 81.3%, and diagnostic accuracy of 97.4%. The final model to predict pCR included six MRI parameters (two clinical, four radiomic) for a sensitivity of 86.5%, specificity of 80.0%, and diagnostic accuracy of 83.9%. The authors concluded that ML models including both clinical and radiomics MRI features can be used to assess HER2 expression level and predict pCR after NAC in HER2-overexpressing breast cancer patients. HER2-positive cancer response was also the focus of another work conducted by Braman and colleagues,[63] where they investigated intra- and peritumoral features on DCE MRI. Their model was able to identify HER2 breast cancer subtype with an AUC of 0.89 and predict NAC response to HER2-targeted therapy in both validation cohorts (AUC = 0.80 and 0.69, respectively).

More recently, Sutton and colleagues[64] developed a model that combined radiomics features, based on both pre- and post- DCE MRI before surgery, with molecular subtypes to predict pCR; the model achieved an AUC of 0.78 on the test set, and the authors noted that these findings are particularly relevant for potentially allowing some breast cancer patients to avoid surgery in the future, in contrast to all breast cancer patients needing to undergo surgery after NAC. Although promising, more work must be done to improve modeling performance for pCR prediction even further to warrant its application for clinical decision making.

Using a radiogenomics approach, Mehta and colleagues[65] associated MR perfusion parameters with early metastasis or with differential gene expression when monitoring anti-VEGF treatment. In another radiogenomics study, Yamamoto and colleagues[66] evaluated a qualitative imaging model including tumor heterogeneity and enhancement for prediction of expression of immune-response genes, and high-level analysis revealed 21 imaging traits that were globally significantly correlated with 71% of the total genes (3717/5231 genes) measured in breast cancer patients.

RECURRENCE SCORES

The prediction of cancer recurrence is another relevant clinical query. Currently, this is clinically assessed through multigene assays (e.g., Oncotype DX, MammaPrint, and PAM50), which have been shown to predict recurrence in early-stage ER-positive/HER2-negative invasive cancers. However, such genetic testing is relatively costly and may not be available for all patients. Thus imaging characteristics have been correlated with assay recurrence scores, which could have important implications in patient management. For example, Woodard and colleagues[67] evaluated breast cancer recurrence in ER-positive patients using Oncotype DX through the association of BI-RADS mammography and MRI features. Indistinct mass margins and fine linear branching calcifications on mammography were associated with a higher recurrence score, whereas breast density on mammography was inversely associated with the recurrence score. Spiculated mass margins and NME on MRI were associated with a lower recurrence score. In DWI, invasive breast cancers with higher Oncotype DX recurrence score exhibit significantly lower ADC values compared with lower-risk lesions[68] and higher signal-to-noise levels on diffusion-weighted images ($b = 800$ s/mm^2).[69]

Extending on these findings, AI-enhanced MRI has shown to be potentially useful for recurrence prediction. Several radiomic imaging models assessing the risk of recurrence given by multigene assays have been developed.[65,66,70–79] Combining imaging and pathology information, Sutton and colleagues[72] developed

a model that was associated with the Oncotype DX recurrence score, which was predictive of recurrence and therapeutic outcome. Li and colleagues[77] found significant associations between computer-extracted imaging phenotypes, including tumor size and enhancement texture, and higher risk for recurrence given by MammaPrint, Oncotype DX, and PAM50/Prosigna. Other studies using radiomics computer-extraction methods besides Li and colleagues[70,78] have also found enhancement heterogeneity to be related to a high risk of recurrence, as given by multigene assays. Apart from enhancement heterogeneity, two studies[70,72] found that rapid contrast uptake predicted high risk of recurrence as given by Oncotype DX. Using a radiogenomics approach, Tokuda and colleagues[80] correlated qualitative and quantitative DCE MRI features with Curebest 95-gene classifier results for recurrence prediction in ER-positive breast cancer. Whereas qualitative parameters were not significant to differentiate low-risk from high-risk groups, high volume ratio of "medium" in initial phase and/or high kurtosis in delayed phase were able to predict high recurrence risk. Ha and colleagues[81] investigated the feasibility of CNN for prediction of low, intermediate, and high risk of recurrence given by Oncotype DX. The CNN algorithm achieved an overall accuracy over 80%, with an AUC of 0.92.

CLINICAL OUTCOMES AND BREAST CANCER RISK PREDICTION

Radiomic features can be combined with other omics and clinical information to predict clinical survival outcomes. Guo and colleagues[82] combined radiomics/radiogenomics features derived from DCE MRI for the prediction of clinical phenotypes in invasive breast carcinomas. Although they found statistically significant associations with clinical outcomes for genomics, radiomics, and radiogenomics data, they did not report any additional value on the prediction performance by combining genomics and radiomics.

Breast MRI has also been proposed as a tool for breast cancer risk prediction, which is relevant, for example, to define screening schemes. Portnoi and colleagues[83] developed an image-based DL model to predict the 5-year breast cancer risk on the basis of a single breast DCE MRI from a screening examination and showed that this model improved individual risk discrimination compared with a state-of-the-art risk assessment model.

Challenges and Future Perspectives

AI-enhanced imaging is a rapidly evolving field that requires continued study. Over the past decade, numerous studies have been published on radiomics and radiogenomics coupled with AI of various cancers including the breast; yet, the implementation of AI-enhanced imaging in clinical practice is still not routinely done. This is due to several limitations associated with AI-enhanced imaging. The main challenges for the implementation of AI techniques in a clinical setting are the lack of standardization and small sample sizes in research studies to date. This is especially relevant for multiparametric MRI studies because of the high cost of MRI and the often limited availability of this imaging modality. In addition, there is no standardized breast MRI protocol, and images are highly variable across different practice sites and MR scanners. These challenges can be actively addressed by assessing the quality of published research (radiomics quality score)[4] or implementing harmonization of the data sets across different sites and scanners.[5,13,14]

To date, AI-enhanced breast MRI has almost exclusively focused on DCE MRI and to some extent DWI and its combination within a multiparametric MRI approach, with most studies having aimed to correlate radiomic features with cancer subtypes, recurrence scores, and treatment outcomes. It can also be expected that the incorporation of multiparametric AI-enhanced MRI will also aid in diagnosis. However, the field of imaging biomarker development with MRI is rapidly growing. In DWI, advanced techniques, such as IVIM and non-Gaussian diffusion (stretched exponential DWI, kurtosis imaging; see Chapter 8), are being investigated and show promise to provide additional robust imaging biomarkers that can be incorporated in radiomics studies.[84] In addition, other emerging MRI techniques that may be useful for radiomics research include spectroscopy (proton, phosphorus, lipid), sodium imaging,[85] chemical exchange saturation transfer imaging,[86] blood oxygenation level–dependent,[87,88] and arterial spin labeling MRI, although obtaining adequate sample sizes for AI-based analysis remains challenging with

such techniques because they are not part of routine imaging.[89]

AI-enhanced MRI in breast cancer is still in its infancy. Larger prospective studies using the full wealth of information that MRI can offer and considerable efforts in standardization and quality control are warranted, especially regarding outcome-related data, in order to meaningfully implement AI-enhanced MRI in the clinical setting.

Conclusion

The field of AI-enhanced breast imaging is rapidly evolving. Because of the noninvasive nature and ubiquitous use of medical imaging in clinical routine, AI-enhanced radiomics is poised to play an important role by adding to our understanding of the etiology of diseases. We anticipate that the implementation of AI-enhanced breast MRI, including DWI, in clinical breast cancer care will further enhance the role of radiology in precision medicine and reshape the way we care for our patients. Although AI-enhanced breast MRI is an unprecedented opportunity to better derive clinical value from imaging, the road to this vision is long and many technical, regulatory, and even ethical problems will have to be addressed.

REFERENCES

1. El Naqa I, Napel S, Zaidi H. Radiogenomics is the future of treatment response assessment in clinical oncology. *Med Phys.* 2018;45(10):4325–4328.
2. Rutman AM, Kuo MD. Radiogenomics: creating a link between molecular diagnostics and diagnostic imaging. *Eur J Radiol.* 2009;70(2):232–241.
3. Bai HX, et al. Imaging genomics in cancer research: limitations and promises. *Br J Radiol.* 2016;89(1061):20151030.
4. Lambin P, Leijenaar RTH, Deist TM, et al. Radiomics: the bridge between medical imaging and personalized medicine. *Nat Rev Clin Oncol.* 2017;14(12):749–762.
5. Johnson WE, Li C, Rabinovic A. Adjusting batch effects in microarray expression data using empirical Bayes methods. *Biostatistics.* 2007;8(1):118–127.
6. Pinker K, et al. Background, current role, and potential applications of radiogenomics. *J Magn Reson Imaging.* 2018;47(3):604–620.
7. Gillies RJ, Kinahan PE, Hricak H. Radiomics: images are more than pictures, they are data. *Radiology.* 2016;278(2):563–577.
8. Sala E, et al. Unravelling tumour heterogeneity using next-generation imaging: radiomics, radiogenomics, and habitat imaging. *Clin Radiol.* 2017;72(1):3–10.
9. Lambin P, et al. Radiomics: extracting more information from medical images using advanced feature analysis. *Eur J Cancer.* 2012;48(4):441–446.

10. Grimm LJ, Breast MRI. radiogenomics: current status and research implications. *J Magn Reson Imaging*. 2016;43(6):1269–1278.
11. Reig B, et al. Machine learning in breast MRI. *J Magn Reson Imaging*. 2020;52(4):998–1018.
12. Tagliafico AS, et al. Overview of radiomics in breast cancer diagnosis and prognostication. *Breast*. 2020;49:74–80.
13. Ibrahim A, Primakov S, Beuque M, et al. Radiomics for precision medicine: current challenges, future prospects, and the proposal of a new framework. *Methods*. 2021;188:20–29.
14. Rogers W, et al. Radiomics: from qualitative to quantitative imaging. *Br J Radiol*. 2020;93(1108):20190948.
15. Zhang L, et al. Accuracy of combined dynamic contrast-enhanced magnetic resonance imaging and diffusion-weighted imaging for breast cancer detection: a meta-analysis. *Acta Radiol*. 2016;57(6):651–660.
16. Dorrius MD, et al. Effect of b value and pre-admission of contrast on diagnostic accuracy of 1.5-T breast DWI: a systematic review and meta-analysis. *Eur Radiol*. 2014;24(11):2835–2847.
17. Chen X, et al. Meta-analysis of quantitative diffusion-weighted MR imaging in the differential diagnosis of breast lesions. *BMC Cancer*. 2010;10:693.
18. Baltzer P, et al. Diffusion-weighted imaging of the breast—a consensus and mission statement from the EUSOBI International Breast Diffusion-Weighted Imaging working group. *Eur Radiol*. 2020;30(3):1436–1450.
19. Goto M, et al. Adding a model-free diffusion MRI marker to BI-RADS assessment improves specificity for diagnosing breast lesions. *Radiology*. 2019;292(1):84–93.
20. Meyer-Base A, et al. Current status and future perspectives of artificial intelligence in magnetic resonance breast imaging. *Contrast Media Mol Imaging*. 2020;2020:6805710.
21. Dalmis MU, et al. Artificial intelligence-based classification of breast lesions imaged with a multiparametric breast MRI protocol with ultrafast DCE-MRI, T2, and DWI. *Invest Radiol*. 2019;54(6):325–332.
22. Eskreis-Winkler S, et al. Using deep learning to improve non-systematic viewing of breast cancer on MRI. *J Breast Imaging*. 2021;3:201–207.
23. Truhn D, et al. Radiomic versus convolutional neural networks analysis for classification of contrast-enhancing lesions at multiparametric breast MRI. *Radiology*. 2019;290(2):290–297.
24. Herent P, et al. Detection and characterization of MRI breast lesions using deep learning. *Diagn Interv Imaging*. 2019;100(4):219–225.
25. Ji Y, et al. Independent validation of machine learning in diagnosing breast cancer on magnetic resonance imaging within a single institution. *Cancer Imaging*. 2019;19(1):64.
26. Bickelhaupt S, et al. Prediction of malignancy by a radiomic signature from contrast agent-free diffusion MRI in suspicious breast lesions found on screening mammography. *J Magn Reson Imaging*. 2017;46(2):604–616.
27. Potsch N, et al. An A.I. classifier derived from 4D radiomics of dynamic contrast-enhanced breast MRI data: potential to avoid unnecessary breast biopsies. *Eur Radiol*. 2021;31(8):5866–5876.
28. Meyer-Base A, et al. AI-enhanced diagnosis of challenging lesions in breast MRI: a methodology and application primer. *J Magn Reson Imaging*. 2021;54(3):686–702.
29. Lo Gullo R, et al. Improved characterization of sub-centimeter enhancing breast masses on MRI with radiomics and machine learning in BRCA mutation carriers. *Eur Radiol*. 2020;30(12):6721–6731.
30. Lo Gullo R, et al. Diagnostic value of radiomics and machine learning with dynamic contrast-enhanced magnetic resonance imaging for patients with atypical ductal hyperplasia in predicting malignant upgrade. *Breast Cancer Res Treat*. 2021;187(2):535–545.
31. Goldhirsch A, et al. Strategies for subtypes-dealing with the diversity of breast cancer: highlights of the St. Gallen International Expert Consensus on the Primary Therapy of Early Breast Cancer 2011. *Ann Oncol*. 2011;22(8):1736–1747.
32. Goldhirsch A, et al. Personalizing the treatment of women with early breast cancer: highlights of the St Gallen International Expert Consensus on the Primary Therapy of Early Breast Cancer 2013. *Ann Oncol*. 2013;24(9):2206–2223.
33. Cancer. Genome Atlas Network Comprehensive molecular portraits of human breast tumours. *Nature*. 2012;490(7418):61–70.
34. Huber KE, Carey LA, Wazer DE. Breast cancer molecular subtypes in patients with locally advanced disease: impact on prognosis, patterns of recurrence, and response to therapy. *Semin Radiat Oncol*. 2009;19(4):204–210.
35. Elias SG, et al. Imaging features of HER2 overexpression in breast cancer: a systematic review and meta-analysis. *Cancer Epidemiol Biomarkers Prev*. 2014;23(8):1464–1483.
36. Grimm LJ, et al. Can breast cancer molecular subtype help to select patients for preoperative MR imaging? *Radiology*. 2015;274(2):352–358.
37. Uematsu T. MR imaging of triple-negative breast cancer. *Breast Cancer*. 2011;18(3):161–164.
38. Grimm LJ, et al. Relationships between MRI Breast Imaging-Reporting and Data System (BI-RADS) lexicon descriptors and breast cancer molecular subtypes: internal enhancement is associated with luminal b subtype. *Breast J*. 2017;23(5):579–582.
39. Yamaguchi K, et al. Intratumoral heterogeneity of the distribution of kinetic parameters in breast cancer: comparison based on the molecular subtypes of invasive breast cancer. *Breast Cancer*. 2015;22(5):496–502.
40. Kim EJ, et al. Histogram analysis of apparent diffusion coefficient at 3.0t: correlation with prognostic factors and subtypes of invasive ductal carcinoma. *J Magn Reson Imaging*. 2015;42(6):1666–1678.
41. Martincich L, et al. Correlations between diffusion-weighted imaging and breast cancer biomarkers. *Eur Radiol*. 2012;22(7):1519–1528.
42. Park SH, Choi HY, Hahn SY. Correlations between apparent diffusion coefficient values of invasive ductal carcinoma and pathologic factors on diffusion-weighted MRI at 3.0 Tesla. *J Magn Reson Imaging*. 2015;41(1):175–182.
43. Mazurowski MA, et al. Radiogenomic analysis of breast cancer: luminal B molecular subtype is associated with enhancement dynamics at MR imaging. *Radiology*. 2014;273(2):365–372.
44. Grimm LJ, Zhang J, Mazurowski MA. Computational approach to radiogenomics of breast cancer: luminal A and luminal B molecular subtypes are associated with imaging features on routine breast MRI extracted using computer vision algorithms. *J Magn Reson Imaging*. 2015;42(4):902–907.
45. Leithner D, et al. Radiomic signatures with contrast-enhanced magnetic resonance imaging for the assessment of breast cancer receptor status and molecular subtypes: initial results. *Breast Cancer Res*. 2019;21(1):106.
46. Sutton EJ, et al. Breast cancer molecular subtype classifier that incorporates MRI features. *J Magn Reson Imaging*. 2016;44(1):122–129.

47. Wu J, et al. Identifying relations between imaging phenotypes and molecular subtypes of breast cancer: model discovery and external validation. *J Magn Reson Imaging.* 2017;46(4):1017–1027.

48. Fan M, et al. Radiomic analysis reveals DCE-MRI features for prediction of molecular subtypes of breast cancer. *PLoS One.* 2017;12(2):e0171683.

49. Leithner D, Bernard-Davila B, Martinez DF, et al. Radiomic signatures derived from diffusion-weighted imaging for the assessment of breast cancer receptor status and molecular subtypes. *Mol Imaging Biol.* 2020;22(2):453–461.

50. Leithner D, Mayerhoefer ME, Martinez DF, et al. Non-invasive assessment of breast cancer molecular subtypes with multiparametric magnetic resonance imaging radiomics. *J Clin Med.* 2020;9(6):1853.

51. Wang Q, et al. Radiomic analysis on magnetic resonance diffusion weighted image in distinguishing triple-negative breast cancer from other subtypes: a feasibility study. *Clin Imaging.* 2021;72:136–141.

52. Sun X, et al. Preliminary study on molecular subtypes of breast cancer based on magnetic resonance imaging texture analysis. *J Comput Assist Tomogr.* 2018;42(4):531–535.

53. Xie T, et al. Differentiation of triple-negative breast cancer from other subtypes through whole-tumor histogram analysis on multiparametric MR imaging. *Eur Radiol.* 2019;29(5):2535–2544.

54. Zhang Y, et al. Invasive ductal breast cancer: preoperative predict Ki-67 index based on radiomics of ADC maps. *Radiol Med.* 2020;125(2):109–116.

55. Iima M, et al. Diffusion MRI of the breast: current status and future directions. *J Magn Reson Imaging.* 2020;52(1):70–90.

56. Bismeijer T, et al. Radiogenomic analysis of breast cancer by linking MRI phenotypes with tumor gene expression. *Radiology.* 2020;296(2):277–287.

57. Ha R, et al. Prior to initiation of chemotherapy, can we predict breast tumor response? deep learning convolutional neural networks approach using a breast MRI tumor dataset. *J Digit Imaging.* 2019;32(5):693–701.

58. Lo Gullo R, et al. Machine learning with multiparametric magnetic resonance imaging of the breast for early prediction of response to neoadjuvant chemotherapy. *Breast.* 2020;49:115–122.

59. Tahmassebi A, et al. Impact of machine learning with multiparametric magnetic resonance imaging of the breast for early prediction of response to neoadjuvant chemotherapy and survival outcomes in breast cancer patients. *Invest Radiol.* 2019;54(2):110–117.

60. Liu Z, et al. Radiomics of multiparametric MRI for pretreatment prediction of pathologic complete response to neoadjuvant chemotherapy in breast cancer: a multicenter study. *Clin Cancer Res.* 2019;25(12):3538–3547.

61. Ha R, et al. Predicting post neoadjuvant axillary response using a novel convolutional neural network algorithm. *Ann Surg Oncol.* 2018;25(10):3037–3043.

62. Bitencourt AGV, et al. MRI-based machine learning radiomics can predict HER2 expression level and pathologic response after neoadjuvant therapy in HER2 overexpressing breast cancer. *EBioMedicine.* 2020;61:103042.

63. Braman NM, et al. Intratumoral and peritumoral radiomics for the pretreatment prediction of pathological complete response to neoadjuvant chemotherapy based on breast DCE-MRI. *Breast Cancer Res.* 2017;19(1):57.

64. Sutton EJ, et al. A machine learning model that classifies breast cancer pathologic complete response on MRI post-neoadjuvant chemotherapy. *Breast Cancer Res.* 2020;22(1):57.

65. Mehta S, et al. Radiogenomics monitoring in breast cancer identifies metabolism and immune checkpoints as early actionable mechanisms of resistance to anti-angiogenic treatment. *EBioMedicine.* 2016;10:109–116.

66. Yamamoto S, et al. Radiogenomic analysis of breast cancer using MRI: a preliminary study to define the landscape. *AJR Am J Roentgenol.* 2012;199(3):654–663.

67. Woodard GA, et al. Qualitative radiogenomics: association between Oncotype DX test recurrence score and BI-RADS mammographic and breast MR imaging features. *Radiology.* 2018;286(1):60–70.

68. Thakur SB, et al. Apparent diffusion coefficient in estrogen receptor-positive and lymph node-negative invasive breast cancers at 3.0T DW-MRI: a potential predictor for an Oncotype DX test recurrence score. *J Magn Reson Imaging.* 2018;47(2):401–409.

69. Amornsiripanitch N, et al. Diffusion-weighted MRI characteristics associated with prognostic pathological factors and recurrence risk in invasive ER+/HER2− breast cancers. *J Magn Reson Imaging.* 2018;48(1):226–236.

70. Ashraf AB, et al. Identification of intrinsic imaging phenotypes for breast cancer tumors: preliminary associations with gene expression profiles. *Radiology.* 2014;272(2):374–384.

71. Siamakpour-Reihani S, et al. Genomic profiling in locally advanced and inflammatory breast cancer and its link to DCE-MRI and overall survival. *Int J Hyperthermia.* 2015;31(4):386–395.

72. Sutton EJ, et al. Breast cancer subtype intertumor heterogeneity: MRI-based features predict results of a genomic assay. *J Magn Reson Imaging.* 2015;42(5):1398–1406.

73. Yamamoto S, et al. Breast cancer: radiogenomic biomarker reveals associations among dynamic contrast-enhanced MR imaging, long noncoding RNA, and metastasis. *Radiology.* 2015;275(2):384–392.

74. Fernandez-Navarro P, et al. Genome wide association study identifies a novel putative mammographic density locus at 1q12–q21. *Int J Cancer.* 2015;136(10):2427–2436.

75. Zhu Y, et al. Deciphering genomic underpinnings of quantitative MRI-based radiomic phenotypes of invasive breast carcinoma. *Sci Rep.* 2015;5:17787.

76. Li H, et al. Pilot study demonstrating potential association between breast cancer image-based risk phenotypes and genomic biomarkers. *Med Phys.* 2014;41(3):031917.

77. Li H, et al. MR imaging radiomics signatures for predicting the risk of breast cancer recurrence as given by research versions of MammaPrint, Oncotype DX, and PAM50 gene assays. *Radiology.* 2016;281(2):382–391.

78. Wan T, et al. A radio-genomics approach for identifying high risk estrogen receptor-positive breast cancers on DCE-MRI: preliminary results in predicting Oncotype DX risk scores. *Sci Rep.* 2016;6:21394.

79. Dialani V, et al. Prediction of low versus high recurrence scores in estrogen receptor-positive, lymph node-negative invasive breast cancer on the basis of radiologic-pathologic features: comparison with Oncotype DX test recurrence scores. *Radiology.* 2016;280(2):370–378.

80. Tokuda Y, et al. Radiogenomics of magnetic resonance imaging and a new multi-gene classifier for predicting recurrence prognosis in estrogen receptor-positive breast cancer: a preliminary study. *Medicine (Baltimore).* 2020;99(16):e19664.

81. Ha R, et al. Convolutional neural network using a breast MRI tumor dataset can predict Oncotype Dx recurrence score. *J Magn Reson Imaging.* 2019;49(2):518–524.

82. Guo W, et al. Prediction of clinical phenotypes in invasive breast carcinomas from the integration of radiomics and genomics data. *J Med Imaging (Bellingham)*. 2015;2(4):041007.

83. Portnoi T, et al. Deep learning model to assess cancer risk on the basis of a breast MR image alone. *AJR Am J Roentgenol*. 2019;213(1):227–233.

84. Mahajan A, Deshpande SS, Thakur MH. Diffusion magnetic resonance imaging: a molecular imaging tool caught between hope, hype and the real world of "personalized oncology." *World J Radiol*. 2017;9(6):253–268.

85. Zaric O, et al. Quantitative sodium MR imaging at 7 T: initial results and comparison with diffusion-weighted imaging in patients with breast tumors. *Radiology*. 2016;280(1):39–48.

86. Kogan F, Hariharan H, Reddy R. Chemical exchange saturation transfer (CEST) imaging: description of technique and potential clinical applications. *Curr Radiol Rep*. 2013;1(2):102–114.

87. Bennani-Baiti B, et al. Non-invasive assessment of hypoxia and neovascularization with MRI for identification of aggressive breast cancer. *Cancers (Basel)*. 2020;12(8):2024.

88. Stadlbauer A, et al. Development of a non-invasive assessment of hypoxia and neovascularization with magnetic resonance imaging in benign and malignant breast tumors: initial results. *Mol Imaging Biol*. 2019;21(4):758–770.

89. Telischak NA, Detre JA, Zaharchuk G. Arterial spin labeling MRI: clinical applications in the brain. *J Magn Reson Imaging*. 2015;41(5):1165–1180.

Diffusion-Weighted Whole Body Imaging With Background Body Signal Suppression (DWIBS)

Taro Takahara, MD, PhD, Toshiki Kazama, MD, PhD, Miho Kita, MD, PhD, and Thomas Kwee, MD, PhD

Basic Concept of Diffusion-Weighted Whole Body Imaging With Background Body Signal Suppression (DWIBS)

Since the 1990s, diffusion-weighted imaging (DWI) has revolutionized the diagnosis of acute cerebral infarction, making it possible for patients to receive thrombolytic agents in emergency situations and escape death or severe chronic invalidity. This life-saving potential prompted manufacturers to rapidly incorporate diffusion magnetic resonance imaging (MRI) into their commercial products. On the other hand, DWI has also shown great potential to manage cancer lesions.[1] Cerebral infarction and cancer have in common a decrease of the apparent diffusion coefficient (ADC, the standard biomarker of diffusion MRI; see Chapter 1), although the mechanisms (reduction of the extracellular space, cell proliferation in cancer, diffusion hindrance increase) are still under investigation. This means that stroke and cancer lesions appear as high-signal areas in DWI. However, DWI is much more difficult to use outside the brain because of its sensitivity to bulk motion. Especially in the torso and the abdomen, cardiac and respiratory motion can be a source of strong artifacts in DWI. Such artifacts can be mitigated in some ways, for instance, by using breath-hold. Therefore DWI of the body was always performed under the limitation of breath-hold and as a result greatly suffered from low signal-to-noise ratio (SNR).

Diffusion-weighted whole-body imaging with background body signal suppression (DWIBS) is the name of a DWI approach that intentionally uses free breathing

scanning rather than breath-holding or respiratory triggering to visualize (moving) visceral organs.[2,3] Similar to standard DWI, DWIBS also uses echo-planar imaging (EPI; see Chapter 12) with a fat-suppression technique, typically short tau inversion recovery (STIR). Another issue in the body is the presence of fat, as fat usually exhibits very low ADC and can contaminate fibroglandular tissue diffusivity measures and be misinterpreted as malignancy. Hence efficient fat suppression must be used in combination with EPI. The multiple signal acquisitions necessary to encode imaging render macroscopic motion incoherent across scans, but single-shot MRI encoding methods such as EPI can alleviate those motion artifacts. In principle, only random motion (incoherent motion) affects the contrast of DWI and not constant linear motion (coherent motion), such as respiratory motion. DWIBS uses this principle. Free breathing scanning allows for the acquisition of a thin-sliced data set (suitable for multiplanar reformats and maximum intensity projections [MIPs]) with a large anatomical coverage within a clinically reasonable scan time.[2,3] Note that these targets cannot be achieved when using a breath-hold or respiratory-triggered DWI acquisition. The advent of DWIBS is similar to that of multislice CT around the year 2000 when arbitrary multiplanar reconstructions and MIPs could be obtained. The DWIBS method also relies on the MIP approach to display the distribution of cancer lesions in 3D or arbitrary multiplanar reformats (Fig. 11.1). The latter is similar to fluorodeoxyglucose (FDG)-positron emission tomography (PET), which also provides a generally high lesion-to-background contrast and where MIP images can be used

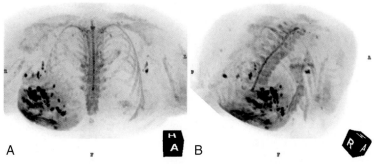

Fig. 11.1 MIP image of DWI from thin-slice (4 mm) data set in a 76-year-old woman with right-sided breast cancer (the images were acquired in 2003). (A) MIP image from the anteroposterior viewpoint. (B) MIP image from the right anterosuperior viewpoint. A large breast cancer located in the right breast is demonstrated as a high-intensity area (appears dark on the black/white inverted display). The associated inflammatory process is seen around the tumor. Axillary lymph node swelling is well visualized. Although the shoulder is one of the frequent sites where fat suppression tends to be insufficient, the effect of STIR-based fat suppression is excellent. Multiple breast cancer foci and the surrounding inflammatory process are well demonstrated three-dimensionally. *MIP*, Maximum intensity projection; *STIR*, short tau inversion recovery. (Reprinted with permission from Takahara T, Imai Y, Yamashita T, Yasuda S, Nasu S, Van Cauteren M. Diffusion weighted whole body imaging with background body signal suppression (DWIBS): technical improvement using free breathing, STIR and high resolution 3D display. *Radiat Med.* 2004;22(4):275–282.)

to detect pathology at a single glance. The use of MIP images can speed up image evaluation and may perhaps increase sensitivity, because they rapidly pinpoint potential lesions that can then be further inspected on 2D source images and other sequences. Reversing the black and white contrast of a DWIBS data set yields an image that resembles the standard (FDG-)PET view (i.e., lesions appear black and background appears white), which may be visually convenient to those readers who are accustomed to the standard (FDG-)PET view. Nevertheless, reversing the black and white contrast is only a matter of habituation and personal taste and is unlikely to affect diagnostic performance.

The DWIBS method has proven versatile and easy to implement. It has been incorporated into clinical protocols and used to identify cancerous lesions,[4] evaluate treatment strategies for bone metastases of prostate cancer,[5] and is part of some imaging evaluation methods such as ONCO-RADS.[6] It is generally less expensive than (FDG-)PET and Positron emission tomography–computed tomography (PET-CT). It does not involve radiation exposure, making it a suitable method for a follow-up study of cancer treatment.[3] Because breast cancer is a disease with a high incidence of bone metastases, DWIBS is often used for screening across the whole body. Recently, ADC color maps have been added to DWIBS to aid in lesion characterization and treatment selection (Fig. 11.2).

The Importance of Fat Suppression in DWIBS

FAT-SUPPRESSION EFFECT

The contrast principle of the DWIBS method is described in the previous section. To obtain a wide coverage of the torso, it is necessary to achieve good fat suppression in any part of the body. In general, in 2D images (e.g., axial images), insufficient fat suppression at the edges of the field of view is rarely a diagnostic problem. However, poorly suppressed superficially located fat can seriously deteriorate the MIP image and obscure lesions.

Among fat-suppression techniques (see Chapter 12), such as STIR, chemical shift selective (CHESS) or spectral attenuated inversion recovery (SPAIR), the use of STIR has shown to be effective for homogeneous fat suppression[2] (Fig. 11.3), although both STIR and SPAIR techniques showed similar diagnostic performances for ADC-based differentiation of malignant from benign breast tumors,[7] and SPAIR is recommended in breast DWI by the latest consensus statement of the European Society of Breast Imaging (EUSOBI).[8]

The breast has a spatially complex shape, and the breast cleavage and nipple area are prone to local magnetic field heterogeneities. The STIR method, which relies on T1 differences between fat and tissues, is

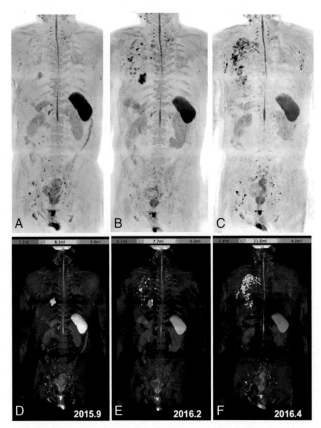

Fig. 11.2 Treatment follow-up of EGFR mutation–positive lung adenocarcinoma in a 65-year-old man using DWI MIP image and ADC color map. (A–C) MIP images. (D–F) ADC color map images (*red, yellow*, and *green* represent ADC values of $\leq 0.5 \times 10^{-3}$ mm²/s, $0.5 \leq 1.0 \times 10^{-3}$ mm²/s, and $\geq 1.0 \times 10^{-3}$ mm²/s, respectively). (A) The primary tumor was found in the right lower lobe and treated with a molecular target drug (gefitinib). (B) Five months later, the primary tumor enlarged, and pleural dissemination occurred. Therefore first-line chemotherapy (CBDCA + PEM) was started. (C) The primary tumor shrank, but pleural dissemination was observed in a larger area. Therefore first-line chemotherapy was considered ineffective, and second-line chemotherapy (DTX) was started. However, the ADC color map (F) at the same time point showed that the ADC values of the pleurally disseminated foci had increased, so it could be inferred that the first-line chemotherapy could have been continued a little longer. *ADC*, Apparent diffusion coefficient; *CBCDA*, carboplatin; *DTX*, docetaxel; *EGFR*, epidermal growth factor receptor; *MIP*, maximum intensity projection; *PEM*, pemetrexed.

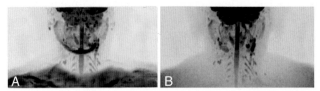

Fig. 11.3 Comparison of STIR-EPI and SE-EPI with CHESS pulse regarding the degree of fat suppression in a 28-year-old man with swollen lymph nodes (pathology unknown). SE-EPI DWI with CHESS pulse (A) shows insufficient fat suppression around the jaw and clavicle. On the other hand, STIR-EPI DWI (B) shows adequate fat suppression. Swollen lymph nodes around the left submandibular gland *(arrow)* are well visualized without interfering artifact. *CHESS*, Chemical shift selective; *DWI*, diffusion-weighted imaging; *SE-EPI*, spin-echo echo-planar imaging; *STIR-EPI*, short tau inversion recovery echo-planar imaging. (Reprinted with permission from Takahara T, Imai Y, Yamashita T, Yasuda S, Nasu S, Van Cauteren M. Diffusion weighted whole body imaging with background body signal suppression (DWIBS): technical improvement using free breathing, STIR and high resolution 3D display. *Radiat Med.* 2004;22(4):275–282.)

more robust than CHESS, which is based on the fat/water frequency difference, particularly for the superficial regions of the breast.[9] Fig. 11.4 shows a DWI of a breast performed with the commonly used fat-suppression method (CHESS). The MIP image looks clear at a first glance (pseudotransparent effect), but it is important to note that the signal intensity of the surface fat is dominant, and the interior is not visible.

Even with STIR, the fat-suppression effect may not be perfect. There are two potential options to enhance fat suppression in STIR: spatial-spectral radiofrequency (SSRF; Fig. 11.5) or slice selective gradient reversal (SSGR). Although SSGR has the advantage of no trade-offs,[10,11] it is susceptible to magnetic field inhomogeneity, and it is generally more prone to failure when used for the breast region, so its use requires extreme caution.

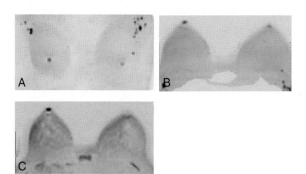

Fig. 11.4 Pseudotransparent effect of surface residual fat signal. (A, B) MIP images (AP and SI, respectively): the images appear to be very uniform. (C) Source 2D image: residual surface fat signal is observed. The SI of fat is higher than that of the mammary glandular tissue. This indicates that only the surface fat is visible on the MIP image, whereas the interior of the breast is not. *AP*, Abbreviated protocol; *MIP*, maximum intensity projection; *SI*, signal intensity.

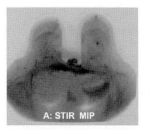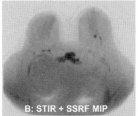

Fig. 11.5 STIR alone versus STIR + SSRF for fat suppression at 3T. (A) STIR alone for fat suppression. (B) STIR + SSRF combined fat suppression. Fat suppression is even better in (B). This combination works particularly well at 3T but can also be useful at 1.5T to obtain robust fat suppression. *MIP*, maximum intensity projection; *SSRF*, water excitation; *STIR*, short tau inversion recovery.

EVALUATION OF FAT SUPPRESSION

The quality of fat suppression in DWIBS of the breast can be evaluated by (1) the evenness in SNR and contrast-to-noise ratio (CNR) between the left and right sides (Fig. 11.6) and (2) the observation of a mammary fibroglandular tissue signal that is higher than that of fat (Fig. 11.7). The latter is especially important, because small cancerous lesions (in the millimeter

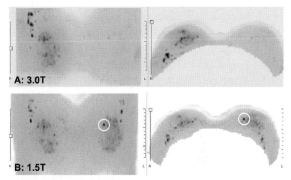

Fig. 11.6 Example of an undetected lesion due to a left-right difference in SNR and CNR. (A) MIP (AP and SI) images (taken with 3T scanner): the left mammary gland and lymph nodes are not well delineated. (B) MIP (AP and SI) image (retaken with 1.5T scanner with same *b*-values and other relevant specs): equal SNR and CNR between the left and right side; a complicated cyst, which was not depicted in (A), is seen in the left breast. It is important to realize that such a difference in SNR and CNR between the left and right sides of the image may cause false negatives. *AP*, Abbreviated protocol; *CNR*, contrast-to-noise ratio; *MIP*, maximum intensity projection; *SI*, signal intensity; *SNR*, signal-to-noise ratio.

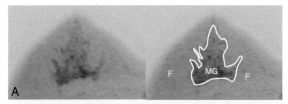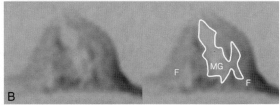

Fig. 11.7 Evaluation of fat and mammary fibroglandular tissue signals. (A) An example of a good image: mammary fibroglandular tissue signal *(MG)* > fat signal *(F)*. (B) An example of a poor image: MG < F. Subtle pathological signal increases within the mammary gland are not detectable on such images. In addition, lesions with a deeper location are not visible on maximum intensity projection images.

range, close to the size of a pixel) may have a relatively lower signal due to partial volume effects, and subtle hyperplastic changes are expected to have a low signal due to lack of high cell density. The detection of such faint lesions can easily be expected to be difficult in images where the fat signal outweighs the mammary fibroglandular tissue signal.

TUMOR/BACKGROUND CONTRAST

In addition to providing good fat suppression, STIR can be used to increase tumor/background contrast. This is because the effects of T1 and T2 prolongation of the lesion on the signal intensity are additive in the STIR method, including STIR-DWI, whereas they have opposite effects in many imaging methods like in a spin-echo (SE) sequence (with a CHESS prepulse).

Fig. 11.8 shows the contrast ratio of breast cancer ([breast cancer − background mammary gland] / background mammary gland) in DWIBS (STIR method) and spin-echo (CHESS method) according to a mathematical simulation.

It can be seen that the contrast is better with DWIBS (STIR method) than with spin-echo (CHESS

method). It is generally believed that the SNR and CNR determine whether an image is good or bad, and STIR-based images are considered to be disadvantageous in this respect compared with spin-echo-based images. However, we should also pay attention that when detecting tumors embedded in the mammary gland, the relative signal intensity to the mammary gland is also important.

A comparison of the CHESS and STIR methods in a breast tumor is shown in Fig. 11.9. A limitation of STIR is that it results in a lower SNR, which requires spending twice as much on acquisition time than with the CHESS method. Nevertheless, total acquisition time of DWIBS with the STIR method can be kept well within clinically acceptable time limits.

Application to Breast Cancer Screening

PERFORMANCE FOR BREAST CANCER DETECTION

The DWIBS method can be used to detect breast cancer, as it provides excellent tumor/background contrast. Two studies[13,14] using DWIBS at 1.5T have shown results comparable to those of contrast-enhanced MRI for both

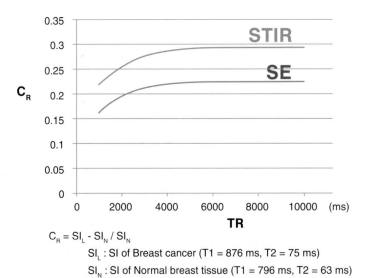

$$C_R = SI_L - SI_N / SI_N$$

SI_L : SI of Breast cancer (T1 = 876 ms, T2 = 75 ms)

SI_N : SI of Normal breast tissue (T1 = 796 ms, T2 = 63 ms)

Fig. 11.8 The CR of breast cancer (SI of breast cancer − SI of background mammary glandular tissue) / SI of background mammary glandular tissue) in DWIBS (STIR method) and SE (CHESS method) according to a mathematical simulation at 1.5T. The signal intensities of the STIR sequence and SE sequence can be simulated by the following equations: $SI_{STIR} = |[1 − 2 \exp(−TI/T1) + \exp(−TR/T1)] \cdot \exp(−TE/T2)|$ is $SI_{SE} = [1 − 2 \exp(−TR−TE/2)T1] + \exp(−TR/T1)] \cdot \exp(−TE/T2)$. Simulation was done with TI of 180 ms, TE of 80 ms, and T1 and T2 values of breast cancer and background mammary glandular tissue of 876, 75, 796, and 63 ms, respectively.[12] The CR is approximately 30% higher for STIR than for SE. *CHESS*, Chemical shift selective; *CR*, contrast ratio; *DWIBS*, diffusion-weighted whole-body imaging with background body signal suppression; *SE*, spin echo; *SI*, signal intensity; *STIR*, short tau inversion recovery; *TE*, echo time; *TI*, inversion time.

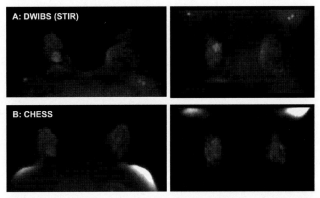

Fig. 11.9 **Comparison of tumor visibility between CHESS and STIR (DWIBS) methods (TNBC).** (A) DWIBS method (STIR), MIP and 2D image. (B) CHESS method, MIP and 2D image. In this case, the difference between the mammary fibroglandular tissue signal and the tumor signal was small in the CHESS method, and the tumor could not be clearly displayed. *CHESS,* Chemical shift selective; *DWIBS,* diffusion-weighted whole-body imaging with background body signal suppression; *MIP,* maximum intensity projection; *STIR,* short tau inversion recovery; *TNBC,* triple negative breast cancer.

screening and diagnostic applications. Telegrafo and colleagues[13] compared screening performance of unenhanced (UE)-MRI with DWIBS ($b = 0$ and $1000 \, s/mm^2$) and contrast-enhanced (CE)-MRI in 280 consecutive patients with suspicious mammographic or ultrasound findings ($n = 110$) and high-risk women with dense breasts ($n = 170$). UE-MRI and CE-MRI were reviewed independently by two radiologists in consensus, with a 2-week washout period in between. UE-MRI sequences obtained sensitivity, specificity, diagnostic accuracy, positive predictive value (PPV), and negative predictive value (NPV) values of 94%, 79%, 86%, 79%, and 94%, respectively. CE-MRI sequences obtained sensitivity, specificity, diagnostic accuracy, PPV, and NPV values of 98%, 83%, 90%, 84%, and 98%, respectively. No statistically significant difference between performance of UE-MRI and CE-MRI was found, suggesting DWIBS could be a valuable noncontrast alternative for breast cancer screening.

In another study, Bickelhaupt and colleagues[14] compared diagnostic performance of two abbreviated protocols (APs) based on MIPs; DWIBS with $b = 0$ and $1500 \, s/mm^2$ (AP1; unenhanced) and T1-weighted subtraction images created from the first postcontrast minus precontrast series (AP2; contrast-enhanced) in 50 patients with suspicious mammographic findings. With unenhanced AP1 (DWIBS), the sensitivity, specificity, NPV, and PPV were 92%, 94%, 93%, and 94%, respectively. With the contrast-enhanced AP2 protocol, the sensitivity, specificity, NPV, and PPV were 85%, 90%, 89%, and 87%, respectively. They found no difference in accuracy between either of the APs and the full diagnostic protocol, suggesting DWIBS could be useful for detecting cancer and ruling out malignancy in BI-RADS category 4 or 5 lesions detected on x-ray screening mammograms.

DWIBS AS A NONCONTRAST MRI SCREENING MODALITY

Breast cancer screening using dynamic contrast-enhanced (DCE) MRI has been proposed by Kuhl and colleagues and has shown outstanding results.[15] The cancer detection rate of DCE MRI is known to be more than twice as high as that of mammography and ultrasound. However, in 2004, it was reported that gadolinium-based contrast agents (GBCAs) could be deposited not only in the brain[16] but also in other organs throughout the body. In addition, the accumulation of excreted gadolinium is becoming an increasingly important environmental issue.[17] Although the harmful effects of repeated administration of GBCAs are not clearly understood, it is ethically challenging to envision repeated administration of GBCAs for screening healthy people. For this reason, screening with noncontrast MRI (DWI) is increasingly considered.[18]

Another noteworthy aspect of Kuhl and colleagues' proposal is that they were conscious of the need for a time-efficient interpretation when using MRI for breast cancer screening. They realized this by creating a single MIP image from subtracted data (i.e., enhanced − unenhanced image) and using this MIP image to rapidly (i.e., in a matter of seconds) exclude the presence of a lesion. If any significant enhancement is present on the MIP image, other sequences can be inspected for further characterization. However, the majority of cases are negative and will not show any significant enhancement, in which a brief inspection of the single MIP image will suffice most of the time. This concept of image interpretation (i.e., availability of one "diagnostic key image" to quickly stratify cases with and without suspicious abnormalities) can be considered an important precondition for breast cancer screening. Applying the acquisition and interpretation approach of a standard diagnostic breast MRI protocol to a screening setting may considerably compromise workflow efficiency. Importantly, the MIP image that can be created from a noncontrast-enhanced DWIBS acquisition parallels the capabilities of a MIP image from subtracted data (i.e., enhanced − unenhanced image; Fig. 11.10),[14] thereby providing the same time efficiency of image interpretation that is necessary for breast cancer screening. For optimal image quality, it is important to overcome the inherent drawback of low SNR of STIR in DWIBS by increasing scan time. This relative increase in scan time can be afforded in a noncontrast screening protocol, because relatively time-consuming DCE sequences are omitted.

Limitations of DWIBS

FALSE POSITIVE FINDINGS

Although the DWIBS method shows excellent tumor detection rates using qualitative interpretation, its specificity is not perfect. Areas with high signal intensity do not necessarily correspond to areas of high cell density. Of critical clinical importance are highly viscous fluid collections, which have both intermediate long T2s and low ADC values and often short T1s. Complicated cysts that fall into this category are extremely frequent and may be misdiagnosed as cancer at DWIBS, potentially eliciting a high number of false positive cases. Therefore it is important to complement signal observations at DWIBS with assessment of the corresponding ADC map and visual appearance of potential lesions on fat saturation T1WI and T2WI to identify complicated cysts and increase specificity. An example is shown in Fig. 11.11. Typical parameters of the sequences

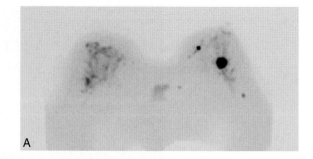
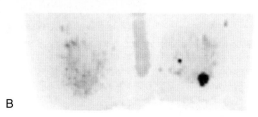

Fig. 11.10 A 41-year-old woman with HER2-positive breast cancer. (A) MIP image in axial direction. (B) MIP image in coronal direction. On the MIP image with DWIBS (STIR) technique, the internal mammary fibroglandular tissue signal can be clearly observed thanks to good fat suppression. The presence or absence of tumor can be relatively straightforwardly determined on the MIP image, which is useful to achieve a reading speed that is required in a mass screening setting. *DWIBS*, Diffusion-weighted whole-body imaging with background body signal suppression; *HER2*, human epidermal growth factor receptor 2; *MIP*, maximum intensity projection; *STIR*, short tau inversion recovery.

are shown in Table 11.1. An ADC measurement may give some direction to the diagnosis. However, ADC values may be subject to variation depending on the system and protocol used, so there is a need for standardization (see Chapter 14).

IMPORTANCE OF IMAGE QUALITY ADJUSTMENT

Traditionally, MRI systems have been believed to produce nearly identical images when using identical acquisition parameters. In reality, however, as shown in Fig. 11.12, there is not infrequently a very large difference in image quality when the same patient undergoes imaging on different scanners. The 1.5 T scanners tend to more easily produce stable image quality, whereas the 3.0 T scanners are often unstable in this respect[19] (see Fig. 11.6). At both field strengths, careful shimming is necessary (Fig. 11.13). It may be helpful to evaluate and solve any differences in image quality if a test patient can be imaged with different systems. Chapter 14 discusses issues regarding standardization.

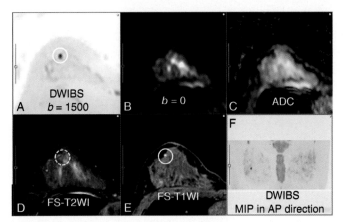

Fig. 11.11 Diagnosis of complicated cyst. (A) DWIBS image (black/white inverted) ($b = 1500\,s/mm^2$). (B) $b = 0$ image. (C) ADC image. (D) Fat-suppressed T2-weighted image. (E) Fat-suppressed T1-weighted image. (F) DWIBS image (MIP in AP direction). DWIBS image (A) shows a high signal intensity nodule in the right breast, and ADC image (C) shows a low value, which may suggest cancer based on DWI alone. Fat-suppressed T1WI (D) shows a round lesion with a high signal, which corresponds to a (complicated) cyst with highly viscous fluid. The signal intensity of complicated cysts is variable, and knowledge of their T1 shortening and T2 shortening that may occur is necessary to establish the correct diagnosis. *ADC*, Apparent diffusion coefficient; *AP*, abbreviated protocol; *DWI*, diffusion-weighted imaging; *DWIBS*, diffusion-weighted whole-body imaging with background body signal suppression; *MIP*, maximum intensity projection.

TABLE 11.1 Typical Sequence Parameters of Breast Cancer Screening at 1.5 T

	DWIBS	FS-T1WI	FS-T2WI
Sequence	STIR-EPI	Vibrant Flex	T2 Flex
Orientation	Transverse	Transverse	Transverse
Scan time	7 minutes 45 seconds	1 minutes 27 seconds	3 minutes 40 seconds
Fat-suppression technique	STIR + SSRF	2-point Dixon	2-point Dixon
FOV (mm)	360 × 360	360 × 360	360 × 360
Acquisition matrix	128 × 128	384 × 256	360 × 288
Reconstruction matrix	256056	512 × 512	512 × 512
Slice thickness/gap (mm)	4/0.4	2 (zip2)	4/0.4
TR (ms)	7053	7	4994
TE (ms)	84.4 (min)	22 / 4.5 (min / full)	102
TI (ms)	180	N/A	N/A
FA (degree)	90	12	90
ETL	48	1	16
Interecho spacing (ms)	0.7	N/A	11.5
NEX	b = 0:2, b = 1500;10	1	1
Postprocess	Rotation MIP, ADC		

Total scan time of the three sequence is 12 minutes 52 seconds.
ADC, Apparent diffusion coefficient; *DWIBS*, diffusion-weighted whole-body imaging with background body signal suppression; *ETL*, echo train length; *FA*, flip angle; *FOV*, field of view; *MIN*, minimum value; *MIP*, maximum intensity projection; *NEX*, number of excitation; *STIR+SSRF*, short tau inversion recovery spatial-spectral radiofrequency; *STIR-EPI*, short tau inversion recovery echo-planar imaging; *TE*, echo time; *TI*, inversion time; *TR*, repetition time.

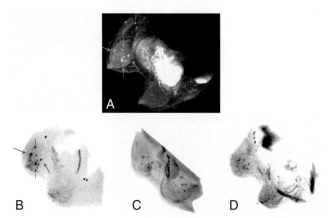

Fig. 11.12 **A 44-year-old woman with multifocal DCIS in the right breast.** (A) Contrast-enhanced MRI (MIP image). (B–D) DWIBS images ($b = 1500 \, s/mm^2$) of the same patient taken at different facilities and with different scanners. Only (B) was taken with advanced shimming and image quality adjustment. (B) shows multifocal lesions in the right breast. (C) and (D) show poor fat suppression and nodular-like signal in the left breast; consequently, in (C) and (D) the perceived signal abnormalities can erroneously be interpreted as either bilateral breast cancer or as bilateral benign nodules without clinical significance. *DCIS,* Ductal carcinoma in situ; *DWIBS,* diffusion-weighted whole-body imaging with background body signal suppression; *MIP,* maximum intensity projection.

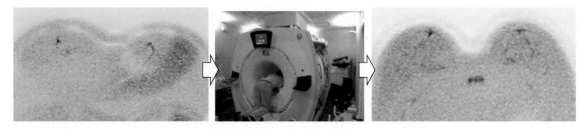

Fig. 11.13 **Importance of equipment adjustment.** *(Left)* DWIBS image ($b = 1500 \, s/mm^2$) performed without equipment adjustment. Sensitivity is generally poor, and strong artifacts are seen in the left breast. *(Middle)* Body coil positioning (submillimeter level) and shimming were performed after the plastic cover of the bore was opened (this is something that an vendor service engineer does, not something that an ordinary operator can do). *(Right)* Image after adjustment. The left-right difference is gone, sensitivity is better, and artifacts have disappeared. It is necessary to make such efforts, and high image quality cannot be obtained by merely copying scan parameters from one to another system. *DWIBS,* Diffusion-weighted whole-body imaging with background body signal suppression.

REFERENCES

1. Iima M, Le Bihan D. Clinical intravoxel incoherent motion and diffusion MRI imaging: past, present, and future. *Radiology.* 2016;278:13–32.
2. Takahara T, Imai Y, Yamashita T, Yasuda S, Nasu S, Van Cauteren M. Diffusion weighted whole body imaging with background body signal suppression (DWIBS): technical improvement using free breathing, STIR and high resolution 3D display. *Radiat Med.* 2004;22(4):275–282.
3. Kwee TC, Takahara T, Ochiai R, Nievelstein RA, Luijten PR. Diffusion-weighted whole-body imaging with background body signal suppression (DWIBS): features and potential applications in oncology. *Eur Radiol.* 2008;18(9):1937–1952.
4. Padhani AR, Liu G, Koh DM, et al. Diffusion-weighted magnetic resonance imaging as a cancer biomarker: consensus and recommendations. *Neoplasia.* 2009;11(2):102–125.
5. Yoshida S, Takahara T, Arita Y, Sakaino S, Katahira K, Fujii Y. Whole-body diffusion-weighted magnetic resonance imaging: diagnosis and follow up of prostate cancer and beyond. *Int J Urol.* 2021;28(5):502–513.
6. Petralia G, Koh DM, Attariwala R, et al. Oncologically relevant findings reporting and data system (ONCO-RADS): guidelines for the acquisition, interpretation, and reporting of whole-body MRI for cancer screening. *Radiology.* 2021;299(3):494–507.
7. Nogueira L, Brandão S, Nunes RG, Ferreira HA, Loureiro J, Ramos I. Breast DWI at 3T: influence of the fat-suppression technique on image quality and diagnostic performance. *Clin Radiol.* 2015;70(3):286–294.
8. Baltzer P, Mann RM, Iima M, et al; EUSOBI International Breast Diffusion-Weighted Imaging Working Group. Diffusion-weighted imaging of the breast: a consensus and mission statement from the EUSOBI International Breast Diffusion-Weighted Imaging Working Group. *Eur Radiol.* 2020;30(3):1436–1450.
9. Kazama T, Nasu K, Kuroki Y, Nawano S, Ito H. Comparison of diffusion-weighted images using short inversion time inversion recovery or chemical shift selective pulse as fat suppression in patients with breast cancer. *Jpn J Radiol.* 2009;27(4):163–167.
10. Park HW, Kim DJ, Cho ZH. Gradient reversal technique and its applications to chemical-shift-related NMR imaging. *Magn Reson Med.* 1987;4(6):526–536.

11. Nagy Z, Weiskopf N. Efficient fat suppression by slice-selection gradient reversal in twice-refocused diffusion encoding. *Magn Reson Med.* 2008;60(5):1256–1260.
12. Merchant TE, Thelissen GR, de Graaf PW, Nieuwenhuizen CW, Kievit HC, Den Otter W. Application of a mixed imaging sequence for MR imaging characterization of human breast disease. *Acta Radiol.* 1993;34(4):356–361.
13. Telegrafo M, Rella L, Stabile Ianora AA, Angelelli G, Moschetta M. Unenhanced breast MRI (STIR, T2-weighted TSE, DWIBS): an accurate and alternative strategy for detecting and differentiating breast lesions. *Magn Reson Imaging.* 2015;33(8):951–955.
14. Bickelhaupt S, Laun FB, Tesdorff J, et al. Fast and noninvasive characterization of suspicious lesions detected at breast cancer x-ray screening: capability of diffusion-weighted MR imaging with MIPs. *Radiology.* 2016;278(3):689–697.
15. Kuhl C, Weigel S, Schrading S, et al. Prospective multicenter cohort study to refine management recommendations for women at elevated familial risk of breast cancer: the EVA trial. *J Clin Oncol.* 2010;28(9):1450–1457.
16. Kanda T, Nakai Y, Oba H, Toyoda K, Kitajima K, Furui S. Gadolinium deposition in the brain. *Magn Reson Imaging.* 2016;34(10):1346–1350.
17. Rogowska J, Olkowska E, Ratajczyk W, Wolska L. Gadolinium as a new emerging contaminant of aquatic environments. *Environ Toxicol Chem.* 2018;37(6):1523–1534.
18. Amornsiripanitch N, Bickelhaupt S, Shin HJ, et al. Diffusion-weighted MRI for unenhanced breast cancer screening. *Radiology.* 2019;293(3):504–520.
19. Mürtz P, Krautmacher C, Träber F, Gieseke J, Schild HH, Willinek WA. Diffusion-weighted whole-body MR imaging with background body signal suppression: a feasibility study at 3.0 Tesla. *Eur Radiol.* 2007;17(12):3031–3037.

Chapter 12

High-Resolution Diffusion-Weighted Breast MRI Acquisition

Brian A. Hargreaves, PhD, Catherine J. Moran, PhD, Jessica A. McKay, PhD, and Bruce L. Daniel, MD

Diffusion-weighted imaging (DWI) is a promising approach for breast magnetic resonance imaging (MRI), both as a way to complement or to replace contrast-enhanced MRI. DWI measures diffusive motion, which is quantified by *diffusivity, D,* often measured in mm²/s. Assuming a Gaussian diffusion model, the measured parameter is called the apparent diffusion coefficient (ADC). DWI uses diffusion gradients to selectively attenuate the signal of water molecules that have greater diffusive motion,[1] and this attenuation is expressed as e^{-bD}, where b is the "b value" of the sequence, typically in s/mm², and indicates the sensitivity of the sequence to diffusion. DWI is useful in the detection of cancers because cancerous tissue often has more restricted diffusion than normal tissue and therefore appears brighter. Numerous groups have explored DWI in the context of breast cancer, with very promising results for detection, diagnosis, and assessment of treatment response. These studies are summarized in several meta-analyses[2–4] and in other chapters of this book. Although DWI remains predominantly a research approach in the context of routine breast MRI, continuous improvements are enabling more robust acquisition of images with greater sensitivity to small lesions.

Breast MRI demands high spatial resolution in order to depict small lesions or to show shape, border, and heterogeneity features. Sufficient contrast-to-noise ratio (CNR) is necessary, particularly to separate potentially malignant lesions from benign lesions or normal tissue. To achieve contrast with DWI requires moderate to high b values (600–800 s/mm² or higher) to create contrast based on typical diffusivities (fibroglandular tissue around 1.6×10^{-3} mm²/s and cancers approximately 1.0×10^{-3} mm²/s), but this

attenuation costs signal-to-noise ratio (SNR), and typically increasing the b value requires greater averaging to recover this SNR. Additionally, due to widely varying breast tissue composition, size, and shape, robust fat saturation is critical, especially in DWI where fat both obscures other signal due to its limited diffusion and may cause artifacts due to its strong signal and chemical shift frequency. High quality radiofrequency (RF) receive coil arrays with consistent patient placement are also important, both for adequate SNR and parallel imaging performance, and again present challenges based on the variation in patient size and breast size and shape. Although scan times are not as critical as in dynamic contrast-enhanced (DCE) imaging, long scans can result in greater patient motion, so imaging efficiency is an important consideration. Furthermore, shorter scans enable greater flexibility to use more advanced diffusion models requiring a higher number of b values and directions. Breast MRI also requires a moderately large field of view (FOV), which means gradient nonlinearities and eddy-current effects can degrade images. Finally, motion and B0 changes due to cardiac and respiratory motion can affect breast MRI. Typically, these challenges are exacerbated in DWI.

This chapter describes many of the acquisition techniques used for DWI in the breast. Fat suppressed single-shot echo-planar imaging (ss-EPI) has been the standard for breast DWI, as it is widely available and overcomes the dominant challenge of motion during DWI; however, it has limited resolution, as well as considerable distortion that results from off-resonance effects that are common in the breast. Techniques including parallel imaging, reduced FOV, and multishot EPI have been demonstrated to overcome some of these challenges. Specifically, multishot imaging variations include readout-segmented EPI (rs-EPI), multiplexed sensitivity encoding (MUSE) and PROPELLER. Other methods have also been explored in research including self-navigated spiral (SNAILS), spatiotemporal encoding (SPEN), and steady-state diffusion. All of these methods typically trade-off between robustness to off-resonance and motion, simplicity, and capability to perform quantitative DWI. These DWI acquisition approaches are generally adaptable to numerous quantitative diffusion approaches, such as diffusion-tensor imaging (DTI),[5] intravoxel incoherent motion (IVIM),[6] diffusion kurtosis imaging (DKI),[7] or restriction spectrum imaging (RSI)[8] (see Chapters 8 and 9).

Standard Echo-Planar Diffusion-Weighted Imaging

A conventional DWI acquisition in the body consists of fat suppression followed by a diffusion encoded spin-echo sequence using a single-shot EPI imaging readout, as shown in Fig. 12.1. The large diffusion-encoding gradients have the adverse effect of making the sequence very sensitive to small bulk motion, which induces unpredictable signal phase variations across the image. The single-shot EPI readout is used to rapidly acquire the *entire* image after a single excitation so that such phase effects can be ignored. Furthermore, single-shot EPI avoids respiratory, cardiac, and random patient motion artifacts resulting from motion between shots. Single-shot EPI typically uses a partial-Fourier approach so that the central k-space signal is acquired before substantial

$T2^*$ signal decay, equivalently reducing the echo time (TE). System calibrations and postprocessing correct for Nyquist ghosting and shading artifacts that can result from imperfections between positive and negative (rightward and leftward) readout lines. Multiple averages are often obtained to improve overall SNR, and typically the number of averages is increased for higher *b* values.

EPI PARAMETER SELECTION

Single-shot EPI is one of the fastest approaches used for image acquisition in MRI, offering images in well under 100 ms and often much faster.[9] Typically, the EPI trajectory is designed to maximize imaging speed. The readout gradient amplitude is maximized given limits on gradient amplitude and sample spacing ($1/FOV_x$). In many cases, sampling occurs on both the readout ramps and plateaus that are shown in Fig. 12.1, with the readout gradient duration sufficient to achieve the desired k_x extent and spatial resolution in *x*. Multiple repeated readout lobes enable sampling of more k-space lines in both directions, which maximizes speed. A phase-encode gradient initially sets the starting k_y location, while "blip" gradients between each readout lobe skip by 1/FOV between k_y to satisfy Nyquist sampling. The number of k_y lines provides sufficient extent in k_y to achieve desired phase-encode resolution. The alternating sampling typically results in ghosts, known as "FOV/2" ghosts or Nyquist ghosts, due to delays or phase differences between the readout gradients of opposite polarity induced by eddy currents or other imperfections. Typically, a reference scan is built into protocols, and enables very good

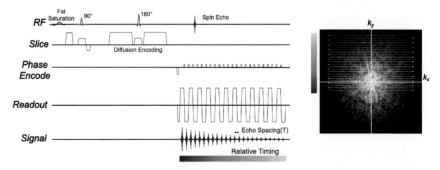

(A) Single-Shot EPI Pulse Sequence   **(B) k-Space Sampling Trajectory**

Fig. 12.1 (A) Single-shot EPI DWI pulse sequence showing fat saturation, diffusion encoding, and EPI acquisition with echo spacing T_{esp}; (B) k-space trajectory shown at right is half-Fourier acquisition. Color scale shows relative timing of acquisition, which determines $T2^*$ blurring and phase evolution that can lead to distortion. *DWI*, Diffusion-weighted imaging; *EPI*, echo-planar imaging; *RF*, radiofrequency.

correction of these ghosts, by measuring any phase and delay variation between all readout lines and correcting data for these before Fourier reconstruction.

LIMITATIONS OF EPI: READOUT DURATION, DISTORTION, AND BLURRING

Single-shot EPI acquires all data for a slice following one excitation. The primary limitations of this approach are that the signal changes in both magnitude and phase during the acquisition. The magnitude change is due to T2* decay and leads to a loss of resolution or blurring in the phase-encode direction. Often half-Fourier acquisitions are used to sample k_y from near the center out to the edge.[10] This reduces the EPI duration and the amount of signal decay, at a cost of minor blurring from the partial-k-space reconstruction. The resulting shortened TE also reduces the inherent T2-weighted contrast that leads to T2 "shine-through" effects. Any off-resonance, caused by B0 inhomogeneity or chemical shift, causes linear phase accrual between k_y lines that depends on the echo spacing (T_{esp}). B0 inhomogeneity leads to spatially varying distortion, especially around the nipple, whereas the chemical shift frequency difference between water and fat causes a *constant* displacement of the fat with respect to water signal. Neither the off-resonance-induced distortion nor the fat/water displacement is affected by the use of half-Fourier sampling, because the k_y velocity described in the next section is unchanged. Phase and amplitude differences along the readout (k_x) are smaller and usually can be ignored.

FOV RELATIONSHIP

To better understand the distortion effects, it is useful to point out the *fundamental* relationship between displacement, the off-resonance effects, and the FOV. To support a given FOV in the phase-encode direction (FOV_y) requires a k-space line separation of $\Delta k_y = 1/FOV_y$. If the echo spacing is T_{esp}, the k_y velocity is $\Delta k_y/T_{esp} = 1/(FOV_y T_{esp})$, and the displacement Δy as a function of off-resonance Δf is $\Delta y = FOV_y \Delta f T_{esp}$. This is a *fundamental* relationship with EPI, that off-resonance-induced distortion is proportional to the frequency offset FOV_y and echo spacing T_{esp}.

For typical parameters of $T_{esp} = 1$ ms, FOV = 20 cm, and a 50-Hz frequency offset, the displacement is 1 cm. At 1.5 T and 3 T, respectively, the fat/water displacement is approximately 4.4 and 8.8 cm, which suggests the importance of fat suppression. Methods to reduce this displacement must reduce FOV_y or T_{esp} and are one of the main advances in breast DWI, as discussed later. Note that many of the approaches to reduce distortion will also reduce blurring, as they tend to shorten the readout duration and thus the amount of T2* decay.

DISTORTION CORRECTION

Image distortion in EPI results primarily from B0 field variations from sources such as air-tissue boundaries or metallic biopsy markers. When the field variation is sufficiently smooth and measurable, the resulting distortion can be corrected by an image "warping" that remaps signal to original pixel locations.[11] More rapid changes in B0 lead to "pile-up" effects, where the signal from multiple locations is mapped to one voxel, and require more advanced correction. Currently a common approach is to repeat the EPI acquisition with the phase encode gradients flipped in reverse polarity directions. Either using the data itself or in combination with a field map, the distortions can then be corrected,[12,13] and the repeated acquisitions can recover more signal than a single acquisition with a field map-based correction, due to averaging. Distortion correction is particularly important when pixel-wise comparisons are desired between different sequences (e.g., to calculate the ADC maps).

NAVIGATOR ACQUISITIONS

Navigator acquisitions are a general approach to acquire additional data to measure and possibly correct for motion during a scan. The large area of diffusion-encoding gradients, on the order of tens of degrees of rotation per micron, means that bulk motion of a few microns between the two gradients can impart substantial phase. In multishot imaging, this phase will modulate the k-space data resulting in different artifacts depending on the order in which k-space lines are acquired. Even in single-shot imaging, if a complex average of images is used (to reduce noise bias), the phase variations must be addressed. One approach to this is to add a second spin echo to the sequence and acquire a low-resolution, full-FOV image that ideally has the same motion-induced phase as the data acquired on the first spin echo.[14,15] The phase of the navigator can then be used to reduce or remove phase variations in the data from the first spin echo of different excitations so that the overall image artifact is reduced or removed. Navigators have been used extensively for different multishot EPI approaches (described shortly) and for non-EPI approaches.[16] Although they can lengthen the scan time per slice, resulting in fewer interleaved slices, they can additionally offer some correction for respiratory motion and other motion that can degrade images.

SUMMARY

Fat-suppressed single-shot EPI is very commonly used for DWI, because the rapid readout avoids motion artifacts that would result in multishot techniques, and most importantly the bulk motion–induced phase can usually be ignored. This sequence is widely available on most MRI systems, with careful corrections built in. The main limitations of distortion and blurring have been studied extensively and are described in detail in the remainder of this chapter. Specifically for breast MRI, the choice of fat suppression is important, and different approaches are described next.

Fat-Suppression Methods

Fat suppression is typically based on frequency differences or T1 differences between fat and water. Chemically selective saturation (CHESS) or inversion pulses precede the sequence. Fat suppression is important to avoid the artifacts that can result from fat, particularly the chemical shift displacement in EPI

that often results in ghosting, especially when parallel imaging is used. In addition, fat has minimal diffusivity and so appears very bright on DWI, which obscures other tissue features and reduces the dynamic range of these features. Fat-suppression approaches may loosely include *reducing* the signal from fat or *separating* the water and fat signal, typically done with Dixon-based methods.[17-19] In DWI in the breast, the former group of approaches is typically used, making use of either T1 differences (STIR)[20] or the chemical shift frequency difference between fat and other tissues, with the schemes shown in Fig. 12.2.

CHEMICALLY SELECTIVE FAT SUPPRESSION

Chemically selective fat suppression, often simply "fat saturation," uses a spectrally selective pulse to selectively excite only the fat signal, as shown at the start of the sequence in Fig. 12.1. An applied gradient then dephases the fat spins so that they contribute no signal. The standard excitation and imaging follow the fat saturation block, with timing unaffected by the fat saturation. Fat saturation is simple and fast but can suffer from sensitivity to B0 and B1 variations. In the breast, susceptibility variations from proximity to the lungs or air-tissue boundaries near the chest wall, axillae, nipple, or the inferior portion of the breast often cause fat suppression to fail. This occurs when the broad spectral fat peak shifts outside the suppression bandwidth of the pulse. Fat saturation can use a simple 90-degree excitation or an inversion followed by an inversion time. Adiabatic spectral inversion recovery (e.g., ASPIR or SPAIR on different systems) is

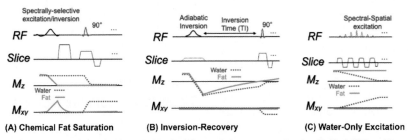

Fig. 12.2 Common schemes to eliminate the fat signal before imaging, and the corresponding longitudinal (Mz) and transverse (Mxy) for water and fat. (A) Chemically selective fat saturation excites a narrow bandwidth around fat before dephasing excited signal to bring transverse fat magnetization to zero. The pulse is played before imaging sequence and has minimal impact on sequence timing or water magnetization. (B) Inversion recovery uses inversion to negate longitudinal signal of water and fat before specified inversion time (TI) to null fat signal. The RF pulse is often adiabatic inversion to improve robustness to B1 variations. TI time can affect sequence timing, and inversion leads to loss of some water signal. (C) Water-only excitation uses multiple short slice-selective excitations scaled to also select only a narrow frequency band around water without affecting fat. Pulse duration can impact sequence timing more than fat saturation. *RF*, Radiofrequency.

sometimes used to reduce sensitivity to off-resonance at a cost of increased RF power.

STIR

Short TI inversion recovery (STIR)[20] suppresses fat based on the shorter T1 (typically 250 ms at 1.5 T and 350 ms at 3.0 T) of fat compared with that of other tissues (typically over 1 second) in the breast. As the name suggests, STIR uses in inversion pulse, which is usually not spatially selective, to invert all signal. After an inversion time (TI) of 150 to 180 ms, normal excitation and imaging proceeds. This time is carefully chosen to null the signal from fat (i.e., based on $e^{-TI/T1} \approx 0.5$). A strength of STIR is the robustness to static magnetic field inhomogeneities, and with the commonly used adiabatic inversion pulses, additional robustness to transmit B1 field variations. The main drawback of STIR is that the inversion-recovery causes a loss in signal of about 30% to 40%, which translates to a need to double the number of averages to achieve adequate SNR. Additionally, it is challenging to interleave other slices within the inversion time, so the number of slices that can be interleaved within one repetition is reduced, which reduces efficiency. Finally, in cases where DWI is performed after DCE, the presence of contrast can result in nulling of other tissue or tumor because of its shortened T1, which can be similar to that of fat.

WATER-ONLY EXCITATION

Water-only excitation or "spectral-spatial" pulses can simultaneously excite a narrow frequency band as well as the imaging slice.[21] As Fig. 12.2C shows, the pulse is a series of slice-selective pulses, with overall scaling that provides selectivity to only the water frequency. The pulse is similar in duration to chemical saturation, and the length can increase the TE (or equivalently the time between excitation and refocusing in a spin-echo sequence). Water-only pulses are typically less prone to residual fat signal than fat saturation, because the water peak (usually narrower than the fat peak) is less likely to shift outside the excitation band. Unlike fat saturation, where B1 variations cause unsuppressed fat, water-only excitations have the same B1 shading/contrast variations as any sequence. The pulse length, typically around 10 to 12 ms at 1.5 T, can be shortened to about 5 to 6 ms at 3 T.

SHIMMING

Regardless of technique, fat suppression is absolutely essential for breast DWI. Aside from different vendor systems and field strengths, the wide range of breast sizes and shapes combined with variations in coils and positioning makes reliable, robust fat suppression a continuous challenge. Because STIR costs time efficiency as well as SNR, chemical-shift-based approaches are most commonly used and rely on careful shimming to minimize the range of B0 variations. Numerous approaches to improving shimming have been studied, with no simple robust approach.[22] Approaches including dual-volume shimming, "smartshim," dynamic per-slice shimming,[23] or even independently shimmed slab excitation over each breast[24,25] have been explored, but applicability to all techniques still remains a challenge, and some shim approaches will add additional examination time. The availability of the aforementioned shimming approaches also varies with different vendor products, so empirical protocol optimization is often the best way to achieve the best results.

SUMMARY

Fat suppression is *critical* for breast DWI, primarily because the fat is much brighter than other tissue owing to its short T1 relaxation, moderately long T2, and limited diffusivity, and therefore it obscures the appearance of lesions. Additionally, the chemical-shift frequency results in a displacement in EPI that causes fat to overlap other parts of the image and causes ghosting when parallel imaging is used without consideration of fat, leading to contamination of tissue diffusivity measures. Multiple approaches can be used for fat suppression, mostly independently of the image acquisition portion of the sequence, each with different trade-offs with respect to timing considerations, sensitivity to B0 and B1 variations, and SNR.

Reducing Distortion, Blurring, and Scan Times With Available Methods

Major limitations of EPI are the distortion and blurring effects that are fundamentally related to the phase-encode FOV and the moderately long scans that are required to achieve adequate slice coverage and SNR. This section explores some of the more readily available improvements to single-shot EPI. One way to mitigate distortion and blurring artifacts in EPI is to speed the k_y traversal of the acquisition. This can be done either by shortening the interecho spacing T or by increasing the spacing between k_y lines. Limitations on gradient amplitudes and slew rates force a reduced k_x traversal extent if T is to be reduced; this is explored later in the section on rs-EPI (rs-EPI). Alternatively, increasing Δk_y results in a reduced acquisition FOV in the y direction that will result in aliasing or wrap artifact. The aliasing can be reduced either by basic approaches that limit the excited FOV along k_y or by using parallel imaging. There is also considerable similarity with interleaved multishot acquisitions, which essentially combine multiple reduced-FOV images, as discussed in more detail later. Finally, simultaneous multislice (SMS) imaging offers improved scan efficiency by acquiring multiple slices together, though it does not shorten echo spacing to reduce either distortion or T2* blurring.

CHOICE OF GEOMETRY

The choice of imaging geometry in breast MRI involves many factors, including the goal of reducing the k_y FOV. Notably, at the resolutions used for DWI, the readout duration is usually limited by the gradient slew rate and amplitude rather than by the sampling rate. This means that the additional FOV in the readout (k_x) direction does not affect the echo spacing T, and therefore ideally the largest FOV dimension could be oriented in the frequency-encode direction and smallest FOV dimension in the phase-encode direction. Artifacts such as aliasing or cardiac or respiratory motion are usually minimized in the readout direction, and often in breast MRI the readout direction is selected as anterior/posterior (A/P) so that cardiac pulsation artifact does not interfere with breast tissue. For axial bilateral breast imaging, often a rectangular FOV is acceptable, with larger coverage needed in the right/left (R/L) direction (typically 32–40 cm) than in the A/P direction. For axial DWI, frequency R/L can therefore enable a smaller FOV than frequency A/P, though the cardiac artifact should be considered. Alternatively, sagittal imaging is sometimes performed with a small FOV in the superior/inferior (S/I) direction. Overall, there are trade-offs to imaging geometry, though most clinical DWI protocols currently use an axial acquisition with readout R/L to limit aliasing from arms or

readout A/P to reduce cardiac pulsation artifact. As described later, phased-array coils enable reduced FOV and parallel imaging. Because it is the reduced FOV rather than the full FOV that determines distortion and T2* blurring, these geometry considerations must be considered together with the coil geometry.

BREAST PHASED-ARRAY COILS

Dedicated breast RF coils (typically receive-only) are essential for high-quality breast MRI. Generally, such coils are designed for robustness across a variety of patient sizes, aiming to provide relatively uniform signal coverage as the number of elements increases. Commercially available 8-channel coils became standard for imaging during 2001 to 2010 and are still widely used. However, 16-channel coils from numerous vendors have become commonplace both for 1.5 T and 3.0 T imaging. The smaller receive elements of higher-channel-count coils offer greater sensitivity based on higher signal as well as lower noise per channel. Additionally, when these sensitivities vary considerably from one element to another, parallel imaging can be used to further improve performance, as described next. Dedicated breast coils have limited sensitivity to signal from tissues deep in the body and from the patient's arms (when imaged with "arms down" along their sides), so it can simplify the selection of geometry and enable reduction of the k_y FOV in different directions.

PARALLEL IMAGING

Parallel imaging was a transformational advance in MRI that uses the varying spatial sensitivity of coil arrays to reconstruct images that are acquired with a reduced FOV, which is of course synonymous with skipping k_y lines. The reduced-FOV images take less time because the k_y spacing is larger, and therefore there are fewer acquired k_y lines. Common reconstruction approaches are to undo aliasing (sensitivity encoding, SENSE)[26] or to fill in missing k-space lines (GRAPPA),[27] though many variants and hybrids of these approaches exist.[28,29] Standard parallel imaging is applied *only* along a phase-encode dimension. A simplistic but intuitive example of breast parallel imaging is that if two coil elements are each sensitive to one breast, then a reduced FOV image of each breast can be simultaneously acquired, and these can be stitched together to form a bilateral image in the same scan time. Note that this example requires the phase-encode direction to be L/R. Although the coil sensitivities overlap, there are advantages to thinking of parallel imaging as "building up" FOV by using multiple coil elements.[30]

PARALLEL IMAGING AND EPI

In EPI, the use of parallel imaging has strong additional benefits: the increased k_y spacing increases the rate of k_y traversal, which reduces both blurring and distortion.[31] These effects are clearly demonstrated in Fig. 12.3, which shows an example of axial DWI with the phase-encode direction R/L and three reduction factors (R = 1, 2, and 4), with reduced distortion and blurring when a greater reduction is used. These benefits arise directly from the FOV relationship described earlier. Parallel imaging must be applied in the phase-encode (k_y) direction and requires a multichannel coil with sensitivity variation in this direction. Theoretically, the reduction factor R should not exceed the number of coil elements in that direction. In practice, in breast imaging, 8-channel coils are typically capable of R = 2 (L/R), and 16-channel coils can achieve R = 4 L/R and R = 2 S/I or A/P. However, the key question for distortion and blurring is the *reduced phase-encode FOV* (phase-encode FOV/R), not only the reduction factor R. For example, it may be possible to use a smaller FOV to cover A/P and use the readout direction to cover the full L/R FOV with better overall performance in spite of a lower R. Another form of parallel imaging, SMS imaging, uses coil sensitivities to speed up acquisition by acquiring multiple slices at the same time. SMS, which is described shortly, generally does not change distortion and resolution in EPI.

LIMITED FOV EXCITATION

Although limited or varying spatial sensitivity of receiver coils can be used to reduce aliasing with a reduced FOV, an alternative approach is to only excite a limited region in the phase-encode direction. This approach is termed reduced-FOV (rFOV) excitation and has been explored specifically for DWI.[32] Here the standard slice-selective excitation is replaced with a 2D selective excitation that excites a limited extent in the slice and phase-encode directions, shown in Fig. 12.4. The result is that the acquisition FOV can be reduced without aliasing, which offers the same benefits of faster k_y traversal described earlier. The 2D excitation has a low effective bandwidth in the slice direction, and careful combination with the refocusing pulse during diffusion encoding can additionally provide fat suppression. However, the same low bandwidth also makes the technique more sensitive to slice distortion/displacement due to varying B0 field. rFOV DWI has been applied to breast MRI in several studies. Singer and colleagues have shown that the higher spatial resolution enabled by rFOV allows

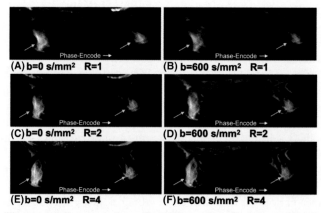

Fig. 12.3 Comparison of DWI at different parallel imaging factors using ASSET on a GE 3.0 T scanner, and the phase-encode direction right-to-left. DWI images with $b = 0$ s/mm[2] (A, C, E) and $b = 600$ s/mm[2] (B, D, E) are both shown, with 8, 16, and 20 averages, respectively. As the parallel imaging factor (R) is increased from 1 (A, B) to 2 (C, D) to 4 (E, F), the distortion is markedly decreased *(yellow arrows)* and the image sharpness improves due to reduced T2* blurring over the longer echo train. A higher number of averages is used to preserve SNR lost due to reduced sampling time and greater parallel imaging. *DWI,* Diffusion-weighted imaging; *SNR,* signal-to-noise ratio.

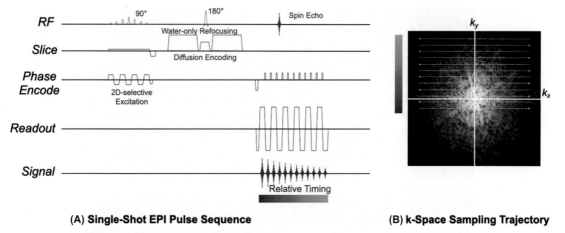

(A) Single-Shot EPI Pulse Sequence   **(B) k-Space Sampling Trajectory**

Fig. 12.4 (A) Reduced-FOV EPI sequence (2x smaller FOV than Fig. 12.1), including 2D-selective excitation to limit phase-encode direction signal extent and refocusing of only water slice location. (B) k-space trajectory shown at right traverses the k_y extent in half the time of the single-shot trajectory. Note that parallel imaging acquisitions and multishot EPI use same acquisition trajectory, though multishot interleaves are offset slightly in k_y and in time. Color scale shows shorter time window used for acquisition compared with Fig. 12.1. *EPI*, Echo-planar imaging; *FOV*, field of view; *RF*, radiofrequency.

improved depiction of heterogeneity,[33] which can be an important marker of malignancy. Similarly, Kang and colleagues showed the presence of a "rim sign" on reduced-FOV DWI images analogous to that seen in DCE.[34] Wilmes and colleagues have shown the promise of rFOV DWI for assessment of the response to neoadjuvant chemotherapy.[35] Finally, Barentsz and colleagues demonstrated better depiction of lesion morphology with rFOV DWI than conventional DWI.[36]

The main limitation of the rFOV approaches is that they zoom in on part of the FOV and may not provide full volumetric coverage and are therefore less useful when the location of a potential lesion or abnormality is unknown. Approaches have been explored to stitch together multiple sub-FOV images using in-plane simultaneous multiband imaging,[37] which is compared with reduced FOV and conventional DWI in Fig. 12.5. Both reduced FOV techniques improve sharpness compared with conventional single-shot EPI, whereas the in-plane multiband approach includes the full L/R volume. Although these approaches may be promising, the multishot techniques described subsequently offer improved SNR efficiency, as they inherently provide averaging over the full volume, whereas exciting only one portion of the FOV at a time does not provide such averaging.

Although the use of a 2D excitation in the rFOV EPI DWI technique has been explored for breast DWI, it is important to note that other reduced FOV approaches are options. Outer-volume suppression pulses are commonly available on most vendor systems, so the FOV can be reduced while suppressing signal from tissue beyond the desired FOV.[38] Although often effective, the additional RF power of these suppression pulses can increase the minimum repetition time (TR) or reduce the number of slices interleaved within the same TR, both effectively reducing the number of slices that can be acquired in a given time. Additionally, these pulses often saturate magnetization in adjacent slices, so may cost some signal. Alternatively, inner-volume excitation techniques use a 90-degree excitation that is limited to a slice, whereas the 180-degree pulse refocuses signal over a limited region in the phase-encode direction or vice versa.[39,40] Although simple, inner-volume approaches are subject to out-of-slice excitation effects and inherently saturate the signal from adjacent slices. However, both outer-volume suppression and inner-volume excitation may be available on systems that do not offer the direct rFOV excitation.

MULTISHOT METHODS

Multishot EPI methods divide the k-space into different regions that are acquired following separate excitations. The reduced k-space coverage of each shot can increase the k_y traversal rate to reduce both distortion and blurring. However, in DWI, the major challenge is

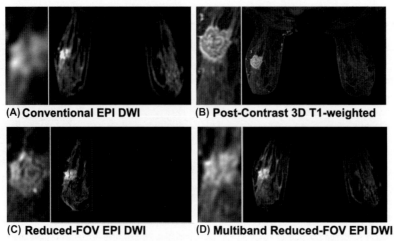

(A) Conventional EPI DWI **(B) Post-Contrast 3D T1-weighted**

(C) Reduced-FOV EPI DWI **(D) Multiband Reduced-FOV EPI DWI**

Fig. 12.5 Comparison of DWI methods with contrast-enhanced Cartesian imaging in patient with TNBC (magnified images of lesion are shown at left in each case). (A) Single-shot EPI DWI with $2.0 \times 2.0 \times 5.0$ mm^3 resolution and 4:24 scan time, parallel imaging factor of 2, and $b = 600$ s/mm^2. (B) Contrast-enhanced gradient-echo T1-weighted image ($0.5 \times 0.5 \times 1.0$ mm^3). (C) Reduced-FOV EPI DWI image, with $0.8 \times 0.8 \times 4.0$ mm^3 resolution and 4:27 scan time, equivalent of R = 4 FOV reduction, and $b = 750$ s/mm^2. (D) In-plane multiband reduced-FOV image with $1.5 \times 1.5 \times 4.0$ mm^3 resolution in 4:50, with R = 4 FOV reduction but full coverage and $b = 600$ s/mm^2. Lesion depiction is much clearer in (C) and (D), where T2* blurring is reduced in comparison to (A). *DWI*, Diffusion-weighted imaging; *EPI*, echo-planar imaging; *FOV*, field of view; *TNCB*, triple negative breast cancer.

that small motion during the diffusion gradients causes inconsistent phase between the shots, which can result in artifacts when the data from different shots are combined. Several multishot acquisition approaches have been explored in the breast, as shown in Fig. 12.6, and remain common. Additionally, there are numerous reconstruction approaches to address shot-to-shot phase inconsistencies. These are described in more detail later, with particular relevance to breast MRI. An important note is that multishot approaches inherently increase the scan time as more excitations are required while also reducing the overall SNR efficiency as the acquisition time per excitation is reduced.

Interleaved Multishot EPI

In multishot EPI, some number N of shots is acquired, whereby every shot acquires the full k-space extent, but skipping by N lines. Typically, the nth shot is delayed very slightly by $(n/N)T$ so that the duration from the excitation to the center of each k_y line varies

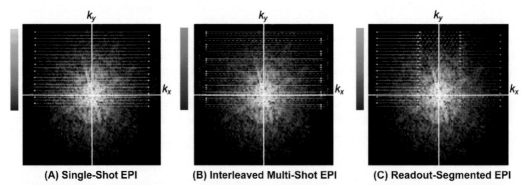

(A) Single-Shot EPI **(B) Interleaved Multi-Shot EPI** **(C) Readout-Segmented EPI**

Fig. 12.6 Comparison of ss-EPI to three-shot interleaved EPI and three-shot rs-EPI. (A) Color scales show the time variation over readout window, including the shorter duration for multishot approaches. rs-EPI (B) would likely have slightly longer readout duration than interleaved multishot (C) due to gradient slew-rate limitations. Generally, the trade-off is that multishot methods divide k-space coverage into multiple shots to improve image quality but lengthen scan time, and may result in ghosting or blurring. *EPI*, Echo-planar imaging; *rs-EPI*, readout-segmented echo-planar imaging; *ss-EPI*, single-shot echo-planar imaging.

perfectly linearly and off-resonance leads only to displacement rather than more complicated artifacts. The image from a single shot is simply a reduced-FOV (FOV/N) image that would have N replicas compared with a full-FOV image. This helps to explain why shot-to-shot phase variations result in replicas or ghosting. Because the k_y traversal is N times faster, distortions and displacements are reduced by a factor of N, and T2* blurring is reduced due to the reduced signal decay period.

Readout-Segmented EPI

In rs-EPI, k-space is divided into patches or blinds with limited extent in k_x, with multiple shots used to acquire different portions of the full k_x space.[41] The *readout lines* are shortened, resulting in smaller echo spacing T_{esp}. The exact relationship between number of shots and T_{esp} depends on the gradient slew rate, whether sampling during ramps is used, and the amount of k-space overlap between shots. However, again the reduced T_{esp} will reduce both distortion and T2* blurring. rs-EPI can be combined with half-Fourier sampling in either the readout or phase-encode direction, and standard parallel imaging is also typically used. Typically, an additional navigator spin-echo is used to correct shot-to-shot phase differences. Notably, the failure mode of such correction is likely a loss in resolution, less serious than the ghosting that may occur with multishot EPI. rs-EPI is available as a product (RESOLVE) and has been applied to breast imaging in numerous studies. Bogner and colleagues showed improvement in diagnostic accuracy of rs-EPI for breast lesions at the same prescribed image resolution as single-shot EPI, owing to reduced T2* blurring effects.[42] Wisner and colleagues found breast lesion-to-background contrast to be higher for rs-EPI than ss-EPI and further demonstrated the use of ADC in rs-EPI to separate benign from malignant lesions.[43] Kim and colleagues showed improvement in resolution and distortion of rs-EPI over conventional single-shot DWI,[44] whereas An and colleagues showed added value of quantitative DWI using rs-EPI compared with DCE.[45] Finally, Baltzer and colleagues showed that, diagnostically, rs-EPI DWI performs similarly to the DCE but with reduced conspicuity.[46] Overall, rs-EPI is a very promising approach with clear improvements over ss-EPI. One study compared rs-EPI to rFOV EPI,

although with substantially different resolution,[47] but showed that both techniques were superior to ss-EPI.

MUSE

MUltiplexed SEnsitivity encoding (MUSE) is a reconstruction approach for DWI EPI that uses coil sensitivity information to simultaneously apply parallel imaging to interleaved multishot EPI,[48] which results in much better inversion conditioning than SENSE. MUSE requires measurement of coil sensitivities, similar to other parallel imaging approaches, but does not require or use a navigator. Therefore the phase correction is inherently calculated from the data itself. A variation called POCS-MUSE iteratively calculates this phase for greater motion robustness.[49] There have been several studies of MUSE for breast DWI. Naranjo and colleagues compared a 2x parallel imaging approach to overall 3x accelerated MUSE (with slightly higher resolution) and demonstrated improved image quality and significant difference in calculated ADC between benign and malignant lesions with MUSE.[50] Similarly, Baxter and colleagues compared these approaches (2× parallel imaging to 1.5× MUSE) but with twice the phase-encode matrix size in MUSE and found that MUSE offered superior contrast and sharpness. Finally, Hu and colleagues compared MUSE to parallel imaging, showing increased sharpness with MUSE.[51] All of these studies include multiple cases, which is critical for assessing robustness to breast size, shape, and the variations in motion across patients.

There are currently no studies directly comparing MUSE or other interleaved EPI methods to rs-EPI, partly because the methods exist as products on different vendor systems. Both are multishot techniques and improve image sharpness and distortion. Residual artifacts on rs-EPI are likely to be blurring in the readout direction, whereas for MUSE they are ghosting in the phase-encode direction. Finally, it should be noted that the two approaches are potentially compatible. However, as the number of shots increases and readout is shortened, SNR efficiency continues to decrease.

Data-Driven MUSE Variants

Tremendous advances in image reconstruction now allow us to exploit redundancies in data to improve reconstruction. As an example, calibrationless parallel imaging notes that over a small spatial patch of an image, there is redundancy in data between channels, and this can be used in place of measured coil sensitivities.[52] Two data-driven variants of MUSE similarly take advantage of the fact that the phase variations between shots have some redundancy across the image. Specifically, if a matrix with columns consisting of phases for each shot at nearby pixels is composed, it is low in rank. When the pixels in a local region are grouped, the method is referred to as locally low rank (LLR). An iterative reconstruction enables minimization of the rank while ensuring data consistency with the acquired data. In Shot-LLR, the shot-to-shot phase is treated just as a coil sensitivity variation. A similar approach applied to DWI is MUSSELS,[53] which performs the low-rank formulation in k-space and has primarily been demonstrated in the brain. Shot-LLR has been shown to improve resolution and residual ghosting artifacts in the breast and compares favorably with MUSE, as shown in Fig. 12.7. Although both MUSE and Shot-LLR improve reconstruction compared with parallel imaging alone, a comparison in the breast shows that Shot-LLR can handle a higher number of shots and improves perceived resolution while also offering some denoising, as is common in model-based reconstructions.[51] Shot-LLR and similar advanced reconstruction methods currently are limited by lengthy reconstruction times, but deep-learning-based reconstructions are offering substantial improvements; for Shot-LLR, the time per slice can be reduced from 20 to 0.5 s,[54] and similar approaches are being explored.[55]

SIMULTANEOUS MULTISLICE (SMS)

SMS imaging refers to exciting and imaging multiple slices at the same time,[56] which typically uses a modulated RF pulse that can excite different slices with control over individual slice phases. SMS offers the ability to take advantage of coil sensitivity variations in the *through-slice* direction[57] to acquire the additional slices with no scan-time penalty, except for additional coil calibration. Controlled aliasing in parallel imaging approaches[58] can shift the aliasing pattern of different slices to improve parallel imaging performance, and these have been applied to EPI using blipped-CAIPI.[59] Whereas SMS necessarily increases the RF heating, in EPI DWI this typically is not a limitation on scan time. Rather, for DWI, SMS can accelerate scans when the number of slices limits the TR, either by enabling shorter TR or avoiding a second acquisition.

SMS has been explored by numerous studies in the breast. Ohlmeyer and colleagues directly compared single-shot DWI EPI to SMS in 69 subjects,[60] where

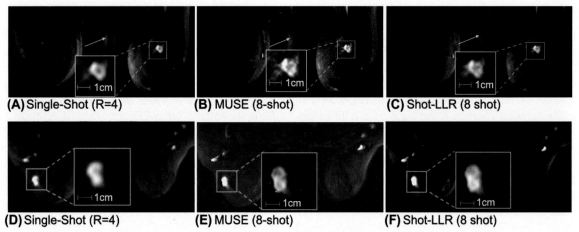

(A) Single-Shot (R=4)   **(B)** MUSE (8-shot)   **(C)** Shot-LLR (8 shot)

(D) Single-Shot (R=4)   **(E)** MUSE (8-shot)   **(F)** Shot-LLR (8 shot)

Fig. 12.7 Comparison of single-shot EPI, MUSE, and Shot-LLR, all with *b* = 600 s/mm², in two patients with lesions (A–C and D–F). Single-shot EPI (A, D) has relatively lower resolution (2.1 × 2.1 × 5.0 mm³ in a scan time of 2:18) than multishot approaches (B, C, E, and F), which are 1.0 × 1.0 × 5.0 mm³ in 2:22. Typically shot-LLR (C, F) outperforms MUSE (B, E) for 8-shot EPI, which exceeds parallel imaging capability of most breast coils. Both MUSE and Shot-LLR improve lesion morphology depiction over single-shot, but residual ghosting *(arrows)* is greater with MUSE. *EPI*, Echo-planar imaging; *LLR*, locally low rank; *MUSE*, multiplexed sensitivity encoding.

SMS reduced the TR from 9 to 4.3s, and correspondingly reduced scan time while maintaining similar image artifact levels and ADC values. Most of the other studies compare rs-EPI with and without SMS. Filli and colleagues compared ADC and SNR with 1×, 2×, and 3x SMS in eight subjects and showed the expected gains in SNR efficiency with no significant other differences, including in ADC.[61] Song and colleagues compared 2x SMS to standard rs-EPI in 134 patients, with the same parameters except no partial Fourier with SMS and 6/8 in regular.[62] They found that although reader-evaluated SNR was not significantly different, lesion contrast, image quality, and lesion conspicuity were higher with SMS. Sanderink and colleagues compared SMS rs-EPI (0.9 × 0.9 × 4.0mm resolution, 2:45 scan) to regular rs-EPI (1.2 × 1.2 × 5mm, 4:23) in 25 subjects with histologically proven breast cancer.[63] Readers scored image quality lower in SMS than non-SMS but scored lesion visibility higher on SMS. Finally, Hu and colleagues looked at 102 lesions in 96 patients, comparing rs-EPI (4:27 scan) to SMS-rs EPI (2:17 scan) with otherwise identical parameters, looking at mean kurtosis, mean diffusion and ADC as well as scoring in numerous categories.[64] They found no significant differences between the techniques. Overall, unsurprisingly, SMS is a straightforward tool to use coil sensitivity to increase the number of acquired slices and therefore improve acquisition efficiency of breast DWI.

Axially Reformatted SMS

An alternative use of SMS has been shown by McKay and colleagues.[65] The axially reformatted SMS (AR-SMS) approach uses a sagittal scan plane with very thin (1.25-mm) slices and an SMS acceleration of 4 to exploit coil sensitivity in the L/R direction. The sagittal acquisition enables the use of a small S/I FOV in-plane (further reduced with 2x in-plane parallel imaging) so that distortion is greatly reduced, whereas thin slices enable reformatting of images into the axial plane with 1.25 × 1.25 mm^2 resolution and essentially no distortion in the axial plane. This approach has been demonstrated in 40 patients with 28 lesions, with higher reader scores for image quality and spatial resolution compared with ss-EPI (R = 3) and rs-EPI (R = 3) imaging. It should be noted that it may be possible to achieve similar overall performance using axial imaging with 2x SMS and a 4x parallel imaging acceleration in the L/R direction, though this has not been demonstrated. However, the AR-SMS approach nicely shows again that the consideration of coil geometry and acquisition FOV is an important consideration in setting up and comparing protocols.

Other Advanced Methods

Most of the methods described earlier are currently readily available on at least one of the major MRI vendor scanners. However, the excitement around DWI for breast and other imaging means that there continues to be extensive research to further improve acquisition. This section describes some of the novel approaches that are being explored for breast DWI, which may not yet be widely available. Additionally, comments are offered regarding some of the more general DWI options that are available but as yet not studied in the breast.

SPATIOTEMPORAL ENCODING (SPEN)

Diffusion-weighted SPatiotemporal ENcoding (SPEN) is an alternative to standard Fourier encoding for MR image acquisition.[66] The refocusing RF pulse is a swept-frequency RF pulse that is played along with a gradient in the "SPEN direction" (which replaces the phase-encode direction). The readout gradient is identical to EPI, performing Fourier encoding in the readout direction. However, a constant gradient in the SPEN direction brings different portions of the image into focus at different times, hence the name "spatiotemporal encoding." Although some distortion from off-resonance effects persists, SPEN may overcome some of the blurring issues with single-shot EPI, especially when the point-spread function (PSF) is accounted for during reconstruction. A more recent technique called X-SPEN may substantially reduce distortions at a small cost of longer TE.[67] SPEN has been investigated for DWI in the breast, showing substantial improvement over ss-EPI in distortion and artifacts from fat suppression, and enabling reliable ADC calculation,[68] though the RF power limitations may limit overall efficiency by increasing the minimum TR or limiting the number of slices per TR.

STEADY-STATE GRADIENT-ECHO DWI

Steady-state DWI approaches take advantage of short TRs to rapidly encode diffusion, typically using 3D image encoding, which offers the potential for improved through-slice resolution without distortion. Unbalanced spoiler gradients provide diffusion weighting through multiple coherence pathways, and diffusion sensitivity can be increased either by increasing gradient size or reducing flip angles so that the mixing time is longer. Unlike standard DWI, the diffusion sensitivity (and the ADC) is dependent on relaxation times T1 and T2 as well as the flip angle, TE and TR.[69] Bulk motion in the presence of diffusion gradients again induces phase, which can cause inconsistencies in data but also can affect the steady state. Therefore the phase effects are even more difficult to compensate than standard nonsteady state (diffusion-prepared) approaches. Navigated approaches have been proposed to mitigate these artifacts,[70] and a real-time phase adjustment could help maintain the steady state, though only compensating for bulk motion.[71]

Multiple approaches have been explored for steady-state breast DWI, aiming at 3D distortion-free images either to align with or replace contrast-enhanced breast MRI. Fat suppression is typically achieved with water-only excitation to avoid disrupting the steady-state. The acquisition of signal before and after the spoiler gradient using double-echo steady state

(DESS) can help with quantitation of diffusion sensitivity.[72,73] DESS has been shown to offer substantial improvements in resolution in the breast while eliminating the distortion of EPI, as shown in Fig. 12.8.[74] Although promising, this approach remains quite sensitive to motion, as described earlier. More recently, the use of center-out non-Cartesian acquisitions, such as 3D cones, has been demonstrated to dramatically reduce motion sensitivity, which enables more robust 3D DWI in the breast.[75] The use of a 3D cones readout (Fig. 12.9) also improves the acquisition efficiency so that $1 \times 1 \times 3$ mm resolution can be obtained in 2 to 3 minutes. Overall, the diagnostic capability of 3D DESS cones was shown to be better than conventional DWI in the breast.[75] Fig. 12.9 shows example images in the breast at $1.4 \times 1.4 \times 3.0$ mm^3 resolution, compared with EPI DWI and Cartesian DCE.

OTHER ADVANCED DWI APPROACHES

Research in diffusion-weighted MRI remains very active, and it should be noted that numerous techniques could be promising for breast DWI, though studies have not been published to date. Diffusion-prepared spin-echo-train imaging offers distortion-free imaging by using a spin-echo-train readout instead of EPI. Although shot-to-shot phase variations affect the spin-echo-train signal, approaches to mitigate this offer robustness, usually at a cost of SNR.[76,77] Diffusion-prepared single-shot spin-echo-train-imaging has been

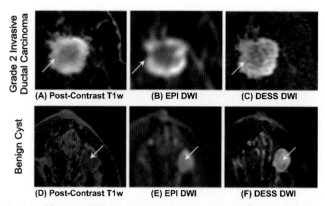

Fig. 12.8 Comparison of (A,D) postcontrast images to (B,E) noncontrast EPI DWI ($b = 600$ s/mm^2) and (C,F) DESS DWI (no exact b value, but equivalent attenuation to approximately $b = 300$ s/mm^2). DESS DWI shows high spatial resolution and lower distortion (near nipple) than EPI DWI. Suspicious rim high signal and spiculation of grade-2 IDC are present on all images. Suspicious irregular tumor margins, as well as smooth margins of cyst, are better seen on DESS than conventional EPI DWI. *DESS*, Double-echo steady state; *DWI*, diffusion-weighted imaging; *EPI*, echo-planar imaging; *IDC*, invasive ductal carcinoma.

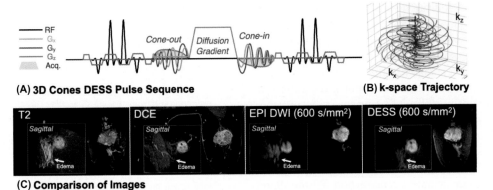

(A) 3D Cones DESS Pulse Sequence

(B) k-space Trajectory

(C) Comparison of Images

Fig. 12.9　Cones DESS sequence. (A) uses water-only excitation to suppress fat, samples outward on first echo, returns to center on second echo, both along surface of different cones, and (B) offers high sampling duty cycle with flexibility to sample k-space more quickly than Cartesian imaging. (C) 3D DWI images show high spatial resolution of cones DESS (equivalent $b = 500\,s/mm^2$, $1.4 \times 1.4 \times 3.0\,mm^3$ resolution, 2:54 scan time) compared with EPI DWI ($b = 600\,s/mm^2$, $2.0 \times 2.0 \times 5.0\,mm^3$ resolution, 1:04 scan time), including sagittal reformatted image in subject with TNBC. Notably, edema is darker than on EPI DWI, as additional T1 weighting of DESS suppresses long-T1 fluids. A standard T2-weighted and postcontrast DCE image ($0.5 \times 0.5 \times 1.0\,mm^3$ resolution) are also shown for comparison. *DCE*, Dynamic contrast-enhanced; *DESS*, double-echo steady state; *DWI*, diffusion-weighted imaging; *EPI*, echo-planar imaging; *RF*, radiofrequency; *TNBC*, triple negative breast cancer.

used in several studies in the breast. Partridge and colleagues used this approach to study ADC variations with menstrual cycle demonstrating the lack of distortion.[78] Baltzer and colleagues compared a single-shot method (HASTE-DWI) to EPI-DWI, showing HASTE-DWI had reduced distortion and comparable ADC to EPI-DWI but greater measurement variance due to the lower SNR.[79] Other studies have shown the expected lack of distortion seen in EPI for discriminating invasive ductal carcinoma from fibroadenoma,[80] as well as for acquisition of IVIM acquisition and analysis.[81]

Similar to diffusion-prepared spin-echo-train methods, diffusion-prepared SSFP offers distortion-free imaging, but instead shot-to-shot *amplitude* variations must be addressed. A widely available DWI method that has yet to be applied in the breast is PROPELLER, where k-space is divided into images with limited phase-encode resolution where the phase-encode direction is *rotated* between shots or blades. For DWI, individual PROPELLER blades can be implemented using FSE[82] or EPI.[83] Each image is full-FOV, and this provides a self-navigator to correct for motion effects including shot-to-shot phase variations. Another variation is short-axis PROPELLER (SAP),[84] which further reduces distortions in individual blades, similar to rs-EPI.[41] In PROPELLER

techniques, the trade-off is that the overlapping central k-space reduces overall efficiency, and acquisition times are typically 2x to 3x longer than for conventional acquisitions. Self-navigated interleaved spirals (SNAILS) is a DWI technique similar to multishot EPI but instead uses a dual-density spiral readout.[85] As with most multishot spiral imaging, multiple spiral interleaves are used to acquire the full image data. However, the inner k-space portion of the spiral is higher density and full-FOV and can be used to phase-correct the remaining portion of the spiral readout so that multiple interleaves can be combined with reduced shot-to-shot motion artifact.

FUTURE IMPROVEMENTS

Aside from other DWI approaches described in this chapter that have yet to be extensively studied for breast MRI, other advances in MRI will likely affect breast DWI. Currently, 16-channel breast coils are common at both 1.5 T and 3 T. At 3 T, the higher frequency and shorter wavelength enables the use of smaller coil elements, and it is likely that higher-channel count coils will become available. Breast MRI has been investigated at 7 T, where higher SNR could allow higher resolution,[86] and even smaller coil elements are possible.[87] Newer methods for distortion correction and simultaneous acquisition of DWI with relaxometry methods are also being explored, for example with echo-planar time-resolved imaging.[88] Magnetic resonance fingerprinting is another efficient quantitative imaging approach that has been shown for T1 and T2 measurements in the breast, but DWI using this approach remains difficult.[89] Advances in reconstruction are likely to continue to improve robustness of EPI, including reduced ghosting and blurring artifacts and denoising. Deep learning has been very successfully applied to image reconstruction,[90] offering both faster and more flexible reconstruction. Furthermore, the ability to denoise images using deep learning will have a tremendous effect on DWI,[91] as SNR remains one of the primary limitations.

SUMMARY

Although DWI has tremendous potential for detection, characterization, and surveillance of breast cancer, the acquisition approaches require careful consideration. Conventional EPI is widely available but is very limited in the breast primarily due to blurring and distortion artifacts. Additionally, consistent fat suppression remains challenging to achieve in breast DWI, though there are multiple options. Over the last decade, some promising approaches have been developed and tested to address blurring and distortion and have demonstrated clear improvements for breast DWI. These include parallel imaging, reduced-FOV EPI, rs-EPI, and interleaved multishot EPI with MUSE reconstruction. SMS has further improved the scan-time efficiency challenges and can offer flexibility. Finally, there is potential for novel approaches to further improve on resolution and robustness of acquisitions.

REFERENCES

1. Stejskal EO, Tanner JE. Spin diffusion measurements: spin echoes in the presence of a time-dependent field gradient. *J Chem Phys*. 1965;42:288–292.
2. Peters NH, Borel Rinkes IH, Zuithoff NP, et al. Meta-analysis of MR imaging in the diagnosis of breast lesions. *Radiology*. 2008;246:116–124.
3. Baxter GC, Graves MJ, Gilbert FJ, et al. A meta-analysis of the diagnostic performance of diffusion MRI for breast lesion characterization. *Radiology*. 2019;291:632–641.
4. Amornsiripanitch N, Bickelhaupt S, Shin HJ, et al. Diffusion-weighted MRI for unenhanced breast cancer screening. *Radiology*. 2019;293:504–520.
5. Basser PJ, Mattiello J, Le Bihan D. MR diffusion tensor spectroscopy and imaging. *Biophys J*. 1994;66:259–267.
6. Le Bihan D, Breton E, Lallemand D, et al. MR imaging of intravoxel incoherent motions: application to diffusion and perfusion in neurologic disorders. *Radiology*. 1986;161:401–407.
7. Lu H, Jensen JH, Ramani A, et al. Three-dimensional characterization of non-gaussian water diffusion in humans using diffusion kurtosis imaging. *NMR Biomed*. 2006;19:236–247.
8. White NS, McDonald CR, Farid N, et al. Diffusion-weighted imaging in cancer: physical foundations and applications of restriction spectrum imaging. *Cancer Res*. 2014;74:4638–4652.
9. Mansfield P. Multiplanar image formation using NMR spin-echoes. *J Phys Chem Solid State Phys*. 1977;10:L55.
10. Noll DC, Nishimura DG, Macovski A. Homodyne detection in magnetic resonance imaging. *IEEE Trans Med Imaging*. 1991;10:154–163.
11. Jezzard P, Balaban RS. Correction for geometric distortion in echo planar images from B0 field variations. *Magn Reson Med*. 1995;34:65–73.
12. Andersson JL, Skare S, Ashburner J. How to correct susceptibility distortions in spin-echo echo-planar images: application to diffusion tensor imaging. *Neuroimage*. 2003;20:870–888.
13. Smith SM, Jenkinson M, Woolrich MW, et al. Advances in functional and structural MR image analysis and implementation as FSL. *Neuroimage*. 2004;23:S208–S219.
14. Ordidge RJ, Helpern JA, Qing Z, et al. Correction of motional artifacts in diffusion-weighted MR images using navigator echoes. *Magn Reson Imaging*. 1994;12:455–460.
15. Anderson AW, Gore JC. Analysis and correction of motion artifacts in diffusion weighted imaging. *Magn Reson Med*. 1994;32:379–387.
16. Norris DG. Implications of bulk motion for diffusion-weighted imaging experiments: effects, mechanisms, and solutions. *J Magn Reson Imaging*. 2001;13:486–495.
17. Dixon WT. Simple proton spectroscopic imaging. *Radiology*. 1984;153:189–194.
18. Reeder SB, Herzka DA, McVeigh ER. Signal-to-noise ratio behavior of steady-state free precession. *Magn Reson Med*. 2004;52:123–130.
19. Ma J. Breath-hold water and fat imaging using a dual-echo two-point Dixon technique with an efficient and robust phase-correction algorithm. *Magn Reson Med*. 2004;52:415–419.
20. Bydder GM, Pennock JM, Steiner RE, et al. The short TI inversion recovery sequence: an approach to MR imaging of the abdomen. *Magn Reson Imaging*. 1985;3:251–254.
21. Meyer C, Pauly J, Macovski A, et al. Simultaneous spatial and spectral selective excitation. *Magn Reson Med*. 1990;15:287–304.
22. Hancu I, Govenkar A, Lenkinski RE, et al. On shimming approaches in 3T breast MRI. *Magn Reson Med*. 2013;69:862–867.
23. Lee SK, Tan ET, Govenkar A, et al. Dynamic slice-dependent shim and center frequency update in 3 T breast diffusion weighted imaging. *Magn Reson Med*. 2014;71:1813–1818.
24. Pauly JM, Cunningham CH, Daniel BL. Independent dual-band spectral-spatial pulses. In: Proceedings of the 11th Annual Meeting of ISMRM. Toronto; 2003:966.
25. Han M, Cunningham CH, Pauly JM, et al. Homogenous fat suppression for bilateral breast imaging using independent shims. *Magn Reson Med*. 2014;71:1511–1517.
26. Pruessmann KP, Weiger M, Scheidegger MB, et al. SENSE: sensitivity encoding for fast MRI. *Magn Reson Med*. 1999;42:952–962.
27. Griswold MA, Jakob PM, Heidemann RM, et al. Generalized autocalibrating partially parallel acquisitions (GRAPPA). *Magn Reson Med*. 2002;47:1202–1210.

28. Larkman DJ, Nunes RG. Parallel magnetic resonance imaging. *Phys Med Biol.* 2007;52:R15–R55.

29. Deshmane A, Gulani V, Griswold MA, et al. Parallel MR imaging. *J Magn Reson Imaging.* 2012;36:55–72.

30. Heidemann RM, Ozsarlak O, Parizel PM, et al. A brief review of parallel magnetic resonance imaging. *Eur Radiol.* 2003;13:2323–2337.

31. Bammer R, Keeling SL, Augustin M, et al. Improved diffusion-weighted single-shot echo-planar imaging (EPI) in stroke using sensitivity encoding (SENSE). *Magn Reson Med.* 2001;46:548–554.

32. Saritas EU, Cunningham CH, Lee JH, et al. DWI of the spinal cord with reduced FOV single-shot EPI. *Magn Reson Med.* 2008;60:468–473.

33. Singer L, Wilmes LJ, Saritas EU, et al. High-resolution diffusion-weighted magnetic resonance imaging in patients with locally advanced breast cancer. *Acad Radiol.* 2012;19:526–534.

34. Kang BJ, Lipson JA, Planey KR, et al. Rim sign in breast lesions on diffusion-weighted magnetic resonance imaging: diagnostic accuracy and clinical usefulness. *J Magn Reson Imaging.* 2014;41:616–623.

35. Wilmes LJ, McLaughlin RL, Newitt DC, et al. High-resolution diffusion-weighted imaging for monitoring breast cancer treatment response. *Acad Radiol.* 2013;20:581–589.

36. Barentsz MW, Taviani V, Chang JM, et al. Assessment of tumor morphology on diffusion-weighted (DWI) breast MRI: diagnostic value of reduced field of view DWI. *J Magn Reson Imaging.* 2015;42:1656–1665.

37. Taviani V, Alley MT, Banerjee S, et al. High-resolution diffusion-weighted imaging of the breast with multiband 2D radiofrequency pulses and a generalized parallel imaging reconstruction. *Magn Reson Med.* 2017;77:209–220.

38. Wilm B, Svensson J, Henning A, et al. Reduced field-of-view MRI using outer volume suppression for spinal cord diffusion imaging. *Magn Reson Med.* 2007;57:625–630.

39. Feinberg DA, Hoenninger J, Crooks L, et al. Inner volume MR imaging: technical concepts and their application. *Radiology.* 1985;156:743–747.

40. Jeong EK, Kim SE, Guo J, et al. High-resolution DTI with 2D interleaved multislice reduced FOV single-shot diffusion-weighted EPI (2D ss-rFOV-DWEPI). *Magn Reson Med.* 2005;54:1575–1579.

41. Porter DA, Heidemann RM. High resolution diffusion-weighted imaging using readout-segmented echo-planar imaging, parallel imaging and a two-dimensional navigator-based reacquisition. *Magn Reson Med.* 2009;62:468–475.

42. Bogner W, Pinker-Domenig K, Bickel H, et al. Readout-segmented echo-planar imaging improves the diagnostic performance of diffusion-weighted MR breast examinations at 3.0 T. *Radiology.* 2012;263:64–76.

43. Wisner DJ, Rogers N, Deshpande VS, et al. High-resolution diffusion-weighted imaging for the separation of benign from malignant BI-RADS 4/5 lesions found on breast MRI at 3T. *J Magn Reson Imaging.* 2013;40:674–681.

44. Kim YJ, Kim SH, Kang BJ, et al. Readout-segmented echo-planar imaging in diffusion-weighted MR imaging in breast cancer: comparison with single-shot echoplanar imaging in image quality. *Korean J Radiol.* 2014;15:403–410.

45. An YY, Kim SH, Kang BJ. Differentiation of malignant and benign breast lesions: added value of the qualitative analysis of breast lesions on diffusion-weighted imaging (DWI) using readout-segmented echo-planar imaging at 3.0 T. *PLoS One.* 2017;12:e0174681.

46. Baltzer PAT, Bickel H, Spick C, et al. Potential of noncontrast magnetic resonance imaging with diffusion-weighted imaging in characterization of breast lesions: intraindividual comparison with dynamic contrast-enhanced magnetic resonance imaging. *Invest Radiol.* 2018;53:229–235.

47. Park JY, Shin HJ, Shin KC, et al. Comparison of readout segmented echo planar imaging (EPI) and EPI with reduced field-of-view diffusion-weighted imaging at 3T in patients with breast cancer. *J Magn Reson Imaging.* 2015;42:1679–1688.

48. Chen Nk, Guidon A, Chang HC, et al. A robust multi-shot scan strategy for high resolution diffusion weighted MRI enabled by multiplexed sensitivity-encoding (MUSE). *Neuroimage.* 2013;72:41–47.

49. Chu ML, Chang HC, Chung HW, et al. POCS-based reconstruction of multiplexed sensitivity encoded MRI (POCSMUSE): a general algorithm for reducing motion-related artifacts. *Magn Reson Med.* 2015;74:1336–1348.

50. Daimiel Naranjo I, Lo Gullo R, Morris EA, et al. High-spatial resolution multishot multiplexed sensitivity-encoding diffusion-weighted imaging for improved quality of breast images and differentiation of breast lesions: a feasibility study. *Radiol Imaging Cancer.* 2020;2:e190076.

51. Hu Y, Ikeda DM, Pittman SM, et al. Multishot diffusion-weighted MRI of the breast with multiplexed sensitivity encoding (MUSE) and shot locally low-rank (Shot-LLR) reconstructions. *J Magn Reson Imaging.* 2021;53:807–817.

52. Trzasko JD, Manduca A. Calibrationless parallel MRI using CLEAR. In: Signals, Systems and Computers (ASILOMAR), 2011 Conference Record of the Forty-Fifth Asilomar Conference on IEEE; 2011:75–79.

53. Mani M, Jacob M, Kelley D, et al. Multi-shot sensitivity-encoded diffusion data recovery using structured low-rank matrix completion (MUSSELS). *Magn Reson Med.* 2017;78:494–507.

54. Hu Y, Xu Y, Tian Q, et al. RUN-UP: accelerated multishot diffusion-weighted MRI reconstruction using an unrolled network with U-Net as priors. *Magn Reson Med.* 2021;85:709–720.

55. Aggarwal HK, Mani MP, Jacob M. MoDL-MUSSELS: model-based deep learning for multishot sensitivity-encoded diffusion MRI. *IEEE Trans Med Imaging.* 2019;39:1268–1277.

56. Glover GH. Phase-offset multiplanar (POMP) volume imaging: a new technique. *J Magn Reson Imaging.* 1991;1:457–461.

57. Larkman DJ, deSouza NM, Bydder M, et al. An investigation into the use of sensitivity-encoded techniques to increase temporal resolution in dynamic contrast-enhanced breast imaging. *J Magn Reson Imaging.* 2001;14:329–335.

58. Breuer FA, Blaimer M, Heidemann RM, et al. Controlled aliasing in parallel imaging results in higher acceleration (CAIPIRINHA) for multi-slice imaging. *Magn Reson Med.* 2005;53:684–691.

59. Setsompop K, Cohen-Adad J, Gagoski BA, et al. Improving diffusion MRI using simultaneous multi-slice echo planar imaging. *Neuroimage.* 2012;63:569–580.

60. Ohlmeyer S, Laun FB, Palm T, et al. Simultaneous multislice echo planar imaging for accelerated diffusion-weighted imaging of malignant and benign breast lesions. *Invest Radiol.* 2019;54:524–530.

61. Filli L, Ghafoor S, Kenkel D, et al. Simultaneous multi-slice readout-segmented echo planar imaging for accelerated diffusion-weighted imaging of the breast. *Eur J Radiol.* 2016;85:274–278.

62. Song SE, Woo OH, Cho KR, et al. Simultaneous multislice readout-segmented echo planar imaging for diffusion-weighted MRI in patients with invasive breast cancers. *J Magn Reson Imaging.* 2021;53:1108–1115.

63. Sanderink WB, Teuwen J, Appelman L, et al. Comparison of simultaneous multi-slice single-shot DWI to readout-segmented DWI for evaluation of breast lesions at 3T MRI. *Eur J Radiol.* 2021;138:109626.

64. Hu Y, Zhan C, Yang Z, et al. Accelerating acquisition of readout-segmented echo planar imaging with a simultaneous multi-slice (SMS) technique for diagnosing breast lesions. *Eur Radiol.* 2021;31(5):2667–2676.

65. McKay JA, Church AL, Rubin N, et al. A comparison of methods for high-spatial-resolution diffusion-weighted imaging in breast MRI. *Radiology.* 2020;297:304–312.

66. Solomon E, Shemesh N, Frydman L. Diffusion weighted MRI by spatiotemporal encoding: analytical description and in vivo validations. *J Magn Reson.* 2013;232:76–86.

67. Zhang Z, Seginer A, Frydman L, Single-scan MRI. with exceptional resilience to field heterogeneities. *Magn Reson Med.* 2017;77:623–634.

68. Solomon E, Nissan N, Furman-Haran E, et al. Overcoming limitations in diffusion-weighted MRI of breast by spatio-temporal encoding. *Magn Reson Med.* 2015;73:2163–2173.

69. Buxton RB. The diffusion sensitivity of fast steady-state free precession imaging. *Magn Reson Med.* 1993;29:235–243.

70. Miller KD. Issues and challenges for antiangiogenic therapies. *Breast Cancer Res Treat.* 2002;75:S45–S50.

71. O'Halloran R, Aksoy M, Aboussouan E, et al. Real-time correction of rigid body motion-induced phase errors for diffusion-weighted steady-state free precession imaging. *Magn Reson Med.* 2015;73:565–576.

72. Staroswiecki E, Granlund KL, Alley MT, et al. Simultaneous estimation of T2 and apparent diffusion coefficient in human articular cartilage in vivo with a modified three-dimensional double echo steady state (DESS) sequence at 3 T. *Magn Reson Med.* 2012;67:1086–1096.

73. Bieri O, Ganter C, Scheffler K. Quantitative in vivo diffusion imaging of cartilage using double echo steady-state free precession. *Magn Reson Med.* 2012;68:720–729.

74. Granlund KL, Staroswiecki E, Alley MT, et al. High-resolution, three-dimensional diffusion-weighted breast imaging using DESS. *Magn Reson Imaging.* 2014;32:330–341.

75. Moran CJ, Cheng JY, Sandino CM, et al. Diffusion-weighted double-echo steady-state with a three-dimensional cones trajectory for non-contrast-enhanced breast MRI. *J Magn Reson Imaging.* 2021;53:1594–1605.

76. Alsop DC. Phase insensitive preparation of single-shot RARE: application to diffusion imaging in humans. *Magn Reson Med.* 1997;38:527–533.

77. Schick F. SPLICE: sub-second diffusion-sensitive MR imaging using a modified fast spin-echo acquisition mode. *Magn Reson Med.* 1997;38:638–644.

78. Partridge SC, McKinnon GC, Henry RG, Hylton NM. Menstrual cycle variation of apparent diffusion coefficients measured in the normal breast using MRI. *J Magn Reson Imaging.* 2001;14(4):433–438.

79. Baltzer PA, Renz DM, Herrmann KH, et al. Diffusion-weighted imaging (DWI) in MR mammography (MRM): clinical comparison of echo planar imaging (EPI) and half-Fourier single-shot turbo spin echo (HASTE) diffusion techniques. *Eur Radiol.* 2009;19(7):1612–1620.

80. Kinoshita T, Yashiro N, Ihara N, Funatu H, Fukuma E, Narita M. Diffusion-weighted half-Fourier single-shot turbo spin echo imaging in breast tumors: differentiation of invasive ductal carcinoma from fibroadenoma. *J Comput Assist Tomogr.* 2002;26(6):1042–1046.

81. Cho GY, Moy L, Kim SG, et al. Evaluation of breast cancer using intravoxel incoherent motion (IVIM) histogram analysis: comparison with malignant status, histological subtype, and molecular prognostic factors. *Eur Radiol.* 2016;26(8):2547–2558.

82. Pipe JG, Farthing VG, Forbes KP. Multishot diffusion-weighted FSE using PROPELLER MRI. *Magn Reson Med.* 2002;47:42–52.

83. Wang FN, Huang TY, Lin FH, et al. PROPELLER EPI: an MRI technique suitable for diffusion tensor imaging at high field strength with reduced geometric distortions. *Magn Reson Med.* 2005;54:1232–1240.

84. Skare S, Newbould RD, Clayton DB, et al. Propeller EPI in the other direction. *Magn Reson Med.* 2006;55:1298–1307.

85. Liu C, Bammer R, Kim D-H, et al. Self-navigated interleaved spiral (SNAILS): application to high-resolution diffusion tensor imaging. *Magn Reson Med.* 2004;52:1388–1396.

86. Umutlu L, Maderwald S, Kraff O, et al. Dynamic contrast-enhanced breast MRI at 7 Tesla utilizing a single-loop coil: a feasibility trial. *Acad Radiol.* 2010;17:1050–1056.

87. van de Bank BL, Voogt IJ, Italiaander M, et al. Ultra high spatial and temporal resolution breast imaging at 7T. *NMR Biomed.* 2013;26:367–375.

88. Wang F, Dong Z, Reese TG, et al. Echo planar time-resolved imaging (EPTI). *Magn Reson Med.* 2019;81:3599–3615.

89. Panda A, Chen Y, Ropella-Panagis K, et al. Repeatability and reproducibility of 3D MR fingerprinting relaxometry measurements in normal breast tissue. *J Magn Reson Imaging.* 2019;50:1133–1143.

90. Hammernik K, Klatzer T, Kobler E, et al. Learning a variational network for reconstruction of accelerated MRI data. *Magn Reson Med.* 2017;79:3055–3071.

91. Lebel RM. Performance characterization of a novel deep learning- based MR image reconstruction pipeline. 2020: arXiv:200806559. Epub ahead of print.

Chapter 13

Clinical Interpretation of Diffusion MRI, ROI Assessment, Common Errors, Pitfalls and Artifacts, Challenges in Acquisition

Gabrielle C. Baxter, PhD, Ramona Woitek, MD, PhD, Andrew J. Patterson, PhD, and Fiona J. Gilbert, MD, FRCR, FRCP

Diffusion-weighted imaging (DWI) is an magnetic resonance imaging (MRI) technique where the mobility of water molecules diffusing in tissue contributes to the image contrast. Sensitivity to diffusion is achieved by adding a pair of symmetrical diffusion sensitizing gradients to a spin-echo sequence. The amount of diffusion weighting is determined by the b value, which is controlled by the strength and timings of the gradients. In a DWI sequence, at least two diffusion-weighted images are acquired, one at a low b value (0, or $<100 \, s/mm^2$ if excluding perfusion effects) and one at a high b value (usually $600-1000 \, s/mm^2$).[1] The higher b value can be chosen to maximize contrast between malignant and benign or fibroglandular tissue. Images are interpreted by observing the difference in signal attenuation on images acquired at different b values (see Chapter 1). In tissue, the diffusion of water is impeded by cell membranes and other cellular structures, sometimes in an anisotropic manner. In addition to the random molecular motion of water, there are a number of other biological processes that contribute to signal attenuation, such as blood and lymphatic flow in the microvasculature and diffusion restriction from microstructures. Bulk flow and motion can also affect the measurement of signal, and therefore the measured diffusion coefficient is referred to as the apparent diffusion coefficient (ADC). Visual assessment of signal attenuation on DWI and measurement of the ADC can be used for tumor detection, characterization, and assessment of response to treatment in patients with breast cancer. Although DWI is an emerging technique alongside dynamic contrast-enhanced (DCE) MRI, it has yet to be incorporated into the American College of Radiology (ACR) Breast Imaging Reporting and Data System (BI-RADS).

A series of diffusion-weighted images is usually acquired using two or more b values, with higher b values indicating higher diffusion weighting. The appearance of low b value images is usually similar to that of T2-weighted images with fat suppression. In contrast, high b value images tend only to show high signal only where diffusion is restricted (with few exceptions, which will be covered later). From these images acquired using two or more different b values, the ADC can be calculated directly or by fitting the decrease in signal between low and high b value acquisitions for each voxel (see Chapter 1). The resulting ADC is then displayed as a parametric map (the ADC map).

When interpreting clinical DWI of the breast, it is recommended to view both, high b *value* images and ADC maps. High b value images can be used for lesion detection as they help with lesion identification, whereas ADC maps are necessary to confirm restricted diffusion in areas with high signal intensity on high b value images. ADC maps can be assessed visually, or the ADC of a tissue can be measured by defining a region of interest (ROI) on an ADC map. Diffusion is restricted in regions that are hyperintense on high b value DWI and correspond to a low measured ADC

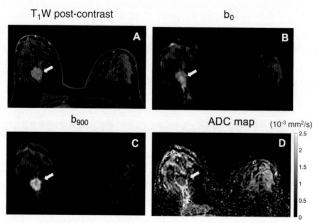

Fig. 13.1 Example breast images acquired with DWI for a 34-year-old woman with invasive ductal carcinoma *(arrows)*. (A) Postcontrast DCE image, (B) low *b* value DWI ($b = 0\,s/mm^2$), (C) higher *b* value DWI ($b = 900\,s/mm^2$), and (D) the corresponding ADC map. The tumor appears hyperintense on DWI (C) and hypointense on the ADC map (D). *ADC*, Apparent diffusion coefficient; *DCE*, dynamic contrast-enhanced; *DWI*, diffusion-weighted imaging.

(Fig. 13.1). However, signal intensity on high *b* value images is not solely dependent on water diffusion but also T2 relaxation. Therefore an area with a high signal intensity may derive from a tissue with a long T2 relaxation time, that is, tissue with a high water content such as cysts or fibroadenoma as opposed to restricted diffusion (known as "T2 shine-through"). Therefore high *b* value images should be interpreted alongside T2-weighted images (or low *b* value images) or together with the ADC map. Conversely, tissues and lesions with a low water content, such as fibrotic parenchyma, scars, and some invasive lobular cancers, will appear as areas of very low signal on DWI (sometimes referred to as T2 blackout) and may be difficult to visualize on the DWI images.

Clinical Interpretation

CLINICAL SEQUENCES

When interpreting full diagnostic protocol MRI of the breast including DWI, it is recommended to review the MRI together with conventional imaging (mammograms, tomosynthesis, and whole breast or hand-held ultrasound). Contrast-enhanced T1-weighted images (ideally including subtractions of unenhanced from enhanced images and maximum intensity projections (MIPs) are usually the first series to be reviewed, as they allow evaluation of the degree of background parenchymal enhancement and whether or not contrast-enhancing lesions can be identified on the scan.

Once enhancing lesions are identified, they need to be further characterized by evaluating their morphology and their enhancement kinetics on dynamic-contrast enhancement. Ideally, kinetic maps are created automatically and overlaid on T1-weighted images to display the type of enhancement for each voxel reaching a set enhancement threshold (type 1, continuous enhancement; type 2, plateau enhancement; type 3, washout; type 3 is the most suspicious; see Chapter 2). Additional review of T2-weighted images is recommended to evaluate the signal intensity of enhancing lesions and to assess for nonenhancing lesions such as cysts. DWI is then reviewed for further lesion characterization. The recommended image review process is summarized in Table 13.1.

Typically, the low and high diffusion sequences will be saved to the picture archiving and communication system (PACS), ready for clinical interpretation. Ideally the slice thickness and location will match the T2W sequence, although often the slice thickness will be greater than the T2W sequence. ADC will be calculated and the ADC maps saved onto the PACS. The quality of the DWI images should be assessed for artifact and movement and a decision made as to whether the images are interpretable. With this relatively new sequence, the DWI is often overlooked by the technicians and is sometimes not repeated when required. The radiologist starts with the high signal on a high *b* value image (with the greatest diffusion weighting) to try and identify abnormalities and correlate them

TABLE 13.1   Recommended Image Review Process

Sequence	Evaluate for
DCE T1-weighted	Background parenchymal enhancement
	Presence of enhancing lesions
	Lesion morphology
	Enhancement kinetics
T2-weighted	Nonenhancing lesions
	Lesion morphology and signal
DWI	Presence of diffusion restriction
	ADC measurements
Unenhanced T1-weighted	Hyperintensities like hematoma

ADC, Apparent diffusion coefficient; *DCE*, dynamic contrast-enhanced; *DWI*, diffusion-weighted imaging.

with the other sequences. Generally, all high signal area in DWI greater than 5 mm should be interrogated. Using the ADC map, regions of lowest signal are also identified and further interrogated. For lesions identified on contrast-enhanced sequences or (if omitted as in unenhanced MRI protocols) on DWI, an ROI should be drawn within the boundaries of the lesion, either encompassing the largest possible region but avoiding any surrounding fat or fibroglandular tissue, or covering a small subregion with the lowest ADC. Meticulous comparison made with DCE images is recommended to ensure the lesion of concern is being included. One must be aware that the spatial position may not spatially map to the DCE sequence, as DWI sequences suffer from distortion, therefore requiring to pick up on anatomical features to make a match. The ROI can either be drawn on the high *b* value DWI images and then transferred onto the ADC map or on the ADC map directly. The ADC should be noted and if a marginal value is obtained then a repeat measurement should be undertaken.

LESION CLASSIFICATION

DWI is increasingly used in the classification of suspicious breast lesions on MRI as an adjunct to DCE MRI to reduce false positive results and avoid unnecessary biopsies. In tumors, the tight cellular packing hinders or restricts diffusion, resulting in signal hyperintensity compared with normal breast tissue on high *b* value diffusion-weighted images, and significantly lower ADC values are measured in malignant breast tumors compared with benign lesions and fibroglandular tissue[2] (Fig. 13.2). A meta-analysis of the diagnostic performance of DWI using the ADC demonstrated a

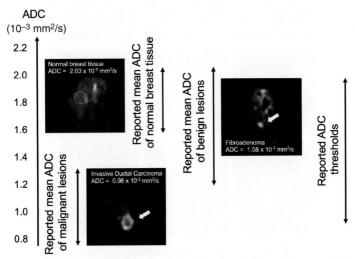

Fig. 13.2 Ranges of reported ADC values for malignant and benign breast lesions and normal breast tissue. There is a large range of reported threshold ADC values used to discriminate between malignant and benign lesions.[1] *ADC*, Apparent diffusion coefficient.

pooled sensitivity of 89% (95% CI 87–91) and specificity of 82% (95% CI 78–85) in 65 studies (6408 cancers in 5892 patients).[3] A threshold ADC value can be used to classify lesions that appear hyperintense on DWI. These thresholds are often found empirically or using receiver operating characteristic curve analysis on a cohort of breast cancer patients. Reported ADC threshold values range from 0.87×10^{-3} mm^2/s to 2×10^{-3} mm^2/s across 65 studies.[3] Variations in MRI technique and lack of standardization to date have prevented the establishment of a generalized ADC threshold. The choice of b value will affect the measured ADC, with ADC decreasing with increasing b value,[4] though there is no evidence that choice of b value affects diagnostic performance.[5] However, this suggests that ADC thresholds must be adjusted depending on chosen acquisition parameters or, better,

that standardization fixes b values to be used so as to homogenize ADC cut-off values across protocols and sites. A sufficiently high ADC threshold can also be chosen to achieve 100% sensitivity, though this may lead to unnecessary biopsies. DWI should always be interpreted alongside supporting morphological and functional information (DCE MRI and unenhanced T2-weighted images) to enable accurate lesion classification. Example DWI images for a range of breast lesions are shown in Fig. 13.3.

MORPHOLOGICAL ASSESSMENT

According to the ACR BI-RADS, lesions can be classified as either foci, masses, or nonmass enhancement (NME). Masses can be ascribed descriptors for shape (round, oval, irregular) and internal signal pattern (homogeneous, heterogeneous, rim), and nonmass

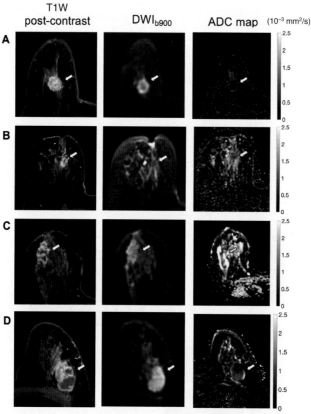

Fig. 13.3 Example breast lesions shown on DCE MRI, DWI, and the ADC map (arrows). (A) An invasive ductal carcinoma with high-grade DCIS (0.84×10^{-3} mm^2/s), (B) invasive lobular carcinoma (1.03×10^{-3} mm^2/s), (C) mucinous carcinoma (2.21×10^{-3} mm^2/s), and (D) metaplastic carcinoma (1.87×10^{-3} mm^2/s). *ADC*, Apparent diffusion coefficient; *DCE*, dynamic contrast-enhanced; *DCIS*, ductal carcinoma in situ; *DWI*, diffusion-weighted imaging.

lesions can be described in terms of distribution (focal, regional, linear, segmental) and internal signal pattern (homogeneous, heterogeneous). The qualitative assessment of the location, size, and morphology of lesions is possible using DWI. However, the low spatial resolution of DWI limits morphological assessment compared with other high resolution anatomical and contrast-enhanced sequences. Morphology as assessed on DWI can be reported when it is discrepant with other sequences.

The majority of DWI literature has focused on enhancing masses. DWI is less sensitive for NMEs,[6–8] with ROI placement significantly affecting the diagnostic accuracy of ADC measurements. NME lesions also have a lower conspicuity on DWI, with one study finding a third of lesions (29/94 NME lesions) could not be evaluated on DWI due to either nonvisibility or poor quality of DWI, suggesting that DCE MRI is required for the detection of all NME lesions.[8]

A number of false positive and false negative findings on DWI can be attributed to the underlying tumor histology of different breast cancer histopathological subtypes. The most commonly reported examples of false positive lesions on DWI are complicated cysts and fibroadenomas, likely due to high cellularity (creating a more restricted environment for diffusion), fibrosis (providing boundaries or obstacles to the free diffusion of water), and chronic inflammatory elements.[9,10] An inverse correlation has been found between ADC and the degree of fibrosis.[11] Atypical ductal hyperplasia and intraductal papilloma are also often misclassified due to increased cellularity[12] and duct ectasia, which has a low measured ADC.[13] Diffusion can also be restricted in regions of high viscosity or intra- or extracellular edema, such as in mastitis, abscesses, and coagulated blood or proteinaceous debris within ducts and cysts.[14]

On the other hand, mucinous carcinoma is a common false negative finding given that its measured ADC is significantly higher than other malignant tumors, due to the low cellularity relative to the abundant mucin and the high extracellular water content.[11] Higher ADC values are also measured in papillary carcinomas due to the distribution of tumor cell batches within stromal spaces, allowing for more free diffusion in the interstitium,[15] and scirrhous adenocarcinoma has a low cellularity and is often misdiagnosed.[13] Lesions with extensive necrosis will also have a higher

TABLE 13.2   Common False Positive and False Negative Findings

Finding	Type of Lesion
False positive	Complicated cysts
	Fibroadenomas
	Fibrosis
	Atypical ductal hyperplasia
	Intraductal papilloma
	Duct ectasia
	Edema
	Mastitis
	Abscess
	Hematoma
False negative	Mucinous carcinoma
	Papillary carcinoma
	Scirrhous adenocarcinoma
	Tumors with central necrosis

ADC due to more free diffusion in the necrotic core.[16] Common false positive and false negative findings are summarized in Table 13.2.

PROBLEM-SOLVING

Whereas DCE-MRI is a highly sensitive technique for the detection of breast cancer, DWI is often used as an adjunct to contrast-enhanced MRI diagnosis of breast cancer to reduce false positive results, with a meta-analysis of 14 studies finding a combined sensitivity and specificity of 92% and 86%, respectively.[17] Breast cancers are generally detected through the observation of suspicious enhancement after the administration of gadolinium contrast, identifying areas of increased vascularity and perfusion. However, benign lesions may also show suspicious enhancement on DCE MRI. The addition of complementary information regarding tissue cellularity provided by DWI can improve the ability of MRI to distinguish between malignant and benign breast lesions. Results from the multicenter ACRIN 6702 trial have shown that the use of ADC values from DWI can significantly reduce the number of benign biopsies prompted by breast MRI without reducing sensitivity.[18]

DWI is also able to overcome some of the shortfalls of mammography. DWI has shown promise for detecting cancer in women with dense breasts for whom mammography has a reduced sensitivity and poor lesion visibility.[19,20] In the detection of mammographically occult cancers, DWI has been shown to be superior to MRI-guided focused ultrasound[21] and comparable to DCE MRI.[22] Although DWI is increasingly investigated in common types of breast lesions, further investigation is needed for the types of lesions that are of interest for problem-solving where DCE MRI is inconclusive, including small lesions, multifocal and multicentric lesions, and NMEs (where no correlate can be found on mammograms or ultrasound, which require MRI guided biopsy).

LYMPH NODES

Early detection of axillary lymph node metastasis may improve breast cancer staging and selection of treatment.[23] Sentinel node biopsy is current standard practice in assessing lymph node involvement with little morbidity compared with the more accurate surgical assessment, which is associated with morbidity including seroma, hematoma, lymphedema, and paresthesia.

On MRI, most normal lymph nodes will exhibit certain imaging features, such as fatty hila, uniform shape, and high T2 signal, which may enable a radiologist to identify them as benign.[12] Abnormal lymph nodes can be enlarged either due to tumor involvement or reactive change. Loss of the kidney-bean oval shape to a rounded appearance, loss of the fatty hilum, and increased or irregular cortical thickness are classic signs of malignancy together with an increase in short axis diameter.

Although mean ADC values of metastatic lymph nodes have been shown to be significantly lower than those of nonmetastatic lymph nodes in a recent meta-analysis,[24] and several studies reported high sensitivity and specificity of DWI in diagnosing metastatic axillary lymph nodes,[25] contrasting results have been reported as well, with the diagnostic accuracy of DWI reported as inferior to T1- and T2-weighted sequences. These results indicate that further research is needed to evaluate the value of DWI for axillary lymph node assessment.[26,27] At present, MRI does not match the accuracy of sentinel lymph node biopsy.

UNENHANCED SCREENING

There is increasing interest in DWI as a stand-alone screening tool (see Chapter 6). DWI has been investigated independently for screening or for the noncontrast detection of cancers through blinded reader studies, reporting sensitivities >85%[10,28–30] or modest sensitivity (50%–77%) and high specificity >90%.[19,31,32] However, the performance of DWI is reduced for small cancers less than 1 cm in size.[19,32] The in-plane spatial resolution of DWI (2×2 mm^2) and slice thickness (3–5 mm) are limiting factors in the detection of these small lesions, as well as the limitations of the overall image quality of DWI. For DWI to be clinically useful in a screening setting, it must be able to detect and characterize a range of cancers at least comparable to that of contrast-enhanced MRI, particularly small, early stage cancers. Further evidence from larger prospective and multicenter studies in a true screening setting is required before the adoption of unenhanced DWI screening into clinical practice.

MONITORING TREATMENT RESPONSE

Neoadjuvant chemotherapy induces changes at a cellular level, significantly altering the histopathologic appearance of tumors[33] (see Chapter 5). Studies investigating cellular changes to tumor specimens after chemotherapy found a significant reduction in tumor cellularity[34] and increased nuclear atypia,[35] with one study finding it difficult to distinguish between residual tumor cells and chemotherapy-induced atypia.[36] Combined with a measurement of residual tumor size, the assessment of response using a measure of tumor cellularity can be more accurate than using tumor size alone.[37]

Changes in tumor ADC as measured using DWI reflect these changes in cellularity. Response to treatment has been associated with changes in ADC as measured after one cycle,[38,39] two cycles,[38] at midtreatment,[40] and at the end of treatment.[40,41] Increases in ADC after chemotherapy have also been associated with the presence of necrosis and increasing cell lysis.[42]

DWI can be a useful tool in the early assessment of response to therapy, as changes in ADC have been shown to occur before reduction in tumor size.[43,44] Studies by Park and colleagues and Iacconi and colleagues found that tumors with lower pretreatment ADC and high cell density responded better to neoadjuvant chemotherapy.[45,46] A meta-analysis by Chu and colleagues found a pooled sensitivity of 88% and specificity of 79% for ADC in the prediction of pathological treatment response (pCR) but with a higher pooled AUC when using the change in ADC during treatment than pretreatment ADC (0.80 vs. 0.63).[47]

REGION OF INTEREST (ROI) ASSESSMENT

DEFINING AN ROI

The ADC of a lesion can be measured by drawing an ROI around the lesion on the higher b value image and transferring it onto the ADC map or drawing on the ADC map directly, often using contrast-enhanced imaging or other anatomical imaging as a guide to provide information about enhancement and lesion morphology. The ROI should encompass the lesion, though care must be taken to avoid cysts, hematoma, or central necrosis (areas with low cellularity and/or a high water content with a high ADC), as well as areas with artifacts, as these will affect the ADC measurement. The ROI should contain at least three voxels, which corresponds to the ADC of lesions roughly 6 mm or larger being quantifiable using ROI analysis. Images with a larger voxel size will be affected by partial volume effect, where voxels that include both pathology and fibroglandular or adipose tissue will result in an artificially higher or lower ADC measurement. To avoid this, the ROI should be drawn within the hyperintense region on DW images or the darkest area of a lesion on ADC maps. The mean ADC value for the lesion should be reported with units of

10^{-3} mm^2/s. 2D ROIs can be drawn on a slice-by-slice basis to generate a 3D ROI from which a volumetric mean ADC and other metrics can be calculated.

There is still no consensus on whether the ROI should encompass the whole lesion or a smaller, focused area of the lesion. The size and positioning of ROIs affects both the measured ADC and the reproducibility of measurements.[48,49] A small "hotspot" ROI, either drawn freehand or using a predefined shape such as a circle or oval, placed on the most hyperintense regions on DWI (or the most hypointense regions on ADC maps) is similar to the analysis suggested for DCE MRI from ACR BI-RADS. This region has been shown to correspond to the most aggressive tissue[50] and the most active part of the lesion.[49,51] The effect of ROI delineation on measured ADC is demonstrated in Fig. 13.4.

A meta-analysis of 61 studies by Wielema and colleagues compared the diagnostic accuracy of the ADC measured using one of four breast tumor tissue selection methods: (1) whole breast tumor; (2) subtracted whole breast tumor avoiding necrosis, cystic, and hemorrhagic areas; (3) circular breast tumor selection (one or more round elliptical ROIs avoiding necrosis, cystic, and hemorrhagic areas); or (4) lowest diffusion breast tumor (the brightest/darkest part of the tumor on DWI/ADC maps).[52] The highest pooled area under the curves (AUCs) were found for studies using the circular tumor and subtracted whole breast tumor

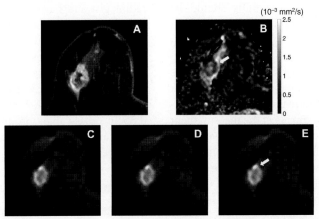

Fig. 13.4 ROI assessment methods. An invasive ductal carcinoma shows central necrosis on DCE-MRI (A). The mean ADC for the lesion measured from the corresponding ADC map (B) was different for an ROI drawn on high b value DWI (C)–(E) encompassing (C) the whole lesion (1.05×10^{-3} mm^2/s), (D) the rim of the lesion avoiding central necrosis (0.97×10^{-3} mm^2/s), and (E) a hotspot in the most intense part of the lesion (0.77×10^{-3} mm^2/s). *ADC*, Apparent diffusion coefficient; *DCE*, dynamic contrast-enhanced; *DCIS*, ductal carcinoma in situ; *DWI*, diffusion-weighted imaging; *ROI*, region of interest.

ROI methods (AUCs of 0.95 and 0.94, respectively). Although it could be argued that the most robust and reproducible method would be the selection of the area with the lowest ADC, this technique finds artificially lower ADC values due to the inclusion of non-suppressed fat.[53]

In terms of the reproducibility of ROIs, Bickel and colleagues showed that the inter- and intrareader agreement was high for both minimum and mean measured ADC and the same for both whole lesion and lowest ADC ROI methods.[51] However, Nogueira and colleagues showed that a small ROI in the area of the highest signal intensity on DWI was more reproducible compared with a whole lesion ROI.[54] Choice of workstation or postprocessing system can also have a systematic but minor effect on ADC measurement.[55]

Defining an ROI for certain types of tumors and NMEs is complicated by the lack of well-defined margins. Though the use of DWI is already limited for nonmass enhancing lesions, the diagnostic accuracy of DWI in NME lesions is significantly affected by ROI method and placement. Furthermore, the intra- and interreader agreement of ADC measurement for these lesions has been shown to be only moderate.[8]

NORMAL TISSUE ROIS

Normal fibroglandular breast tissue can also be evaluated and quantitative ADC measurements taken. Reported mean ADCs of breast parenchyma range from 1.51×10^{-3} to 2.09×10^{-3} mm^2/s when using $b = 600$ s/mm^2.[56] Normal tissue ROIs should be placed on areas of normal-appearing fibroglandular tissue avoiding fat, areas with high T2 signal such as cysts and fibroadenomas, and regions with abnormal enhancement as seen on DCE MRI, ideally in the ipsilateral breast. This technique may be an issue for women without sufficient normal-appearing fibroglandular tissue. Breast density can affect the measurement of the ADC in fibroglandular tissue, as lower ADC values will be found in fatty breasts compared with dense breasts, likely due to the partial volume averaging with fat.[56] Hormonal and physiological changes such as menopause, the menstrual cycle, and lactation may also affect the ADC of breast parenchyma (see Chapter 7). A normalized ADC value can be calculated by dividing the lesion ADC by the fibroglandular tissue ADC.

ALTERNATIVE ADC METRICS

The ADC is generally reported as a mean over an ROI; however, a number of alternative histogram-derived metrics, such as minimum, maximum, percentiles, and standard deviation have been investigated, which can account for intratumoral cellular and microstructural heterogeneity. McDonald and colleagues found that the 25th percentile of ADC achieved the best performance for distinguishing malignant and benign breast lesions (AUC 0.79, 95% CI 0.70–0.88).[57]

Radiomics analysis is increasingly investigated in breast MRI, involving the extraction of quantitative textural features that provide a measure of intratumoral heterogeneity, an established biomarker of poor prognosis[58] that is not visually perceivable by a radiologist. A small number of studies have investigated the use of texture features derived from DWI and ADC maps to differentiate between malignant and benign breast lesions,[59,60] identify triple negative breast cancer,[61] and assess receptor status and molecular subtype[62] (see Chapter 4). Given the large voxel sizes of DWI, the assessment of intratumoral heterogeneity is limited compared with the high spatial resolution of DCE MRI.

SEMIAUTOMATED AND AUTOMATED SEGMENTATION

Manual delineation of tumors may introduce a level of user dependency. Semiautomated or automated techniques using segmentation algorithms can remove the time-consuming need for annotation by a breast radiologist and have been shown to be more reproducible.[63] Semiautomated voxel selection tools that exclude voxels below a dynamically specified signal threshold can improve the interreader reproducibility of ADC measurements.[63] Although automated whole-breast segmentation of DWI using deep-learning models has shown promise (dice scores of 0.85 in cross-validation and 0.72 for external testing),[64] automated segmentation of breast tumors has yet to be investigated.

Common Errors, Pitfalls, Artifacts

COMMON ERRORS AND PITFALLS

A common pitfall in DWI is T2 shine-through. Certain types of lesion, such as cysts and fibroadenoma, and hematoma after biopsy, may appear bright

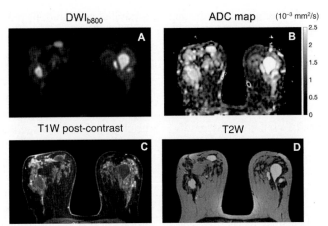

Fig. 13.5 **T2 shine-through.** Lesions with high signal intensity on DWI (A) do not correspond to regions of abnormal enhancement on contrast-enhanced MRI (C) and correspond to regions with a high ADC on the ADC map (B). Reference to T2-weighted images (D) shows that these lesions have a high fluid content and were identified as cysts. *ADC*, Apparent diffusion coefficient; *DWI*, diffusion-weighted imaging.

due to their high water content given the T2 weighting of DWI and may lead to potential misinterpretation (Fig. 13.5). This effect may be reduced by choice of a short echo time (TE) and higher *b* value. Use of an ADC map may provide a more meaningful interpretation of a lesion. Abscesses and pus show diffusion restriction and can mimic malignant lesions on MRI if not evaluated carefully together with other sequences.

The directionality of diffusion must also be accounted for when interpreting DWI. In biological tissue, diffusion is anisotropic. For DWI acquired with diffusion sensitization obtained along one direction, the degree of diffusion restriction leading to observed diffusion contrast will depend on the orientation of tissues being imaged along that direction. The interpretation of this image will be different from the interpretation of an image acquired with diffusion sensitization in a different direction. Thus DWI should be acquired in multiple directions, often in three orthogonal directions, and an average or "trace" image obtained to find a directionally invariant measure of diffusion. Whereas a true trace image calculated from the eigenvalues of the diffusion tensor requires the acquisition of a six-gradient direction scheme often used for diffusion tensor imaging (DTI; see Chapters 1 and 9 and), the three-direction scheme is more commonly available and provides approximate isotropic diffusion contrast.

ARTIFACTS (SEE CHAPTERS 12 AND 14)

Gradient Artifacts

As the strong diffusion-weighting gradients are switched on and off, the time-varying magnetic fields of the gradients induce eddy currents in conductive metallic structures of the magnet, such as the cryostat, main coils, and magnet housing. These eddy currents in turn produce magnetic fields that combine with the applied gradients, affecting the gradient shape and therefore the magnetic field experienced by the objects being imaged. When the images are reconstructed, these errors manifest as geometrical distortions in the diffusion-weighted images as the signal misplaced, resulting in contracted or sheared images. The rapid switching of the frequency encoding gradients can also produce eddy currents (see Chapter 12).

Eddy currents produced by diffusion sensitizing gradients vary with the direction of diffusion sensitization such that combined or trace diffusion-weighted images will contain contributions from different eddy current effects that can reduce image quality and sensitivity for the detection of small lesions. Given that *b* value is proportional to the square of the gradient strength, distortion will be more severe at large *b* values where the gradient amplitude is high. Distortion will also vary between images of different *b* value, resulting in blurred ADC maps and inaccurate quantification of the ADC.

Gradient preemphasis and specialized hardware such as secondary coils that dynamically cancel magnetic flux changes in the main magnet structure are often used to mitigate the effect of eddy currents. Gradient preemphasis changes the shape of the diffusion-weighting gradients to compensate for the contributions of eddy currents.[65] Most modern MR scanners use secondary actively shielded, or self-shielded, gradient coils that are placed between the primary gradient coils and the magnet to minimize stray gradient fields. Opposing currents are driven through these coils to dynamically cancel the changing magnetic fields and minimize eddy currents. The use of specialized radiofrequency (RF) coils for breast imaging assures that gradients are played out further away from the main magnet and other metallic structures. MR scanners can also be designed with fewer conductive surfaces to limit eddy currents.

Other nonuniformities of the magnetic field gradients can also cause artifacts. Strong and stable diffusion-weighting gradients are vital to achieve high *b* values, requiring high performance gradient coils. Given the quadratic relationship between diffusion gradient strength and diffusion attenuation, any deviations from the desired gradients can cause significant errors.[66]

Echo-Planar Imaging Artifacts

DWI is conventionally acquired using single-shot echo-planar imaging (ss-EPI) to maintain a high signal-to-noise ratio (SNR) efficiency while minimizing the effects of patient motion. However, ss-EPI suffers from detrimental image artifacts and distortions, particularly at higher field strengths. The main artifacts are blurring caused by T2* decay during the readout, geometrical distortion, N/2 ghosting, and chemical shift artifacts.

A single "shot" acquisition refers to the acquisition of all of k-space, the imaging data, from one RF excitation. During an EPI readout, the frequency encoding gradient switches rapidly between positive and negative amplitude as the small phase encoding gradient is repeatedly blipped until each line of k-space and all the imaging data for one slice is acquired. During this long acquisition, signal decays due to T2* relaxation, reducing the signal at the edges of k-space that correspond to fine spatial detail, resulting in a blurred image. Advanced acquisition techniques such

as parallel acceleration, reduced field of view (FOV), and multishot imaging can improve this blurring by shortening the readout.

As the bandwidth of EPI in the phase encoding direction is low, EPI is susceptible to artifacts caused by local frequency shifts and inhomogeneities in the magnetic field in the phase encoding direction. Due to the chemical shift between fat and water and the large proportion of fat tissue in breast, this is of particular importance for breast imaging. The chemical shift between fat and water increases with field strength, which is why this effect is larger at 3 T than 1.5 T but can be avoided with good fat suppression. Robust fat suppression is essential for DWI, as any residual fat signal will be superimposed and spatially offset over the image (Fig. 13.6), which could mask underlying pathology (Fig. 13.7).

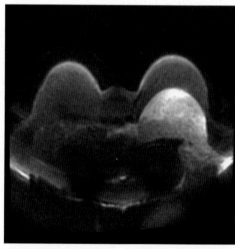

Fig. 13.6 Fat-suppression failure has resulted in a chemical shift artifact. Signal from fat is displaced and appears shifted in the anterior/posterior direction.

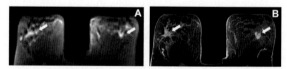

Fig. 13.7 Fat-suppression failure and geometrical distortion affect the visibility of the pathology on DWI (A) compared with the undistorted contrast-enhanced magnetic resonance imaging (MRI) **(B)** for an invasive lobular carcinoma in both left and right breasts. *DWI,* Diffusion-weighted imaging.

In addition to gradient effects, geometrical distortions also occur in areas where the static magnetic field is not homogeneous, caused by poor shimming and variations in magnetic susceptibility (the magnetic properties of tissue), particularly at the interface between air and tissue. This is of particular interest in breast imaging given the large area of the breast/air interface. These field inhomogeneities affect the accuracy of the small phase encoding gradients, resulting in phase shift errors and signal being mapped to the wrong location.

During an EPI readout, the back-and-forth trajectory through k-space results in the accumulation of phase shift from eddy currents, off-resonance frequencies, and other sources such as inadequate shimming and gradient nonlinearity. This affects the signal acquired differently in each direction as the readout direction changes. In the Fourier-transformed image, the signal is displaced and appears as a replicate reduced intensity image in the phase encode direction shifted by half the FOV, known as "N/2 ghosting."

A number of techniques have been investigated for distortion correction in EPI to improve the image quality of DWI and quantification of the ADC, applied either retrospectively or prospectively. Postprocessing techniques focus on generating maps of B_0 field inhomogeneity to correct for distortion, either through the acquisition of a dedicated gradient echo sequence[67] or a second DWI sequence with a reversed gradient polarity, exploiting the symmetry of distortion.[68,69] From these maps, a deformation field map describing pixel shift due to B_0 inhomogeneities can be calculated and a correction applied to the distorted image to shift the signal back to the correct location. Prospective distortion correction can be carried out using B_0 field maps acquired before the DWI sequence as previously described to find slice-dependent optimal shim gradients and RF center frequencies that reduce the effects of distortion, which are adjusted before the acquisition of the DWI sequence.[70] Prospective distortion correction has an advantage over postprocessing in that signal dropout in regions of strong distortions are avoided. Acquisition techniques that reduce the echo train length (such as parallel imaging or multishot imaging) reduce the amount of phase shift and therefore can reduce geometrical distortion due to field inhomogeneities.

Challenges in Acquisition

The European Society of Breast Imaging (EUSOBI) has published a set of guidelines on hardware, sequences and parameters to use for DWI.[1] Breast DWI is recommended using a closed bore magnet with a field strength of at least 1.5 T, gradient hardware that is capable of reaching a maximum gradient strength of 30 mT/m, and a dedicated breast coil with at least four channels. The minimum requirements for a breast DWI sequence are given in Table 13.3. Axial orientation is recommended for ease of interpretation, with the FOV chosen to ensure adequate anatomical coverage of the area of interest (extending from the clavicle to the inframammary fold, ideally including the axilla, though this is not mandatory).

Although the administration of contrast agent before the acquisition of DWI does not significantly affect

TABLE 13.3 Minimum Requirements for DWI Protocols[1]

Parameter	Minimum Requirement
Type of sequence	EPI based
Orientation	Axial
FOV	Covering both breasts
In-plane resolution	$\leq 2 \times 2$ mm^2
Slice thickness	≤ 4 mm
Number of b values	2
Lowest b value	0 s/mm^2
High b value	800 s/mm^2
Fat saturation	Required (SPAIR recommended)
TE	Minimum possible by system and choice of parameters
TR	≥ 3000 ms
Parallel acceleration	Parallel imaging factor ≥ 2
Postprocessing	Generation of ADC maps

ADC, Apparent diffusion coefficient; *DWI,* diffusion-weighted imaging; *EPI,* echo-planar imaging; *FOV,* field of view; *SPAIR,* spectral attenuated inversion recovery; *TE,* echo time; *TR,* repetition time.

the measurement of the ADC or the accuracy of the discrimination of malignant/benign breast lesions.[5,52] DWI should be performed before DCE MRI where possible to avoid any possible detrimental effects.

CHOICE OF *b* VALUE

At least two *b* values are required in a DWI sequence. A higher *b* value of 800 s/mm^2 has been recommended, which has been established theoretically[71] and empirically.[5] The use of a higher *b* value may better distinguish between malignant and benign breast lesions and therefore improve specificity,[72] but SNR will be reduced. Increasing the number of *b* values acquired can improve the fitting of signal decay and allow for advanced modeling techniques to be used at the cost of increased scan time (see Chapters 1 and 8), though it has yet to be shown that this offers an additional improvement in the differentiation of malignant and benign breast lesions.[3,4,57,73] Furthermore, use of nonzero minimum *b* value has not been shown to improve performance.[3,57]

SIGNAL-TO-NOISE RATIO (SNR)

Diffusion weighting inherently reduces signal. However, sufficient SNR is required to visualize tissues and anatomical features of interest. There is generally a trade-off between SNR, resolution, and acquisition time. To increase signal, DWI can be acquired with multiple excitations and averaged, particularly for high *b* values. Increasing the number of averages will improve SNR at the cost of increased acquisition time. Increasing the voxel size will improve the SNR at the expense of spatial resolution. Choice of appropriately short TE will also maximize signal. Scanning a higher field strength (3 T) will improve SNR, though the appearance of certain artifacts may be worsened. Fast acquisition using ss-EPI to acquire images before signal decays limits the achievable resolution of DWI. At high *b* values, the ADC may be underestimated due to low SNR, with ADC decreasing with increasing *b* value,[4] as demonstrated in Fig. 13.8. Sufficient SNR can be achieved with a *b* value of approximately 1.1/ADC.[74] This corresponds to optimal diffusion weighting in the range $b = 700$ to 1200 s/mm^2 for typical mean ADC values for measured malignant and benign breast lesions of 0.9 to 1.7 mm^2/s.[1] Although increased diffusion weighting will increase signal attenuation, due to the presence of background noise the MRI signal will never go to 0. At high *b* values, signal will remain above a certain level close to the "noise floor." Thus the signal attenuation will not reflect the true attenuation expected due to diffusion, resulting in an underestimation of the ADC. For measured ADC values around the threshold ADC for the differentiation of malignant and benign breast lesions, this will lead to false positive results.

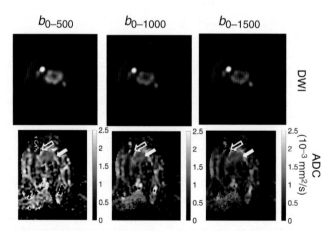

Fig. 13.8 Effect of *b* value on ADC measurement. A 62-year-old woman with invasive ductal carcinoma *(closed arrows)* and a hematoma *(open arrows)*. ADC maps generated using each b_0 and high *b* value combination result in different measured mean ADC values, with ADC decreasing with increasing *b* value. The mean ADC for the invasive ductal carcinoma is 1.18×10^{-3} mm^2/s at b_{500}, 1.03×10^{-3} mm^2/s at b_{1000}, and 0.91×10^{-3} mm^2/s at b_{1500}. *ADC,* Apparent diffusion coefficient; *DWI,* diffusion-weighted imaging.

Qualitatively, sufficiently high SNR such that fibro-glandular tissue (if present) should be visible on low b value images is required.[1] However, in terms of quantitative measurement, there is still no consensus on a universal method of measuring SNR clinically. Noise estimation using the standard deviation of pixel values for an ROI defined in a signal-free area (such as the air) is complicated in DWI by the use of parallel acceleration, which uses combinations of receiver coil sensitivities and the Rician bias of "magnitude" signals. "Multiple acquisition" methods allow for the measurement of SNR on a pixel-by-pixel basis through the repeated acquisition of multiple images with identical scan parameters, however this is generally impractical for clinical imaging. A "difference method" approach to measuring SNR with parallel imaging has been proposed by Reeder and colleagues that can be performed through the acquisition of two identical images, measuring SNR in an ROI using the difference of the two images.[75] Another technique proposed by Kellman and McVeigh reconstructs an image in SNR units using prescan noise.[76]

Denoising of breast DWI has also been investigated to overcome SNR limitations. Denoising techniques generally seek to differentiate between true signal and noise using iterative optimization techniques. Although these techniques can improve image quality and SNR, their use of spatial kernels can result in spatial smoothing and reduced spatial resolution.[77,78] Advanced denoising techniques have been applied to multi-b valued diffusion acquisition without trade-offs in terms of spatial resolution but with increased computational complexity that may be difficult to implement clinically.[79]

FAT SUPPRESSION

Fat suppression is essential for the acquisition of diffusion-weighted breast images to suppress signal from fat and improve the conspicuity of breast lesions. Insufficient fat suppression will result in ghosting, chemical shift artifacts, and inaccurate measurement of the ADC. There are two main methods of fat suppression. Inversion recovery techniques such as short tau inversion recovery (STIR)[80] use a 180-degree RF prepulse applied to invert the longitudinal magnetization and a short inversion time (TI) is chosen such that the signal from fat is nulled at the time the signal generation for the rest of the sequence takes place

(typically 160 ms at 1.5 T and 250 ms at 3 T). Spectral selective techniques include chemical shift selective (CHESS),[81] where 90-degree RF pulses with a narrow bandwidth centered on the resonant frequency of fat are applied to saturate the fat signal, and water only fat suppression,[82] where only water nuclei are excited. Hybrid techniques such as spectral presaturation with inversion recovery (SPIR)[83] and spectral attenuated inversion recovery (SPAIR)[84] combine both frequency-selective and inversion-recovery methods.

SPAIR and STIR are commonly used in breast DWI, and although choice of technique affects image quality and ADC quantification,[53,85,86] it has been shown that diagnostic performance was comparable.[86] Spectrally selective methods generally suppress fat better than inversion-recovery techniques, with the most effective being the water-only excitation technique, which achieved the highest SNR and lowest signal intensity in fatty tissue in a head-to-head comparison of techniques, though it was not significantly different from SPAIR.[53] STIR offers advantages, as it is insensitive to B_0 inhomogeneity at a cost of lower SNR.[85] However, fat-suppression techniques are unable to eliminate all fat signal, such that voxels can be contaminated with fat signal and affect ADC measurement.[53,56]

SHIMMING

Image distortion and poor fat suppression using spectral selective techniques in breast DWI can often be attributed to poor B_0 inhomogeneity.[87] Although geometrical distortion can be partially corrected using postprocessing techniques, these techniques are unable to recover lost SNR due to intravoxel dephasing. Spectrally selective fat suppression requires a relatively homogeneous field. Ensuring that B_0 inhomogeneity is reduced as much as possible before image acquisition is desirable. In axial breast imaging, the large air-tissue susceptibility interface is the main contributor to the B_0 gradient in the anterior-posterior direction, with the nipple creating a local region of high static field within the breast.[88] Susceptibility of the heart, lungs, and liver contribute to B_0 gradients in the left-right direction. Given the variation in size and shape of tissue composition in the breast, there is significant variability of B_0 inhomogeneity between individuals, though a common feature traceable to generic anatomy exists in the linear gradient.[89]

Shimming is a technique that involves the adjustment of field gradients to improve local B_0 homogeneity. Low-order whole body shim coils can be used to correct for linear variations in B_0 but will not correct for higher-order nonlinear field patterns localized within the breast.[88] In bilateral breast MRI, dual shim ROIs can be placed over each breast, with each shim value and center frequency tuned for each of the two breasts. Higher-order shimming techniques enable personalized shimming for each patient, though these techniques add time to the scanning process. Localized arrays of shim coils[90] and susceptibility padding[91] have been shown to further improve B_0 variation; however, these require additional hardware or materials.

PATIENT FACTORS

Patient Motion

Patient motion includes both physiological motion (due to respiration or pulsation of the blood vessels) and the movement of the patient (voluntary or involuntary). Motion artifacts are generally observed in the phase-encoding direction. Although EPI is a rapid acquisition technique that can minimize the effects of physiological motion, bulk patient motion between the acquisition of the low and high *b* value images will result in spatial mismatch between the images, affecting the accuracy of the calculation of ADC maps. Correction via registration before the calculation of ADC maps is required for accurate quantification of the ADC. However, although postprocessing can be used to correct for patient motion, a study by Partridge and colleagues found spatial mismatch for 11% of images that could not be corrected by a spatial registration algorithm.[92] Improving patient comfort is essential to reduce motion, as is reminding the patient to remain still.

Patient Positioning

Patients must be positioned in the breast coil such that the breasts can hang freely in the two holes in the bilateral breast coil to avoid signal distortion and ensure homogeneous fat suppression. For women with large breasts, incorrect positioning will lead to compression against the coil, which results in errors in signal intensity where the breasts are in contact with the coil or if there is compression or folding of the breast tissue itself.

Metal Artifacts

Metallic objects made up of certain ferromagnetic (iron, nickel, cobalt) and nonferromagnetic (titanium) materials, such as biopsy clips, surgical clips, piercings or jewelry, tattoos, and metallic parts of clothing will result in signal distortion due to their higher magnetic susceptibility. Metallic objects should be removed where possible or a lower field strength scanner used (1.5 T vs. 3 T). Surgical clips and percutaneous biopsy clips can cause considerable distortion depending on the materials used. Metallic susceptibility artifacts may also be seen due to the deposition of metal fragments from the core biopsy needle or from electrocautery devices during surgery.[93]

REFERENCES

1. Baltzer P, Mann RM, Iima M, et al; EUSOBI International Breast Diffusion-Weighted Imaging Working Group. Diffusion-weighted imaging of the breast: a consensus and mission statement from the EUSOBI International Breast Diffusion-Weighted Imaging Working Group. *Eur Radiol.* 2020;30:1436–1450.
2. Tsushima Y, Takahashi-Taketomi A, Endo K. Magnetic resonance (MR) differential diagnosis of breast tumors using apparent diffusion coefficient (ADC) on 1.5-T. *J Magn Reson Imaging.* 2009;30:249–255.
3. Baxter GC, Graves MJ, Gilbert FJ, Patterson AJ. A meta-analysis of the diagnostic performance of diffusion MRI for breast lesion characterization. *Radiology.* 2019;291:632–641.
4. Bogner W, Gruber S, Pinker K, et al. Diffusion-weighted MR for differentiation of breast lesions at 3.0 T: how does selection of diffusion protocols affect diagnosis? *Radiology.* 2009;253:341–351.
5. Dorrius MD, Dijkstra H, Oudkerk M, Sijens PE. Effect of b value and pre-admission of contrast on diagnostic accuracy of 1.5-T breast DWI: a systematic review and meta-analysis. *Eur Radiol.* 2014;24:2835–2847.
6. Kul S, Eyuboglu I, Cansu A, Alhan E. Diagnostic efficacy of the diffusion weighted imaging in the characterization of different types of breast lesions. *J Magn Reson Imaging.* 2014;40:1158–1164.
7. Pinker K, Moy L, Sutton EJ, et al. Diffusion-weighted imaging with apparent diffusion coefficient mapping for breast cancer detection as a stand-alone parameter. *Invest Radiol.* 2018;53:587–595.
8. Avendano D, Marino MA, Leithner D, et al. Limited role of DWI with apparent diffusion coefficient mapping in breast lesions presenting as non-mass enhancement on dynamic contrast-enhanced MRI. *Breast Cancer Res.* 2019;21:136.
9. Moschetta M, Telegrafo M, Rella L, Capolongo A, Stabile Ianora AA, Angelelli G. MR evaluation of breast lesions obtained by diffusion-weighted imaging with background body signal suppression (DWIBS) and correlations with histological findings. *Magn Reson Imaging.* 2014;32:605–609.
10. Telegrafo M, Rella L, Stabile Ianora AA, Angelelli G, Moschetta M. Unenhanced breast MRI (STIR, T2-weighted TSE, DWIBS): an accurate and alternative strategy for detecting and differentiating breast lesions. *Magn Reson Imaging.* 2015;33:951–955.

11. Woodhams R, Kakita S, Hata H, et al. Diffusion-weighted imaging of mucinous carcinoma of the breast: evaluation of apparent diffusion coefficient and signal intensity in correlation with histologic findings. *Am J Roentgenol.* 2009;193:260–266.

12. Parsian S, Rahbar H, Allison KH, et al. Nonmalignant breast lesions: ADCs of benign and high-risk subtypes assessed as false-positive at dynamic enhanced MR imaging. *Radiology.* 2012;265:696–706.

13. Guo Y, Cai Y-Q, Cai Z-L, et al. Differentiation of clinically benign and malignant breast lesions using diffusion-weighted imaging. *J Magn Reson Imaging.* 2002;16:172–178.

14. Lee SH, Shin HJ, Moon WK. Diffusion-weighted magnetic resonance imaging of the breast: standardization of image acquisition and interpretation. *Korean J Radiol.* 2021;21(1):9–22.

15. Bozkurt TB, Koç G, Sezgin G, Altay C, Gelal MF, Oyar O. Value of apparent diffusion coefficient values in differentiating malignant and benign breast lesions. *Balkan Med J.* 2016;33:294–300.

16. Youk JH, Son EJ, Chung J, Kim JA, Kim EK. Triple-negative invasive breast cancer on dynamic contrast-enhanced and diffusion-weighted MR imaging: comparison with other breast cancer subtypes. *Eur Radiol.* 2012;22:1724–1734.

17. Zhang L, Tang M, Min Z, Lu J, Lei X, Zhang X. Accuracy of combined dynamic contrast-enhanced magnetic resonance imaging and diffusion-weighted imaging for breast cancer detection: a meta-analysis. *Acta Radiol.* 2016;57:651–660.

18. Rahbar H, Zhang Z, Chenevert TL, et al. Utility of diffusion-weighted imaging to decrease unnecessary biopsies prompted by breast MRI: a trial of the ECOG-ACRIN Cancer Research Group (A6702). *Clin Cancer Res.* 2019;25:1756–1765.

19. Kazama T, Kuroki Y, Kikuchi M, et al. Diffusion-weighted MRI as an adjunct to mammography in women under 50 years of age: an initial study. *J Magn Reson Imaging.* 2012;36:139–144.

20. Bu Y, Xia J, Joseph B, et al. Non-contrast MRI for breast screening: preliminary study on detectability of benign and malignant lesions in women with dense breasts. *Breast Cancer Res Treat.* 2019;177:629–639.

21. Amornsiripanitch N, Rahbar H, Kitsch AE, Lam DL, Weitzel B, Partridge SC. Visibility of mammographically occult breast cancer on diffusion-weighted MRI versus ultrasound. *Clin Imaging.* 2018;49:37–43.

22. Partridge SC, DeMartini WB, Kurland BF, Eby PR, White SW, Lehman CD. Differential diagnosis of mammographically and clinically occult breast lesions on diffusion-weighted MRI. *J Magn Reson Imaging.* 2010;31:562–570.

23. Li L, Mori S, Kodama M, Sakamoto M, Takahashi S, Kodama T. Enhanced sonographic imaging to diagnose lymph node metastasis: importance of blood vessel volume and density. *Cancer Res.* 2013;73:2082–2092.

24. Xing H, Song CL, Li WJ. Meta analysis of lymph node metastasis of breast cancer patients: clinical value of DWI and ADC value. *Eur J Radiol.* 2016;85:1132–1137.

25. Kuijs VJL, Moossdorff M, Schipper RJ, et al. The role of MRI in axillary lymph node imaging in breast cancer patients: a systematic review. *Insights Imaging.* 2015;6(2):203–215.

26. Scaranelo AM, Eiada R, Jacks LM, Kulkarni SR, Crystal P. Accuracy of unenhanced MR imaging in the detection of axillary lymph node metastasis: study of reproducibility and reliability. *Radiology.* 2012;262:425–434.

27. Schipper R-J, Paiman M-L, Beets-Tan RGH, et al. Diagnostic performance of dedicated axillary T2- and diffusion-weighted MR imaging for nodal staging in breast cancer. *Radiology.* 2015;275:345–355.

28. Baltzer PAT, Benndorf M, Dietzel M, Gajda M, Camara O, Kaiser WA. Sensitivity and specificity of unenhanced MR mammography (DWI combined with T2-weighted TSE imaging, ueMRM) for the differentiation of mass lesions. *Eur Radiol.* 2010;20:1101–1110.

29. Rotili A, Trimboli RM, Penco S, et al. Double reading of diffusion-weighted magnetic resonance imaging for breast cancer detection. *Breast Cancer Res Treat.* 2020;180:111–120.

30. Kang H, Hainline A. Combining multiparametric MRI with receptor information to optimize prediction of pathologic response to neoadjuvant therapy in breast cancer: preliminary results. *J Med Imaging (Bellingham).* 2018;5(1):011015.

31. Yabuuchi H, Matsuo Y, Okafuji T, et al. Enhanced mass on contrast-enhanced breast MR imaging: Lesion characterization using combination of dynamic contrast-enhanced and diffusion-weighted MR images. *J Magn Reson Imaging.* 2008;28:1157–1165.

32. Belli P, Bufi E, Bonatesta A, et al. Unenhanced breast magnetic resonance imaging: detection of breast cancer. *Eur Rev Med Pharmacol Sci.* 2016;20:4220–4229.

33. Moll UM, Chumas J. Morphologic effects of neoadjuvant chemotherapy in locally advanced breast cancer. *Pathol Res Pract.* 1997;193:187–196.

34. Rajan R, Poniecka A, Smith TL, et al. Change in tumor cellularity of breast carcinoma after neoadjuvant chemotherapy as a variable in the pathologic assessment of response. *Cancer.* 2004;100:1365–1373.

35. Briffod M, Spyratos F, Tubiana-Hulin M, et al. Sequential cytopunctures during preoperative chemotherapy for primary breast carcinoma. Cytomorphologic changes, initial tumor ploidy, and tumor regression. *Cancer.* 1989;63:631–637.

36. Kennedy S, Merino MJ, Swain SM, Lippman ME. The effects of hormonal and chemotherapy on tumoral and nonneoplastic breast tissue. *Hum Pathol.* 1990;21:192–198.

37. Kumar S, Badhe BA, Krishnan K, Sagili H. Study of tumour cellularity in locally advanced breast carcinoma on neo-adjuvant chemotherapy. *J Clin Diagnostic Res.* 2014;8:FC09–13.

38. Yuan L, Li JJ, Li CQ, et al. Diffusion-weighted MR imaging of locally advanced breast carcinoma: the optimal time window of predicting the early response to neoadjuvant chemotherapy. *Cancer Imaging.* 2018;18(1):38.

39. Pereira NP, Curi C, Osório CABT, et al. Diffusion-weighted magnetic resonance imaging of patients with breast cancer following neoadjuvant chemotherapy provides early prediction of pathological response—a prospective study. *Sci Rep.* 2019;9(1):16372.

40. Partridge SC, Zhang Z, Newitt DC, et al. Diffusion-weighted MRI findings predict pathologic response in neoadjuvant treatment of breast cancer: the ACRIN 6698 multicenter trial. *Radiology.* 2018;289:618–627.

41. Park SH, Moon WK, Cho N, et al. Comparison of diffusion-weighted MR imaging and FDG PET/CT to predict pathological complete response to neoadjuvant chemotherapy in patients with breast cancer. *Eur Radiol.* 2012;22:18–25.

42. Partridge SC, Nissan N, Rahbar H, Kitsch AE, Sigmund EE. Diffusion-weighted breast MRI: clinical applications and emerging techniques. *J Magn Reson Imaging.* 2017;45:337–355.

43. Pickles MD, Gibbs P, Lowry M, Turnbull LW. Diffusion changes precede size reduction in neoadjuvant treatment of breast cancer. *Magn Reson Imaging.* 2006;24:843–847.

44. Sharma U, Danishad KKA, Seenu V, Jagannathan NR. Longitudinal study of the assessment by MRI and diffusion-weighted imaging of tumor response in patients with locally advanced breast cancer undergoing neoadjuvant chemotherapy. *NMR Biomed*. 2009;22:104–113.

45. Park SH, Moon WK, Cho N, et al. Diffusion-weighted MR imaging: pretreatment prediction of response to neoadjuvant chemotherapy in patients with breast cancer. *Radiology*. 2010;257:56–63.

46. Iacconi C, Giannelli M, Marini C, et al. The role of mean diffusivity (MD) as a predictive index of the response to chemotherapy in locally advanced breast cancer: a preliminary study. *Eur Radiol*. 2010;20:303–308.

47. Chu W, Jin W, Liu D, et al. Diffusion-weighted imaging in identifying breast cancer pathological response to neoadjuvant chemotherapy: a meta-analysis. *Oncotarget*. 2018;9(6): 7088–7100.

48. Lambregts DMJ, Beets GL, Maas M, et al. Tumour ADC measurements in rectal cancer: effect of ROI methods on ADC values and interobserver variability. *Eur Radiol*. 2011;21:2567–2574.

49. Arponent O, Sudah M, Masarwah A, et al. Diffusion-weighted imaging in 3.0 Tesla breast MRI: diagnostic performance and tumor characterization using small subregions vs. whole tumor regions of interest. *PLoS One*. 2015;10(10):e0138702.

50. Costantini M, Belli P, Rinaldi P, et al. Diffusion-weighted imaging in breast cancer: relationship between apparent diffusion coefficient and tumour aggressiveness. *Clin Radiol*. 2010;65:1005–1012.

51. Bickel H, Pinker K, Polanec S, et al. Diffusion-weighted imaging of breast lesions: region-of-interest placement and different ADC parameters influence apparent diffusion coefficient values. *Eur Radiol*. 2017;27:1883–1892.

52. Wielema M, Dorrius MD, Pijnappel RM, et al. Diagnostic performance of breast tumor tissue selection in diffusion weighted imaging: a systematic review and meta-analysis. *PLoS One*. 2020;15(5):0232856.

53. Baron P, Dorrius MD, Kappert P, Oudkerk M, Sijens PE. Diffusion-weighted imaging of normal fibroglandular breast tissue: influence of microperfusion and fat suppression technique on the apparent diffusion coefficient. *NMR Biomed*. 2010;23(4):399–405.

54. Nogueira L, Brandão S, Matos E, et al. Region of interest demarcation for quantification of the apparent diffusion coefficient in breast lesions and its interobserver variability. *Diagn Interv Radiol*. 2015;21:123–127.

55. Clauser P, Marcon M, Maieron M, Zuiani C, Bazzocchi M, Baltzer PAT. Is there a systematic bias of apparent diffusion coefficient (ADC) measurements of the breast if measured on different workstations? An inter- and intra-reader agreement study. *Eur Radiol*. 2016;26:2291–2296.

56. Partridge SC, Singer L, Sun R, et al. Diffusion-weighted MRI: influence of intravoxel fat signal and breast density on breast tumor conspicuity and apparent diffusion coefficient measurements. *Magn Reson Imaging*. 2011;29:1215–1221.

57. McDonald ES, Romanoff J, Rahbar H, et al. Mean apparent diffusion coefficient is a sufficient conventional diffusion-weighted MRI metric to improve breast MRI diagnostic performance: results from the ECOG-ACRIN Cancer Research Group A6702 Diffusion Imaging Trial. *Radiology*. 2021;298(1):60–70.

58. Ashraf AB, Daye D, Gavenonis S, et al. Identification of intrinsic imaging phenotypes for breast cancer tumors: preliminary associations with gene expression profiles. *Radiology*. 2014;272:374–384.

59. Bickelhaupt S, Paech D, Kickingereder P, et al. Prediction of malignancy by a radiomic signature from contrast agent-free diffusion MRI in suspicious breast lesions found on screening mammography. *J Magn Reson Imaging*. 2017;46:604–616.

60. Parekh VS, Jacobs MA. Integrated radiomic framework for breast cancer and tumor biology using advanced machine learning and multiparametric MRI. *NPJ Breast Cancer*. 2017;3:43.

61. Xie T, Zhao Q, Fu C, et al. Differentiation of triple-negative breast cancer from other subtypes through whole-tumor histogram analysis on multiparametric MR imaging. *Eur Radiol*. 2019;29:2535–2544.

62. Leithner D, Bernard-Davila B, Martinez DF, et al. Radiomic signatures derived from diffusion-weighted imaging for the assessment of breast cancer receptor status and molecular subtypes. *Mol Imaging Biol*. 2020;22:453–461.

63. Rahbar H, Kurland BF, Olson ML, et al. Diffusion-weighted breast magnetic resonance imaging: a semiautomated voxel selection technique improves interreader reproducibility of apparent diffusion coefficient measurements. *J Comput Assist Tomogr*. 2016;40:428–435.

64. Zhang L, Mohamed AA, Chai R, Guo Y, Zheng B, Wu S. Automated deep learning method for whole-breast segmentation in diffusion-weighted breast MRI. *J Magn Reson Imaging*. 2020;51:635–643.

65. Papadakis NG, Martin KM, Pickard JD, Hall LD, Carpenter TA, Huang CL-H. Gradient preemphasis calibration in diffusion-weighted echo-planar imaging. *Magn Reson Med*. 2000;44:616–624.

66. Bammer R, Markl M, Barnett A, et al. Analysis and generalized correction of the effect of spatial gradient field distortions in diffusion-weighted imaging. *Magn Reson Med*. 2003;50:560–569.

67. Jezzard P, Balaban RS. Correction for geometric distortion in echo planar images from B_0 field variations. *Magn Reson Med*. 1995;34:65–73.

68. Holland D, Kuperman JM, Dale AM. Efficient correction of inhomogeneous static magnetic field-induced distortion in echo planar imaging. *Neuroimage*. 2010;50:175–183.

69. Teruel JR, Fjøsne HE, Østlie A, et al. Inhomogeneous static magnetic field-induced distortion correction applied to diffusion weighted MRI of the breast at 3T. *Magn Reson Med*. 2015;74:1138–1144.

70. Lee SK, Tan ET, Govenkar A, Hancu I. Dynamic slice-dependent shim and center frequency update in 3 T breast diffusion weighted imaging. *Magn Reson Med*. 2014;71:1813–1818.

71. Xing D, Papadakis NG, Huang CLH, Lee VM, Carpenter TA, Hall LD. Optimised diffusion-weighting for measurement of apparent diffusion coefficient (ADC) in human brain. *Magn Reson Imaging*. 1997;15:771–784.

72. Iima M, Kataoka M, Kanao S, et al. Intravoxel incoherent motion and quantitative non-gaussian diffusion MR imaging: evaluation of the diagnostic and prognostic value of several markers of malignant and benign breast lesions. *Radiology*. 2018;287(2):432–441.

73. Pereira FPA, Martins G, de Vasconcellos Carvalhaes de Oliveira R. Diffusion magnetic resonance imaging of the breast. *Magn Reson Imaging Clin N Am*. 2011:95–110.

74. Jones DK, Horsfield MA, Simmons A. Optimal strategies for measuring diffusion in anisotropic systems by magnetic resonance imaging. *Magn Reson Med*. 1999;42:515–525.

75. Reeder SB, Wintersperger BJ, Dietrich O, et al. Practical approaches to the evaluation of signal-to-noise ratio performance with parallel imaging: application with cardiac

imaging and a 32-channel cardiac coil. *Magn Reson Med.* 2005;54:748–754.

76. Kellman P, McVeigh ER. Image reconstruction in SNR units: a general method for SNR measurement. *Magn Reson Med.* 2005;54:1439–1447.

77. Lam F, Babacan SD, Haldar JP, Weiner MW, Schuff N, Liang Z-P. Denoising diffusion-weighted magnitude MR images using rank and edge constraints. *Magn Reson Med.* 2014;71:1272–1284.

78. Haldar JP, Wedeen VJ, Nezamzadeh M, et al. Improved diffusion imaging through SNR-enhancing joint reconstruction. *Magn Reson Med.* 2013;69:277–289.

79. Tan ET, Wilmes LJ, Joe BN, et al. Denoising and multiple tissue compartment visualization of multi-b-valued breast diffusion MRI. *J Magn Reson Imaging.* 2021;53:271–282.

80. Bydder GM, Pennock JM, Steiner RE, Khenia S, Payne JA, Young IR. The short TI inversion recovery sequence: an approach to MR imaging of the abdomen. *Magn Reson Imaging.* 1985;3:251–254.

81. Frahm J, Haase A, Hanicke W, Matthaei D, Bomsdorf H, Helzel T. Chemical shift selective MR imaging using a whole-body magnet. *Radiology.* 1985;156:441–444.

82. Schick F, Forster J, Machann J, Huppert P, Claussen CD. Highly selective water and fat imaging applying multislice sequences without sensitivity to B1 field inhomogeneities. *Magn Reson Med.* 1997;38:269–274.

83. Foo TKF, Sawyer AM, Faulkner WH, Mills DG. Inversion in the steady state: contrast optimization and reduced imaging time with fast three-dimensional inversion-recovery-prepared GRE pulse sequences. *Radiology.* 1994;191:85–90.

84. Bernstein MA, King KF, Zhou XJ. *Handbook of MRI Pulse Sequences.* Elsevier, Inc; 2004.

85. Nogueira L, Brandão S, Nunes RG, Ferreira HA, Loureiro J, Ramos I. Breast DWI at 3 T: influence of the fat-suppression technique on image quality and diagnostic performance. *Clin Radiol.* 2015;70:286–294.

86. Brandão S, Nogueira L, Matos E, et al. Fat suppression techniques (STIR vs. SPAIR) on diffusion-weighted imaging of breast lesions at 3.0 T: preliminary experience. *Radiol Med.* 2015;120:705–713.

87. Harvey JA, Hendrick RE, Coll JM, Nicholson BT, Burkholder BT, Cohen MA. Breast MR imaging artifacts: how to recognize and fix them. *Radiographics.* 2007;27(suppl 1):S131–S145.

88. Maril N, Collins CM, Greenman RL, Lenkinski RE. Strategies for shimming the breast. *Magn Reson Med.* 2005;54:1139–1145.

89. Lee S-K, Hancu I. Patient-to-patient variation of susceptibility-induced B_0 field in bilateral breast MRI. *J Magn Reson Imaging.* 2012;36:873–880.

90. Juchem C, Nixon TW, McIntyre S, Rothman DL, de Graaf RA. Magnetic field homogenization of the human prefrontal cortex with a set of localized electrical coils. *Magn Reson Med.* 2010;63:171–180.

91. Lee GC, Goodwill PW, Phuong K, et al. Pyrolytic graphite foam: a passive magnetic susceptibility matching material. *J Magn Reson Imaging.* 2010;32:684–691.

92. Partridge SC, DeMartini WB, Kurland BF, Eby PR, White SW, Lehman CD. Quantitative diffusion-weighted imaging as an adjunct to conventional breast MRI for improved positive predictive value. *Am J Roentgenol.* 2009;193:1716–1722.

93. Genson CC, Blane CE, Helvie MA, Waits SA, Chenevert TL. Effects on breast MRI of artifacts caused by metallic tissue marker clips. *Am J Roentgenol.* 2007;188:372–376.

Multiplatform Standardization of Breast DWI Protocols: Quality Control and Test Objects

Dariya Malyarenko, Lisa J. Wilmes and Thomas L. Chenevert

Overview of Breast Diffusion-Weighted Imaging Standardization Efforts

Given the rapid advances in diffusion-weighted imaging (DWI) technology and the multiple parameters influencing quality of breast DWI acquisition and analysis, harmonization of breast DWI protocols necessitates coherent standardization efforts by physicians, researchers, and MR vendors. These standardization efforts will likely include trade-offs between practicality and diagnostic yield.[1,2]

RATIONALE AND NEED FOR STANDARDIZATION FOR CLINICAL TRANSLATION

Clinical translation of developed breast DWI technologies requires design and implementation of standardized acquisition and analysis workflows to improve overall robustness and reduce dependency on site imaging protocols and vendor platforms. Standardization improves reproducibility and accuracy of derived DWI metrics and enables practical application in the clinical setting. Despite great potential and promise of contrast-free imaging sensitive to tissue microstructure, DWI is often being used only qualitatively in the clinic to increase conspicuity of impeded diffusion tissues on high diffusion-weighting images ($b > 700\,s/mm^2$). The typical breast DWI protocol is an auxiliary to the high-resolution contrast-enhanced T1 weighted (T1w) scan that continues to serve as the primary diagnostic driver in breast magnetic resonance imaging (MRI) (see Chapters 2 and 13).

Unlike conventional qualitative DWI based on subjective impressions, the utilization of quantitative DWI metrics derived from biophysical models potentially enables objective thresholds for disease detection and treatment response monitoring.[3,4] Rich quantitative DWI research conducted to date has uncovered major sources of technical bias and variability in breast DWI. Improvement of accuracy and precision via amelioration of bias and unnecessary variability is the focus of ongoing DWI standardization efforts.[1,2] Characterization and reduction of technical errors are prerequisites to define meaningful thresholds for derived quantitative DWI parameters (e.g., apparent diffusion coefficient [ADC], kurtosis, compartment fractions) and for successful widespread translation of DWI technology improvements (see Chapter 12 for multishot, reduced field of view [rFOV], and other advanced acquisition techniques) into the clinical environment.

The common technical errors in breast DWI stem from inherent hardware properties, acquisition protocol, and data analysis workflow. Among acquisition parameters, applied b value sensitization in terms of DWI gradient strength, duration, ranges, and spatial uniformity is the most important and challenging factor for reproducible results.[1–4] Current clinical systems with moderate gradient strength (<50 mT/m) do not routinely provide control over diffusion gradient pulse duration. Diffusion gradient timing is nominally set by the minimum echo time (TE) for the highest b value acquired in a sequence. Therefore ensuring consistent TE and b range across scanners is a reasonable first standardization step to constrain diffusion encode-time bias. TE setting also determines T2 weighting and is a major driver of signal-to-noise ratio (SNR) at high *b* values. It is important to consider potential Rician noise bias in both protocol design and applied diffusion model as it may impact quantitative results (see also Chapters 1 and 8).[5,6] Additionally, due to spatial gradient nonlinearity, applied *b* values possess finite spatial nonuniformity, typically higher than nominal (isocenter value) at anatomical breast locations for horizontal bore scanners. This gradient system-dependent bias requires correction to reduce variability in multicenter, multisystem studies.[7,8]

Use of single-shot (ss) echo-planar imaging (EPI) acquisitions for reasonably short scan duration (<5 minutes) makes clinical breast DWI susceptible to multiple artifacts, including those that stem from imperfect fat suppression, B_0 field inhomogeneity, and eddy currents (see Chapter 13). These issues become particularly challenging for advanced DWI techniques that target more subtle signal features, for example, in diffusion kurtosis via increased high *b* value range (see Chapters 1 and 8) or fractional anisotropy obtained from diffusion tensor imaging (DTI) with at least six diffusion sensitizing directions (see Chapter 9).[9,10] Generation of quantitative DWI metrics based on different biophysical models relies on availability of sequence parameters (e.g., *b* values and DWI gradient orientation) retained in image metadata. This information is often stored in nonstandard structures (vendor-specific "private" metadata fields) in image headers or is not routinely available. Visualization and interpretation of DWI results in clinical picture archive and communication system (PACS) requires adherence to imaging and metadata standards provided by Digital Imaging and Communications in Medicine (DICOM) and imaging insight toolkit (ITK), including intensity scaling and units for quantitative parametric maps.[11]

Most of the DWI standardization issues are common across different organs, but some are particularly acute for breast DWI (e.g., sensitivity to imperfect fat suppression; Fig. 13.6). The ultimate goal of breast DWI protocol standardization is to implement acquisition parameters and image postprocessing that minimize the variability across scanner platforms due to artifacts and technical biases.[1,2]

STANDARDIZATION INITIATIVES AND GUIDELINES

Standardization is a dynamic process, because as new MRI scanners and acquisition sequences are developed, the improved DWI protocols become available on a subset of systems or over subject enrollment interval (e.g., high-resolution DWI with rFOV and segmented EPI acquisition; see Chapter 12).[12–14] DWI biomarker standardization efforts have been initiated to various degrees by multiple organizations (Table 14.1): Radiologic Society of North America (RSNA) Quantitative Imaging Biomarkers Alliance (QIBA) DWI, European Society of Breast Imaging (EUSOBI), National Institute of Standards and Technology (NIST), ACR Imaging Network (ACRIN), National Clinical Trial Network (NCTN), and Medical Imaging Technology Alliance (MITA). The QIBA DWI and EUSOBI groups aim to establish consensus recommendations, based on published data, to specifically inform breast DWI protocol implementation for reproducible results. They also promote rigorous quality assurance (QA) for clinical trials that use DWI as an imaging readout and seek clinical translation of discovered DWI-based biomarkers.

The NIST imaging division develops and calibrates DWI reference standards[15] for acquisition optimization and quantitative evaluation of technical biases. This institute also currently provides the quantitative MRI phantom loan library (see Table 14.1) for clinical trials and validation. The MITA division of the National Electrical Manufacturers Association has developed DICOM standards for DWI metadata and generated parametric maps to ensure compatibility with clinical PACS used by radiologists and to facilitate interoperability of analysis results. These standards require that critical parameters for DWI acquisition (*b* values, diffusion gradient directions) and analysis (algorithm, output scales, units) are archived with and accessible from the metadata for DWI images and quantitative parametric maps (e.g., ADC).

In practice, dominant MR manufactures implement these requirements to variable degrees, for example, routinely storing *b* values, diffusion gradient directions and scale/units in optional "private" tags,[11,16] which can change format between scanner software versions. On the other hand, multiframe 32-bit precision storage of the parametric DICOM volumes is not routinely supported by clinical PACS vendors and DICOM viewer workstations. They also do not routinely support segmentation DICOM for region of interest (ROI) definition. Therefore for implementation of advanced offline

TABLE 14.1   Standardization Organizations and Breast-DWI Relevant Resources

Organization	Resource	URL
European Society of Breast Imaging (EUSOBI)	Optimization of breast DWI protocols	https://www.eusobi.org
RSNA Quantitative Imaging Biomarkers Alliance (QIBA)	DWI profile outlining specifications to achieve baseline ADC precision	https://qibawiki.rsna.org/images/6/63/QIBA_DWIProfile_Consensus_Dec2019_Final.pdf
American College of Radiology Imaging Network (ACRIN)	Supports multicenter oncology clinical trials that use imaging end-points	https://ecog-acrin.org
NCI National Clinical Trial Network (NCTN)	Clinical trial QC requirements for cancer centers	https://www.cancer.gov/research/infrastructure/clinical-trials/nctn
National Comprehensive Cancer Network (NCCN)	Global cancer care, research and imaging standards	https://www.nccn.org/
National Institute of Standards and Technology (NIST)	Ground-truth DWI phantom calibration and lending	https://www.nist.gov/programs-projects/nistnibib-medical-imaging-phantom-lending-library
Medical Imaging Technology Alliance (MITA)	Performance standards for diagnostic imaging	https://www.medicalimaging.org/standards
Digital Image and Communications in Medicine (DICOM)	Image database and archival metadata standards for DWI and ADC parametric maps	https://www.dicomstandard.org/current https://dicom.nema.org/medical/dicom/current/output/chtml/part03/sect_C.8.13.5.9.html
Food and Drug Administration (FDA)	Imaging device specifications and safety for clinical use	https://www.fda.gov/medical-devices
FDA Biomarkers, EndpointS, and Other Tools (BEST)	Clinical imaging biomarker requirements	https://www.ncbi.nlm.nih.gov/books/NBK326791/ https://www.fda.gov/media/99221/download
NCI The Cancer Imaging Archive (TCIA)	Sharing annotated cancer imaging DICOM data	https://www.cancerimagingarchive.net/collections
RSNA Quantitative Imaging Data Warehouse (QIDW)	Sharing DWI phantom data, QC tools and DROs	http://qidw.rsna.org/#collections

ADC, Apparent diffusion coefficient; *DICOM,* Digital Imaging and Communications in Medicine; *DRO,* digital reference object; *DWI,* diffusion-weighted imaging; *QC,* quality control.

DWI analysis, the onus currently remains with the MR scientists/physicists to update DWI DICOM interpretation dictionaries according to vendor-provided DICOM conformance statements distributed with the scanner software that list the available metadata fields and formats. Furthermore, many relevant parameters, including DWI gradient waveform (e.g., single spin-echo [SSE] vs. double spin-echo [DSE], or bipolar) and timing (pulse duration and separation) are commonly missing from metadata. These issues need to be resolved to facilitate harmonization and integration of advanced DWI methods into clinical application workflow.

In the United States, the Food and Drug Administration (FDA) and National Cancer Institute (NCI) NCTN provide general regulations for quality control (QC) requirements in imaging device applications and clinical trials (e.g., FDA "Biomarkers, EndpointS, and Other Tools" [BEST]; see Table 14.1). Several imaging accreditation programs address standardization across multiple imaging modalities and include DWI guidelines to a variable degree. The American College of Radiology (ACR) accredits sites and scanners based on submitted test images, site protocols, and personnel qualifications. Accreditation specific to clinical trials using imaging is performed by both for-profit imaging contract research organizations (iCROs) and core labs associated with cooperative therapy groups. One example of the latter is the Eastern Cooperative Oncology Group (ECOG) ACRIN (see Table 14.1), which has supported studies to evaluate ADC use for breast cancer therapy response prediction (ACRIN 6698) and diagnosis (ACRIN 6702). Related groups also offer accreditation for clinical trials, with the objective of certifying select sites as "trial ready" in terms of their imaging performance. The National Comprehensive Cancer Network (NCCN) provides disease-based clinical practice guidelines for oncology, which is a primary target of current clinical DWI applications.

The EUSOBI organization recently launched an international initiative dedicated to breast-specific DWI protocol optimization to generate consensus guidelines and promote routine clinical implementation as a part of multiparametric MRI evaluation.[1] These guidelines focus on achieving objective description of impeded tissue water mobility across multiple vendor platforms, including specifications on b values, spatial resolution, repetition and echo times, and ROI placement. This work summarizes consensus on assessment of lesion location and morphology using DWI and ADC, and reflects broad ADC ranges (in $\mu m^2/ms$) for malignant (0.8–1.3), benign (1.2–2.0), and normal (1.7–2) breast tissue cited in current literature. The work also highlights the shortcomings of present nonstandard protocols in defining diagnostically meaningful ADC thresholds by potentially broadening observed ADC ranges.

Another international standardization initiative by QIBA DWI biomarker committee, formed by the RSNA, has developed a DWI profile (see Table 14.1) that provides guidelines to establish confidence intervals for interpretation of meaningful biological changes in quantitative ADC metrics for multiple organs, including the breast.[2] As with any quantitative metrics, the confidence intervals of derived breast DWI parameters rely on evaluation of precision (scan-rescan repeatability, cross-platform reproducibility), and technical accuracy (measurement bias).[17] The ultimate goal is to achieve confidence intervals tighter than the measured biological effect. The current QIBA DWI profile contains recommendations for standardization of breast DWI acquisition and analysis and quantitative system performance evaluation to address common technical issues for ADC measurements in multicenter, multiplatform environments. These guidelines ensure that harmonized baseline performance is achieved across multivendor platforms using a DWI phantom, and recommend application of an ADC digital reference object (shared via the RSNA Quantitative Imaging Data Warehouse [QIDW]; see Table 14.1) to confirm that image analysis does not introduce substantial technical bias.

STANDARDIZATION TOOLS AND WORKFLOW: REPEATABILITY AND TECHNICAL BIAS

Practical clinical translation workflow ideally starts from good correlation of pathological findings to the given DWI metric. Then optimization of the acquisition protocol is performed in conjunction with the DWI model constraints to minimize measurement uncertainty and bias, and maximize diagnostic performance, which is ultimately tested in multicenter clinical trials. Presence of system-dependent technical bias increases variability in data collated from multicenter trials leading to inconclusive results and/or necessitating large subject recruitment.[17,18] Characterization and reporting of the acquisition and fit model parameters, as well as bias and repeatability, is critical for quantitative DWI metrics. The latter define confidence intervals to establish reproducible diagnostic thresholds[17,18] and enable emerging radiomics and artificial intelligence (AI) applications.[19–21]

Diffusion scans typically have lower spatial resolution compared with clinical T1- and T2-weighted sequences, and corresponding DWI are ideally coregistered to high-resolution images for (or used to guide) lesion segmentation and characterization. This image processing may introduce additional error sources.[22] Finally, the confidence intervals for diagnostic thresholds are determined by assessing precision and accuracy of the DWI scan protocol and entire analysis workflow.[2,17,18] According to QIBA metrology recommendations,[2,17,18] the assessment of measurement precision for the chosen quantitative DWI metric relies on test-retest repeatability studies,[2,23] which use the same scan protocol over a relatively short time interval to ensure negligible change in breast biological condition. The reproducibility studies, on the other hand, evaluate variation across sites or scanner platform[8] and acquisition protocols.[24] The quantitative measurement accuracy (bias) is assessed with a phantom that provides ground-truth values,[7] and platform-dependent bias should be corrected, when possible, or accounted for in the metric confidence intervals.[17]

Repeatability Analysis Guidelines

Test-retest repeatability studies are usually performed using repeated scans with the same protocol parameters for acquisition and analysis on a group of patients. The repeatability coefficient (RC) is assessed from the within-subject standard deviation (wSD) or coefficient of variance (wCV, when wSD scales with mean parameter value). RC provides an estimate for measurement precision, and can be used directly to establish 95% confidence intervals (CIs) for the longitudinal studies (e.g., treatment response monitoring), assuming constant technical bias across serial imaging time points.

QIBA metrology papers offer guidelines for design and sufficient powering of repeatability studies.[17,18,25] In general, it is desirable to obtain test-retest scans on 30 or more subjects (preferably on different days, or at least with repositioning the patient if on the same day) with consistent acquisition and analysis parameters for derived breast DWI metrics (e.g., ADC mean, percentiles, or cold spot volume). Repeatability analysis, based on Bland–Altman statistics (see Fig. 14.1), assumes that biological tissue characteristics do not change between test and retest, and measurement noise is the main contributor to the disagreement between two results. Due to inherently varying optimal DWI protocols for tissue diffusion properties, different repeatability may be observed for normal tissue versus lesions. Hence, distinct CIs are expected for biologically dissimilar lesion ROIs. The majority of breast DWI repeatability studies performed to date have focused on different characteristics of the ADC histograms (see Fig. 14.1) for lesion ROIs, including

mean, skew, percentiles, and histogram volumes (e.g., dense lesion volume defined as quantity of voxels with ADC up to a given threshold times the voxel volume).

Breast DWI Metric Repeatability

Based on the recently published (sufficiently powered) multiplatform test-retest studies,[23] the current QIBA DWI profile includes a longitudinal claim suggesting that meaningful changes in mean ADC of a breast lesion beyond 13% can be detected with 95% confidence. Similar good repeatability was observed for low ADC histogram percentiles[22] (RC < 20%); however, histogram volumes showed generally poor repeatability (RC > 80%), likely due to high sensitivity to ROI segmentation errors. Higher ADC histogram moments and radiomic features also tend to show higher variability (e.g., 24% for "cold spot" ADC[26] and 85% for entropy).[27] These metrics are apparently more sensitive to noise, although generally less test-retest repeatability data is available[2] for evaluation. Several small repeatability studies for advanced DWI metrics (intravoxel incoherent motion [IVIM] perfusion fraction, kurtosis, fractional anisotropy) similarly report lower repeatability compared with that of the mean ADC.[4,28] This is also consistent with observation of lower reproducibility (e.g., 38%–48% for kurtosis and D*) between different acquisition protocols.[24] More comprehensive studies are needed to characterize effect of lesion size and biological condition on DWI measurement precision. The general challenges of improving precision and accuracy, and minimizing scan time, should be addressed by acquisition protocol optimization[24,29] and advanced image processing (e.g., denoising)[30,31] to allow clinical application of these promising quantitative breast DWI metrics.

Bias Analysis and Correction Guidelines

For cross-sectional diagnostic comparisons (e.g., to differentiate malignant from benign breast conditions), confidence intervals will include both precision and bias. Technical bias evaluation is performed with respect to a phantom with known DWI parameter values. Ideally, these values are chosen to mimic biophysical characteristics of breast diffusion supplied by in vivo observations and in silico modeling. Bias can be evaluated as a function of different acquisition parameters, including resolution, fat suppression, and

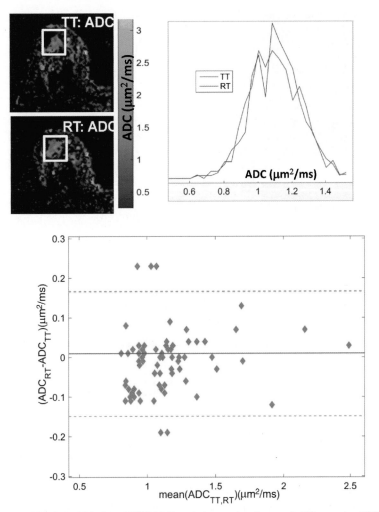

Fig. 14.1. **ADC test-retest repeatability for multisite breast DWI trial.** The color images show the example ADC maps of an ACRIN 6698 patient with invasive breast cancer for test (TT) and retest (RT) scan after coffee break with table repositioning. The white box outlines the lesion with low ADC region tracing the viable tumor before treatment. The quantitative ADC scale is provided in the color bar. Normalized ADC histograms (bin size, 0.04 μm2/ms) are plotted for the full multislice tumor ROI (*red:* RT, *blue:* TT). Bland–Altman plots are shown for histogram mean ADC values across 70 ACRIN 6698 repeatability study subjects (delta = 0.025, LOA = 0.16 μm2/ms, wCV = 5% [CI: 4%–7%]). *ADC,* Apparent diffusion coefficient; *DWI,* diffusion-weighted imaging; *LOA,* limits of agreement; *ROI,* region of interest; *RT,* retest; *TT,* test; *wCV,* within-subject coefficient of variance.

spatial uniformity of b value (Fig. 14.2). A set of physical phantoms has been developed to test acquisition and analysis of breast DWI.[8,32,33] Diffusion properties of phantoms are usually confirmed by reference scans where bias is known to be negligible (e.g., high resolution, artifact free, at magnet isocenter), although reference scans are often not practical for daily clinical applications. The bias of the desired clinical protocol under evaluation is then established by measuring the

difference for measured DWI metrics with respect to phantom reference values. Additionally, for appropriate statistical derivation of the CIs, the linearity test needs to be performed to ensure that measured metric is linearly correlated to the true values[17,18] over the tissue-relevant range.

Evaluation of bias for advanced quantitative models and fit algorithm fidelity may be performed based on virtual phantoms termed digital reference objects

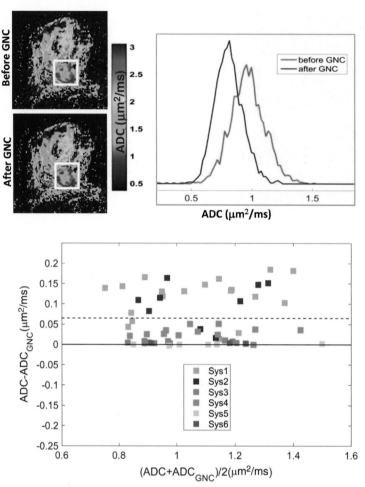

Fig. 14.2 Gradient system-dependent ADC bias for multiscanner breast DWI study. The color images show ADC maps for an ACRIN 6698 patient with invasive breast cancer before *(top)* and after *(bottom)* correction of GNC bias in *b* value. The quantitative ADC scale is provided in the color bar. The corresponding normalized ADC histograms (bin size, 0.04 μm²/ms) are plotted for the full multislice tumor ROI (*magenta*, before GNC; *blue*, after GNC). Bland–Altman-like plot for mean ADC illustrates effects of correction depending on gradient system (color-coded in the legend). The observed (positive) ADC bias before correction ranged from 0 to 0.2 μm²/ms across gradient systems. *ADC*, Apparent diffusion coefficient; *DWI*, diffusion-weighted imaging; *GNC*, gradient nonlinearity correction; *ROI*, region of interest.

(DROs, e.g., for ADC SNR; see Table 14.1), which provide true parameter values from forward modeling of DWI signals and acquisition conditions. DWI DRO intensities are simulated for physical ranges of tissue diffusion parameters (e.g., ADC, D_a, K_a, D* and IVIM fraction).[34] The tested fit algorithm results are then compared with the input DRO parameters to assess bias. Another option for DRO generation is to acquire high-resolution images free of artifact and bias using a long acquisition (e.g., high-resolution turbo-spin-echo [TSE]) that is not clinically viable, and impose known

artifacts (e.g., partial volume averaging due to reduced resolution) to test postprocessing ability to eliminate them with respect to reference images. Sharing acquired test-retest DICOM DWI data (e.g., via the NCI Cancer Imaging Archive [TCIA] collections; see Table 14.1) is also a valuable resource to the breast DWI community to field test emerging denoizing,[30,31] segmentation and classification algorithms.[19–21] These tools are particularly susceptible to overtraining on small available data sets, resulting in poor generalization. Notably, shared and pooled test-retest data is an economical means to benchmark improved performance of new algorithms via improved repeatability statistics (reduced technical variability).

Optimization and Standardization of Breast DWI Acquisition and Analysis

CHALLENGES OF BREAST DWI PROTOCOL STANDARDIZATION FOR CLINICAL TRANSLATION

Protocol optimization for breast DWI is based on maximizing the diagnostic yield, and minimizing the acquisition time and complexity for practical implementation in the clinical environment. Because DWI is sensitive to a variety of breast microstructural and physiological characteristics, optimization of clinical workflow should ideally start with evaluation of cellular histology for target pathology and its correlation to research DWI findings, for example, changes in vascular fraction probed by low b value ranges versus cellular density at intermediate b values versus impeded cellular diffusion at high b values (Chapters 1 and 8; Figs. 1.1–1.4 in Chapter 1). The clinical DWI protocol should then be adjusted to query pathology-specific tissue microstructure and suppress other (unwanted) components by choosing scan parameters that emphasize DWI contrast-to-noise ratio (CNR).[35]

The standardization challenge is in finding parameter ranges (TE, b values, fat suppression) that can be implemented across a variety of clinical scanners and be effective for the study population to probe the distribution of breast tissue diffusivity parameters.[1,35] Standardization and optimization of breast DWI protocols typically involve establishing consistent b values and TE range, as well as ensuring efficient fat suppression and reduction of EPI artifacts (eddy current and shim distortions; Chapter 13) either by acquisition or image postprocessing and registration.

For instance, acquisition of multiple high b values ≥ 800 s/mm^2 for breast DWI could be more informative for impeded diffusion[10,13]; however, it requires prolonged examinations for sufficient SNR and may compromise simultaneous quantification of high ADC tissues.[3] Improved spatial resolution and SNR, reduced distortion, and scan time are common goals of breast DWI protocol optimization and implementation of advanced acquisition techniques (Fig. 14.3).

Clinical Implementation Considerations (See Also Chapter 13)

For practical consideration, adding DWI to an existing breast MRI protocol that typically contains T2w and dynamic contrast-enhanced MRI (DCE-MRI)

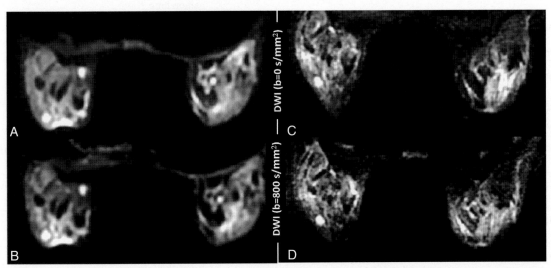

Fig. 14.3 Example breast DWI for ss-EPI versus MUSE. The DWI acquisition for the breast of a normal volunteer using standard ss-EPI (2.7 × 2.7 × 4 mm^3, 7:51 minutes) in (A) and (B) is compared with multishot MUSE (1.7 × 1.7 × 2 mm^3, 5:49 minutes) with inversion recovery fat-suppression in (C) and (D) for $b = 0$ *(top)* and $b = 800$ s/mm^2 *(bottom)*. Reduced geometrical distortions are achieved by MUSE with ~60% higher resolution and ~30% saving in acquisition time with finite SNR trade-off for normal breast tissue. *DWI,* Diffusion-weighted imaging; *MUSE,* multiple sensitivity encoding; *SNR,* signal-to-noise ratio; *ss-EPI,* single-shot spin echo-planar imaging.

acquisitions should strive to minimize disruption to the clinical workflow. Therefore it is important to keep the DWI acquisition time within a reasonable range (ideally <5–7 minutes) while maintaining adequate image quality, CNR, and SNR for radiologists to read the images. This is often difficult to accomplish within the limited time of the clinical breast MRI examination if complete breast coverage in the axial slice (S/I) direction is desired. Additionally, DWI should be acquired before DCE-MRI because gadolinium contrast agent has been shown in some studies to adversely affect the ability to calculate robust tissue ADC statistics, and this effect may be time dependent.[36] The timing of the DWI acquisition needs to be set forth in the imaging protocol, and for multisite clinical trials, ideally controlled for by the central data processing site. Another practical consideration is that DWI images should not interfere with clinical reading; that is, if directional diffusion images are being acquired

for offline ADC analysis (e.g., calculation of ADC map for *b* value subset or eddy current correction), radiologists may request that these images are not sent to PACS; if so, directional DWI data may need to be sent to a separate offline processing computer.

Quantitative Considerations

For multisite quantitative MRI studies, protocol consistency across multiple imaging platforms is important to allow data pooling for statistical analysis.[2,18,24,37] This requires a consistent DWI acquisition protocol (see important factors in Table 14.2) that is implementable across different MRI vendor platforms and software versions. The harmonized DWI protocol should specify values (or ranges) for basic/standard DWI acquisition parameters such as repetition time (TR), TE, *b* values, acquisition time, etc. The *b* values must be consistent across multiple imaging sites and

TABLE 14.2   DWI Acquisition Standardization Factors

Acquisition Property	Examples	Effect
Fat suppression	Shim quality, technique, e.g., spectral vs. inversion recovery (SPAIR vs. STIR)	ADC bias, chemical shift artifact, lesion segmentation, geometrical accuracy, image quality, acquisition time
Acquisition timing	TR, TE, receiver bandwidth	SNR, T2-weighting, ADC accuracy, acquisition time
Pulse sequence class	Type, e.g., ss-EPI vs. ms-EPI vs. ssTSE, Cartesian vs. radial	SNR, T2-weighting, image distortion, motion artifact, resolution, acquisition time
Diffusion gradient waveform	DWI pulse width and separation; gradient amplitude (*b* value) and polarity (e.g., DSE vs. SSE vs. bipolar)	SNR, T2-weighting, ADC value, eddy-current distortion
b Value dependent averaging	Increase number of averages at high *b* values	Acquisition time, SNR, ADC accuracy
Effective echo spacing	Parallel imaging acceleration factor, multi-shot, receiver bandwidth	Degree of distortion, ghosting, SNR, acquisition time
Geometry	FOV, acquired voxel size, slice thickness, fold-over direction	Spatial resolution, SNR, quantitative accuracy, acquisition time, breast coverage
Multi-*b* value sampling	IVIM, ADC, DKI protocols	Quantitative parameter bias, acquisition time
Scan duration	Sequence class, geometry, fat suppression, *b* value sampling and averaging	Image quality, quantitative accuracy, and clinical feasibility

ADC, Apparent diffusion coefficient; *DKI*, diffusion kurtosis imaging; *DSE*, double spin-echo; *DWI*, diffusion-weighted imaging; *FOV*, field of view; *IVIM*, intravoxel incoherent motion; *ms-EPI*, multi-shot echo planar imaging; *ss-EPI*, single-shot echo-planar imaging; *SNR*, signal-to-noise ratio; *SPAIR*, spectral attenuated inversion recovery; *SSE*, single spin-echo; *ssTSE*, single shot turbo spin echo; *STIR*, spectral presaturation with inversion recovery; *TE*, echo time; *TR*, repetition time.

multiple imaging time points for the same patients. Longitudinal DWI data should ideally be acquired on the same MRI scanner using the same breast coil. DWI data must have sufficient SNR to allow derivation of quantitatively accurate model metrics, with the growing emphasis and effort in the field directed toward evaluation of accuracy of breast ADC values. Accurate and reproducible ADC measurements require that TR and TE are within certain ranges to ensure no significant loss of signal (e.g., TR > 4000 ms; TE = 50–100 ms).[1,2] Another acquisition parameter to stipulate is the range of acceleration factors (high enough to allow acquisition time reduction but low enough to minimize SNR loss). The critical metadata information relevant for downstream analysis and not routinely preserved in DICOM (e.g., actual *b* value, diffusion encoding direction, and sequence variant) should be recorded.

Acquisition Considerations

The goal of breast DWI protocol optimization and standardization is to reconcile the clinical and quantitative imaging constraints to achieve a compromise acquisition that accommodates both as much as possible (see Table 14.2). Reconciling the different goals and needs of diagnostic versus treatment response studies using breast DWI includes determining whether different DWI sequences should be used for each or finding a trade-off or hybrid approach (to acquire more data using a standardized DWI sequence). Relevant protocol parameters include fat suppression, sequence class, diffusion gradient waveform, and *b* value range (see Table 14.2). The optimized protocol must be implementable on a variety of MRI scanners of different field strengths (1.5 T, 3 T), manufactured by multiple MRI vendors and equipped with variable hardware configurations (gradient strength and slew rate). The DWI protocol should further be viable across multiple software versions, using a variety of breast coil designs manufactured by different vendors, and comprising a range of coils/channel count (typically 8 or 16).[1,2,37]

Using standard, commercially available product sequences (which may have vendor-specific names and implementations) means that no special research keys or in-house custom options are required, so breast DWI protocols can be uniformly implemented on all/most clinical scanners. Scanner hardware differences and specific software versions may require that a sequence be adapted across diverse systems to achieve results in a comparable way; for example, acquiring a multi-*b* value DWI as multiple sets of 2-*b* value DWI acquisitions holding other parameters constant.[24,37] The acquisitions must be repeatable with a high level of consistency in image quality and calculated ADC values.[16,23] This can be challenging in the breast due to factors such as variability of patient position, shimming, and fat suppression.[4,36,38] The choice of EPI phase-encode direction fold-over depends on higher numbers of coil elements and patient habitus; for example, spatial distortion in phase-encode direction and degree of fat-shift varies between vendors making it hard to prospectively standardize across systems and patients.[38,39] Furthermore, limitations on gradient slew rates determine minimum TE and effective echo spacing that affects the amount of spatial distortion and degree of spatial shift of unsuppressed fat (obscuring parenchyma; see Fig. 13.7). This intra- and intersite variability between DWI acquisitions further highlights the need for MRI phantoms and QA/QC protocols to help with multisite DWI data evaluation.[8,33,40]

The standardized protocol must be flexible enough to acquire comparable DWI data for patients of different sizes and weights. A wide range of FOVs needs to be used to accommodate the full range of patient body habitus (e.g., FOV from 260 mm up to 400 mm). In addition, a different quantity of slices may be required for full breast coverage, which can impact breast DWI scan duration. Variable patient weights also affect the allowable number of slices per unit time (due to specific absorption rate [SAR] calculations) in a given acquisition, which may necessitate modifying TR for required number of slices/breast coverage. Therefore typical multisite protocols necessitate specification of allowable ranges of DWI scan parameters[41–43] (Table 14.3).

Technical Limitations of Standard ss-EPI DWI

Single-shot echo-planar imaging (ss-EPI) has been the DWI sequence of choice for multicenter imaging trials evaluating breast diffusion biomarkers because it is robust to motion and is a standard product sequence on most clinical scanners. However, ss-EPI DWI acquisitions have lower spatial resolution and SNR than clinical T1w sequences (limiting anatomical

TABLE 14.3   Standardized I-SPY 2, ACRIN 6698 and 6702, and DWI Sequence Parameters

Parameter	I-SPY 2	ACRIN 6698/6702	DWI Phantom
Sequence type	Diffusion-weighted 3-orthogonal axes, spin echo, single-shot echo-planar imaging (DW ss-EPI)	Diffusion-weighted 3-orthogonal axes, spin echo, single-shot echo-planar imaging (DW ss-EPI)	Diffusion-weighted 3-orthogonal axes, spin echo, single-shot echo-planar imaging (DW ss-EPI)
Field strength	1.5 T or 3 T	1.5 T or 3 T	1.5 T or 3 T
Slice orientation	Axial 2D multislice	Axial 2D multislice	Axial 2D multislice
Laterality	Bilateral	Bilateral	Bilateral
Frequency direction	A/P (R/L)	A/P	A/P
Phase direction	R/L (A/P)	R/L	R/L
FOV frequency (mm)	260–360	260–360[a]	320
FOV phase (mm)	260–360	300–360[a]	320
Acquired matrix—frequency	128–192	128–192	160
Acquired matrix—phase	128–192	128–192	160
Half-scan factor	NA	>0.65	>0.6
Acquired in-plane (mm)	≤1.9	1.7–2.8	2
Fat suppression	Active fat-sat recommended	Active fat-sat	Active fat-sat
TR (ms)	≥4000	≥4000	≥8000
TE (ms)	Minimum: 50–100	Minimum: 50–100	75–100
b Values (s/mm^2)	0, 800	0, 100, 600, and 800	0, 100, 600, and 800
Slice thickness (mm)	3–5	4–5	4
Number of slices	Variable; complete bilateral coverage	Variable; full bilateral coverage; adjust to keep within single acquisition	30
Slice gap (mm)	≤1.0	No gap	No gap
Parallel imaging factor	≥2	≥2	2 (on 1.5 T); 3 (on 3 T)
No. of excitations/averages	≥2 (to achieve approx. 4-min scan duration)	≥2	1
Receiver bandwidth	NA	>1000 Hz/voxel	1400–1600 Hz/voxel
Sequence acquisition time	≤5 min	minutes	≤3 min/pass × 4 passes[b]

[a]Adjust up to 400 mm to accommodate for large body habitus if necessary.
[b]For phantom, acquire four sequential DWI passes in 4 × 3 min = 12 min or less.
ACRIN, American College of Radiology Imaging Network; *DWI*, diffusion-weighted imaging; *I-SPY 2, Investigation of Serial studies to Predict Your therapeutic response 2*; *ss-EPI*, single-shot echo-planar imaging; *TE*, echo time; *TR*, repetition time.

and morphological evaluation). Furthermore, ss-EPI also suffers from multiple artifacts (see Chapter 13, Figs. 13.6 and 13.7) that adversely affect DWI quantification, such as poor/inadequate shimming, incomplete fat suppression, phase wrap, and parallel imaging "halo" artifact. On some older scanners the automatic center frequency function may mis-assign fat as water peak in subjects with fatty breasts (see Fig. 13.6). These issues can be especially problematic for longitudinal studies: inconsistent acquisition parameters across multiple visits and artifacts may cause one of multiple time points to be unusable/unanalyzable.

Consistent DWI Data Analysis

Recent multicenter studies suggest that centralized image analysis and QC is preferred to ensure reproducible image processing.[16,22,26] DWI and parametric map DICOM standards[11,16] have to be used for metadata storage to insure reproducible analysis. The DWI acquisition site should record and share metadata critical for downstream image analysis. In contrast to qualitative analysis (reader study), quantitative DWI analysis requires calculation of parametric maps and definition of ROIs, typically done using manual or semiautomated approaches. Each additional analysis step can introduce variability due to specific algorithm implementation, parameter choices, and reader biases. Benchmarking analysis on shared, curated data sets is the most efficient way to evaluate performance for emerging tools, models, and algorithms. For instance, using test-retest repeatability DWI DICOM shared through the TCIA (see Table 14.1) can help evaluate the efficacy of the denoizing techniques or automated segmentation by comparison to and improvement of baseline wCV.

RECOMMENDATIONS FOR STANDARD OPERATING PROCEDURES OF BREAST DWI ACQUISITION AND ANALYSIS

The QIBA DWI profile provides a compilation of standard parameters currently used in multicenter breast imaging trials that evaluate ADC for prediction of breast cancer therapy response. Repeatability studies adhering to a standard protocol are essential to establish precision of the derived DWI biomarker.[22,23,26,44] For example, previous studies of ADC changes in breast tumors measured during neoadjuvant chemotherapy have found significant increase in responders' tumor ADCs

ranging from 9% to 60%, depending on treatment and measurement time point. The significance of detected treatment-related ADC changes needs to be evaluated in the context of the underlying technical variability of the tumor ADC measurements, which have been found in a multisite repeatability study (see Fig. 14.1) to have an RC = 0.16 μm^2/ms (13%). Consensus recommendations and precision thresholds summarized by QIBA and EUSOBI are actively sought by commercial trial iCROs (e.g., INVICRO, Bioclinica) and managing core labs (e.g., ACRIN, CQIE) to improve diagnostic yield and reduce the cost of future imaging trials.

Table 14.3 includes versions of the DWI protocols implemented by breast imaging (ISPY-2),[41] therapy response (ACRIN 6698),[42] and diagnostic (ACRIN 6702),[43] multisite trials that evaluated breast ADC. Suggested essential parameter ranges were implemented across multiple clinical scanner platforms to minimize technical variability. Once the parameters for a specific patient were established, they were kept the same for that patient for subsequent scans in longitudinal studies. The parameters for a standard 2-b value DWI acquisition were implemented at all imaging sites. The parameters for a more advanced 4-b value DWI acquisition were evaluated in a substudy (ACRIN 6698) of the main ISPY-2 imaging trial at select imaging sites, which had qualified for participation by submitting phantom and volunteer DWI that passed the QC standards set forth in the protocol. A subset of 89 subjects from the ACRIN 6698 trial participated in test-retest study to establish repeatability of breast DWI protocol and derived ADC (see Fig. 14.1). Phantom scans for ACRIN 6698 and 6702 were used to ensure acceptable DWI technical performance in terms of ADC bias and linearity.

Approaches to Maximize Protocol Compliance

The following methods have been used in multisite clinical trials to date to increase adherence to MRI data acquisition protocols: written documentation of procedures, regular calls with investigators, and comparison of acquired data DICOM header parameter information to study protocol parameters. A DWI ice-water phantom has been used to assess scanner performance (bias, linearity, and precision) and SNR for site qualification. Qualitative review of clinical patient image quality was implemented for evaluation of wrap and ghosting artifacts, fat suppression SNR, and DWI SNR. Distribution of a scanner-specific protocol necessitated parallel definition for multiple clinical scanner platforms with parameters expressed in terms familiar to users of each system. When possible, a software version of the protocol should be provided for direct import into the scanner examination database as a starting point. Centralized monitoring for protocol compliance of DWI acquired from multiple imaging sites is important, because higher protocol compliance may improve predictive power of MRI biomarkers.[24,37]

STANDARDIZATION AND OPTIMIZATION OF EMERGING BREAST DWI METHODS

The breast DWI field is rapidly evolving toward acquisition methods allowing higher spatial resolution, faster imaging, improved fat suppression, and reduced geometric distortion artifacts. Emerging novel protocols require standardization for application in the clinical trial setting. Centralized image analysis and QC is preferred to ensure reproducible image processing.[16] DWI and parametric map DICOM standards[11,16] must be used for metadata storage to support reproducible analysis. For the purpose of clinical translation, it is important to consider the benefits brought by advanced breast DWI methods in terms of enhanced sensitivity (detection and diagnostic differentiation) and improved repeatability (CIs) with respect to clinically implemented benchmark methods. For instance, advanced metrics derived from a non-Gaussian diffusion model (and requiring prolonged multi-*b* DWI acquisition) may be correlated to the ADC, and thus provide redundant clinical information (similar diagnostic contrast), whereas its error bars (CIs) might exceed those of an ADC benchmark. On the other hand, for a specific clinical question (e.g., in relation to molecular HER2 status or tumor vascularity), a given advanced DWI metric (kurtosis or IVIM fraction) may provide unique information, substantiating the need for an advanced acquisition protocol implementation. Furthermore, the selected acquisition protocol should be optimized to minimize acquisition time and boost SNR. For instance, recent work by McDonald and colleagues[29] indicated that breast lesion mean ADC derived from a 2-*b* value DWI acquisition provides similar diagnostic power to that of 4-*b* ADC.

Evaluation of acquisition protocols for emerging techniques should be performed with respect to the current clinical standard, ss-EPI, using a phantom to estimate technical bias (see Fig. 14.4), as well as radiologist assessment for clinical image quality. Testing of the novel diffusion analysis model is typically carried out using DROs or physical phantoms that provide ground truth parameter values. For example, for in vivo implementation of multishot DWI techniques, such as multiple sensitivity encoding (MUSE)[12] and readout segmented long variable echo train (RESOLVE),[13,14] the relevant parameters for breast DWI standardization would include number of shots, receiver band-width, and acceleration to minimize echo spacing and maintain clinically feasible acquisition time less than 6 minutes while ensuring adequate SNR. The viable protocol should also achieve the efficiency of fat suppression compared with clinical standard (e.g., inversion recovery-based vs. spectral saturation) and improve phase correction to effectively reduce ghosting (see Fig. 14.3). For ultimate protocol refinement and practical implementation in the clinical environment, both acquisition and analysis workflow need to be evaluated and standardized in multicenter clinical trials.

T1-w gradient echo	single-shot (ss)-EPI DWI 2b-value	multi-shot EPI DWI 2b-value (MUSE)

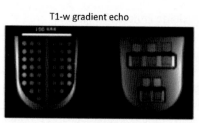 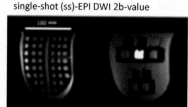 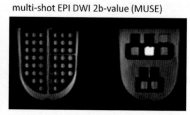

Fig. 14.4 **Breast phantom DWI comparison for ss-EPI versus MUSE.** Representative T1w 3D gradient echo images, standard ss-EPI DWI, and multishot EPI DWI *b* = 0 images were acquired with the commercial NIST/CaliberMRI breast MRI phantom on a 3T MRI scanner. Compared with nominally distortion-free T1w reference images *(left)*, reduced susceptibility induced geometrical distortions are achieved by multishot EPI multiplexed sensitivity encoding, (MUSE, *right*) versus standard ss-EPI *(middle)* with prominent distortion in the right-left (phase) direction. *DWI,* Diffusion-weighted imaging; *EPI,* echo-planar imaging; *MUSE,* multiple sensitivity encoding; *NIST,* National Institute of Standards and Technology; *ss-EPI,* single-shot echo-planar imaging.

Advanced Acquisition and DWI Distortion Correction Techniques

Some examples of typical DWI correction techniques include reversed polarity phase-encode gradients (RPG), limited phase-FOV, and multishot segmented EPI to reduce spatial distortion. For diffusion gradients, bipolar waveforms and/or DSE are used to effectively mitigate eddy currents observed for SSE. Gradient nonlinearity correction (GNC) ensures spatial uniformity of diffusion weighting. However, advanced DWI sequences and imaging options often require longer acquisitions compared with ss-EPI. Furthermore, different vendors' implementations of multishot approaches have distinct constraints and limitations that require harmonization in multisite studies. For instance, the minimum echo spacing time for a RESOLVE[13] approach may differ from MUSE.[12] Additionally, optimized sequence/vendor-specific protocols need to be developed with the goal of maintaining comparable SNR to standard ss-EPI DWI despite lower voxel size with improved spatial resolution (see Figs. 14.3 and 14.4). To assess influence of nondiffusion related factors and improve related performance (e.g., resolution, fat suppression, shim), the corresponding method may be initially evaluated using phantoms (see Fig. 14.4), without need for costly patient repeatability studies. Phantoms also allow assessment of platform-dependent bias of different implementations by vendors and longitudinal performance monitoring during multisite clinical trials.

Advanced DWI Modeling Techniques

In vivo implementation of advanced modeling approaches requires specific protocol considerations. For instance, optimization of a kurtosis imaging protocol should start with proper choice of gradient strength set (b values) to enhance accuracy and detection sensitivity of derived diffusion kurtosis model parameters.[6,10] Minimizing required acquisition time by finding an optimal subset of b values, introducing undersampling (e.g., deep learning reconstruction) with advanced image processing[24,30,31] that does not adversely impact diagnostic performance based on the derived diffusion model metrics is a practical first step toward implementation in the clinical setting. To mitigate the errors introduced by low SNR and reduce required scan time for multi-b acquisitions, denoizing[31,45] can be applied to improve accuracy and

precision of derived diffusivity metrics (e.g., reduce bias in fractional anisotropy [FA] and IVIM fraction estimates and decrease the wCV for mean diffusivity).

In summary, the benefit of advanced breast DWI techniques should be assessed through their ability to improve diagnostic or predictive power (e.g., differentiation of intraductal carcinoma and fibroadenoma or therapy response prediction) of a target breast imaging biomarker with respect to its basic technical repeatability for patient population in a clinical trial. In general, the effect of advanced methods and optimizations need to be evaluated to ensure they do not introduce artifactual image features or reduce precision and accuracy of quantitative diffusion parameter values with respect to standard clinical protocols. To better understand biases and errors introduced by advanced models and protocols, the first step is to assess them with appropriate imaging reference objects (phantoms). The advanced protocol performance should be evaluated in terms of DWI SNR, artifacts, scan time, and related bias in diffusion model parameters with respect to the standard ss-EPI ADC benchmark.

Test Objects and Quality Control for Breast DWI

ROLE OF PHANTOMS FOR STANDARDIZATION AND QC

Physical phantoms are essential tools used as test objects at multiple levels by a variety of stakeholders interested in delivering consistent high-quality imaging services. At the time of scanner installation, manufacturers rely on an array of phantoms for hardware calibration and to demonstrate each scanner meets vendor-specified performance benchmarks. Site physicists/engineers/scientists use phantoms to confirm that a system meets their expectations for initial acceptance testing, as well as for periodic scanning in QC programs often mandated by accreditation organizations (like ACR or ECOG-ACRIN; see Table 14.1). Phantoms also are typically the starting point for solving image quality issues, as well as in development of new technologies (e.g., Fig. 14.4). Finally, phantom scans often serve as the basis for objective performance evaluation across imaging platforms[2,15,33] and institutions as a prerequisite for site certification and participation in multiinstitutional clinical trials that use image-based readouts to pursue study aims.

MRI breast phantoms are typically designed to evaluate one or multiple traditional image quality features including spatial resolution, geometrical accuracy, contrast, signal-to-noise and signal uniformity, and quantitative metrics such as T1, T2, and ADC. Advanced system phantoms (NIST)[46] incorporate multiple aspects allowing protocol optimization, evaluation of resolution, and artifact characterization. Morphology phantoms are also important for AI and radiomics.[47] As with other target organs, breast phantoms are typically not designed for anatomical realism, which for the breast would be particularly challenging to mimic the wide range of parenchyma-to-fat ratios, sizes, and amorphic shapes routinely encountered in practice.

Breast MRI quality, especially DWI, is critically dependent on main magnetic and transmit field uniformity (i.e., B_0 and B_1) and proper identification of spectral constituents essential for good fat suppression.[38,39] Automated shim and spectral peak identification algorithms are challenged by breast asymmetry, irregular shapes/folds, and (silicone) implants when present. Commercial breast phantoms do not contain large fat-mimic zones to adequately evaluate fat suppression uniformity (e.g., CaliberMRI), although one can construct "qualitative" water-fat breast phantoms

that resemble human breast distributions with subcutaneous fat and central parenchyma.

An example of this design is illustrated in Fig. 14.5, constructed from approximately liter-sized cylindrical containers lined with an intentionally irregular thick layer of shortening material (i.e., fats solid at room temperature) and then filled with aqueous gel to simulate parenchyma.

Although these homemade water-fat phantoms are not useful as quantitative test objects, they are very instructive in protocol development to demonstrate sensitivity of fat suppression techniques to choice of shim routine, center frequency (i.e., spectral peak identification) and fat-suppression tune parameters, as well as to illustrate adverse effects of poor fat suppression on DWI and derived ADC maps (see Fig. 14.5F). The impact of residual lipid signal spatially encoded using the default DWI sequence (i.e., ss-EPI) is particularly destructive owing to fat's extremely low mobility (over an order of magnitude relative to water) and chemical shift (~3.5 parts per million [PPM] relative to water), which manifests as large spatial displacement (several centimeters) from its true spatial location (see Fig. 14.5G). This spatially displaced, low mobility residual fat signal superimposed onto parenchyma

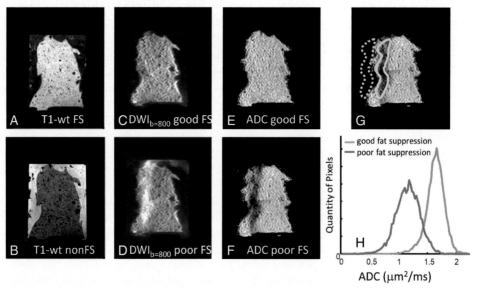

Fig. 14.5 Impact of FS failure on ADC using a water-fat phantom. "Anatomy" of the phantom on T1w MRI (A) with and (B) without FS; $DWI_{b=800}$ (C) with good FS and (D) poor FS; resultant ADC maps via (E) good FS and (F) poor FS; (G) solid line shows ROI location, whereas dotted line shows true location of unsuppressed fat signal displaced 29 mm by chemical shift to severely bias ADC within the ROI, as illustrated in (H) by histograms of pixel ADC values within the ROIs with good FS (green) and poor FS (red). *ADC,* Apparent diffusion coefficient; *DWI,* diffusion-weighted imaging; *FS,* fat suppression; *ROI,* region of interest.

signal creates a strong negative ADC bias, as clearly demonstrated in Fig. 14.5H.

EXAMPLES OF PHANTOMS SPECIFICALLY DESIGNED FOR DIFFUSION

A variety of phantoms comprising materials exhibiting stable mobility properties have been explored and are good candidates to serve as reference standards in breast DWI applications. Two complementary approaches (based on polyvinylpyrrolidone (PVP) and temperature control) are particularly popular for DWI phantoms used in site certification as a prerequisite for participation in multicenter quantitative DWI trials.[23,42,43] It is well known that molecular mobility is a function of temperature. Presumably, in vivo diffusivity is controlled by body temperature regulation processes, whereas phantom diffusion measurement requires knowledge of internal temperature and its control during DWI scanning. Use of an ice-water bath surrounding measurement samples has been a popular and economical solution where one desires an absolute universal diffusion reference standard.[32,40] An alternative is to include an internal validated temperature readout along with calibration table mapping temperature to known diffusivity values for each reference standard. The temperature readout device must be MRI compatible and preferably accurate to less than 1°C because change in water diffusion coefficients is approximately 2% to 3% per °C.

Mono-Exponential/Gaussian Diffusion Phantoms

Temperature-Controlled Ice-Water Phantom. The simple phantom design shown in Fig. 14.6 of a central thin-walled plastic measurement tube of water at thermal equilibrium with surrounding ice-water slurry was used in both ACRIN 6702 and ACRIN 6698 (substudy of the I-SPY 2) North American breast MRI trials for site certification and periodic QC.[23,42,43] The outer container of the cylindrical phantom was flexible plastic by design because the container must deform as the ice melts, otherwise a strong vacuum would be created in a rigid phantom, making it difficult to reopen. Given this, geometrical features (e.g., spatial distortion) of this breast ice-water phantom design are not well controlled and not evaluated in system testing. Obviously, the ice-water phantom requires on-site preparation and detailed filling/use

instructions, which adds some inconvenience for the user. Nevertheless, once the breast ice-water phantoms are filled, the central measurement tube (insulated at both ends) reaches ~0°C within 1 hour and holds this thermal equilibrium for several hours. High precision (~1%) of this design afforded measurement of absolute system ADC bias at representative right and left offsets from iso-center, as illustrated in Fig. 14.6, due to gradient nonlinearity encountered in breast MRI[7,8] (see Fig. 14.2). Other system performance metrics evaluated with this phantom for site certification include ADC spatial uniformity (limited to space within measurement tubes), artifactual b value dependence in ADC values, ADC random error, DWI SNR, and conformance to the specified scan protocol by survey of key DICOM tags.[11,16]

PVP-Based Phantoms. System "linearity" is simply measurement of bias as a function of the magnitude of the metric being studied.[17,18] Although the ice-water phantom described earlier is economical, widely available, and can evaluate absolute system bias, it contains only one material (water) and thus cannot be used to assess system linearity over a range of ADC values. Diffusion phantoms consisting of aqueous dilutions of PVP[15,48] have been developed and have proven to be an excellent platform for tunable monoexponential diffusion values. PVP-based phantoms designed to accommodate ice-water slurry surrounding vials containing 50% to 0% PVP concentrations at 0°C equilibrium have been used to assess absolute system bias and linearity over the range 0.12 μm²/ms to 1.10 μm²/ms, respectively. This spans roughly half the breast tissue ADC range. The same PVP concentrations at room temperature span the full tissue ADC range, but internal phantom temperature must be known to within ~1°C to achieve reasonable accuracy in measured ADC values. Then again, not only must temperature be known, but it must be accompanied by a calibration table or functional form that quantitatively links temperature to diffusion reference ADC values for each PVP sample.[49]

The commercially available (CaliberMRI, Boulder, CO) room temperature PVP-based breast DWI phantom illustrated in Fig. 14.7 is designed with a novel MR-visible LCD readout of internal temperature.[50] This bilateral phantom is permanently sealed with lateral spacing adjustment to fit within multiple breast

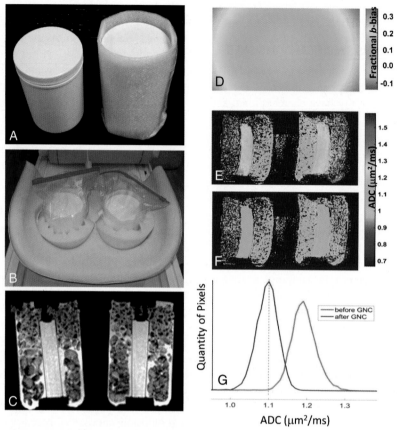

Fig. 14.6 Breast ice-water DWI phantom. Phantom container is shown in (A) with and without insulation used to extend thermal hold time; (B) phantoms in breast coil and (C) internal view of bilateral phantoms on T1w MRI. GNL typically creates positive bias in *b* value with right-left and anterior-posterior distance from iso-center as shown in (D), leading to overestimation of ADC in (E). Spatial GNC functions derived from GNL tensor effectively remove this bias in corrected ADC map shown in (F) and in histograms (G) of ADC values within measurement tubes before and after GNC. Vertical *dashed line* at ADC = 1.1 µm²/ms is the correct value for water at 0°C. *ADC*, Apparent diffusion coefficient; *GNL*, gradient nonlinearity; *GNC*, GNL correction.

coil sizes. This phantom also contains precise machining of high-contrast target plates for objective assessment of geometrical metrics such as distance, spatial distortion, resolution, and lesion (size) detectability limits.[46] These plates are in planes orthogonal to PVP tube arrays, although each breast phantom may be rotated 90 degrees on the support plate to effectively swap PVP and geometrical targets between axial and sagittal acquisition planes. The current version of the phantom also contains one tube housing a fat-mimic material to evaluate fat suppression over a limited spatial zone. In terms of breast DWI protocol optimization and system evaluation, this breast phantom combines multiple advanced features including traditional geometrical metrics with ADC linearity and

potentially absolute ADC bias, assuming the requisite temperature calibration/correction is available.[50]

Non-Gaussian Diffusion Phantoms

As described in Chapter 1, water diffusion in tissue is generally not free and thus can be denoted as "non-Gaussian" (NG). Empirically, NG signal as a function of *b* value does *not* adhere to a mono-exponential decay. For our interest in phantoms, we can (overly) simplify NG diffusion behavior to originate from three sources: (1) blood microcirculation in the capillary networks (i.e., perfusion); (2) nonwater tissue constituents, such as cell membranes and macromolecules that impede water mobility through complex interactions; and (3) the noise floor.

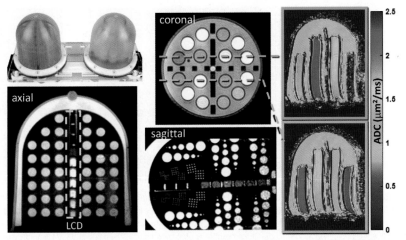

Fig. 14.7 Commercial bilateral DWI phantom based on NIST design. Central orthogonal planes on T1w MRI show high-contrast geometrical features to measure spatial distortion and resolution. Axial and sagittal views also show LCD thermometer (outlined by *yellow dashed line*) used to estimate internal temperature by counting MR-visible cells. Axial color ADC maps display tubes through PVP at 0%, 10%, 14%, 18%, 25%, and 40% concentrations plus one containing oil (short tube, *upper right*) to assess fat suppression. *ADC,* Apparent diffusion coefficient; *DWI,* diffusion-weighted imaging; *NIST,* National Institute of Standards and Technology; *LCD,* liquid crystal display; *PVP,* polyvinylpyrrolidone.

IVIM Perfusion Phantoms. Signal decay due to perfusion in randomly oriented capillary may mimic diffusion (indicated by pseudodiffusion coefficient D*), though numerically D* is much higher than thermally driven water motion in tissue (by an order of magnitude) and is not purely random because D* is linked to cardiac pulsation. Static materials exhibiting hypermobility comparable to perfusion D* levels do not exist, thus phantoms designed to emulate perfusion for application of IVIM model require forced flow (e.g., pump-driven) of minority signal through a dispersive network.[51] Sophisticated IVIM phantoms have been developed in the academic research space[51–54] but are technically difficult to generalize for reproducible widespread use at many centers for QA/QC site-certification applications; therefore they are not discussed further here.

DKI Phantoms. Multiexponential signal decay and various metrics used to model NG signal decay features, ostensibly due to tissue microstructure, are being investigated as quantitative image biomarkers (QIBs) in multicenter trials.[55,56] Given this, stable phantom materials able to emulate nonmonoexponential signal decay (without perfusion) are in demand. Complex interactions between water and nonwater impediments to otherwise free mobility have been developed

in a variety of phantom platforms.[57–59] Of the NG diffusion models discussed in Chapters 1 and 8, the heuristic diffusion kurtosis model is particularly popular. Diffusion kurtosis imaging (DKI) model is defined by an apparent diffusivity parameter, D_a (or ADC_0, for distinction from ADC), plus an additional apparent kurtosis fit parameter, K_a, to account for second-order DWI signal behavior with increasing b value[60]:

$$S(b) = S_o \exp\left[-b \cdot D_a + \frac{K_a}{6}(b \cdot D_a)^2\right].$$

Although phantoms based on "natural" materials like dairy cream and asparagus have been proposed and shown to exhibit kurtosis, they are not easily tunable over the range of kurtosis values seen in tissue and are certainly not stable over time. Polyethylene particle suspensions and microbead impregnated gels are more stable but have limited range in D_a, K_a metrics.[59] More recently, novel kurtosis phantoms have been developed based on lamellar vesicles (fluid-filled microsacs).[57] These are created by combining long-chain fatty alcohols and surfactants to mimic tissue cellularity by forming reasonably regular-spaced membranous units called mesostructures. The prototype phantom shown in Fig. 14.8 was constructed using this variable

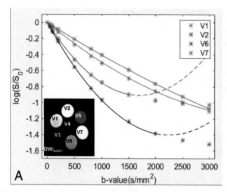 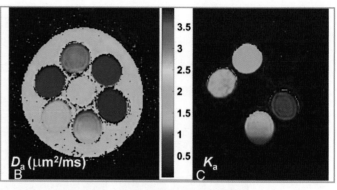

Fig. 14.8 Diffusion kurtosis phantom. Lamellar vesicle materials in vials V1, V2, V6, and V7 (marked on the inset DWI at $b = 3000$ s/mm^2) exhibit multiexponential DWI signal decay (A) due to impeded diffusion leading to strong sustained DWI signal (see inset). Asterisks show the measured data. Solid lines correspond to the fit to the kurtosis model subject to constraint only include data up to "b_{max}," where $b_{max} < 3/D_aK_a$. The *dashed lines* illustrate extrapolation for unconstrained fit where the kurtosis model becomes nonphysical. The model fit for negative control (zero kurtosis) samples in V3, V4, and V5 was also constrained to b_{max} above noise floor. The phantom parametric maps that share a common scale-bar on the right illustrate (B) D_a (μm^2/ms) and (C) K_a (dimensionless) values typical of tumors. The negative control (monoexponential diffusion) samples in V3 (PVP20%), V4 (water), and V5 (PVP40%) appropriately show $K_a \approx 0$. *DWI*, Diffusion-weighted imaging; *PVP*, polyvinylpyrrolidone.

lamellar vesicle size and density platform and could potentially be applicable to breast DKI studies. As illustrated in Fig. 14.8A, data fit to the kurtosis model needs to be constrained for model convergence such that the product ($b_{max} \times D_a \times K_a$) less than 3, where b_{max} is the maximum b value included in the fit.[60] Note that "b_{max}" is allowed to vary for each voxel. Data beyond this constraint should not be fit to the kurtosis model because it would predict increasing DWI signal beyond b_{max}, which is not physically possible, as illustrated by dashed lines in Fig. 14.8A.

Synthetic Diffusion Phantoms

As one increases b value to gain sensitivity to true kurtotic diffusion behavior, one increases risk of false kurtosis due to measured signal being buoyed by the noise floor (see Figs. 1.1–1.4). Artifactual noise-induced curvature to signal decay depends not only on b value choice and scanner noise floor (see Figs. 11.1–11.11) but also the true diffusion properties of the tissue. That is, within a given multiple b value DWI series, there may be high ADC (or Da) tissue regions negatively biased by noise (i.e., mobility is underestimated), whereas low ADC (or Da) tissues remain unbiased. In DWI/DKI protocol optimization to maximize diffusion contrast while minimizing noise bias, it is beneficial to understand this trade-off between

target diffusion properties, inherent system noise, and acquisition parameters (e.g., b values, voxel size, averaging) by synthetic phantom simulations[34] (see Table 14.1: ADC SNR DRO).

Armed with target diffusion properties and reasonable estimates of base system signal and noise levels, one may predict random and bias error in fit diffusion model parameters by numerical simulation of the idealized diffusion model and stochastic noise. Fig. 14.9 illustrates simulation of noise impact for true monoexponential diffusion studied by two DWI protocols: $b = [0, 400, 800]$ s/mm^2 (top panels) versus $b = [0, 800, 1600]$ s/mm^2 (bottom panels), assuming baseline (i.e., measured at $b = 0$) SNR $= 25$ (left panels) versus SNR $= 50$ (right panels). Simulation indicates the higher b value protocol reduces random error (displayed as vertical error bars) for low ADC tissues but increases negative bias error (displayed as deviation from the horizontal dashed line) for high ADC tissues. This tradeoff should be considered within the context of the specific desired breast DWI application. For example, if the application is to detect and/or characterize exclusively low ADC lesions (below ~0.7 μm^2/ms), then it may be reasonable to use high b values (~1600 s/mm^2) even though signals from higher ADC tissues (e.g., cystic or necrotic) are driven into the noise floor, thus not reliably quantified.

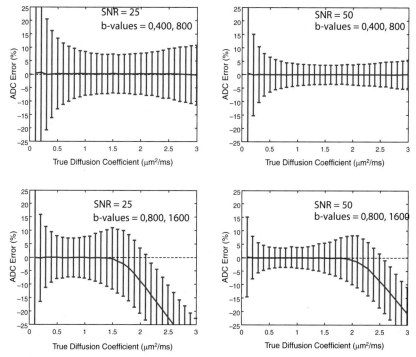

Fig. 14.9 Numerical simulation of percent ADC random and bias errors. ADC errors due to DWI signal approaching the noise floor are quantified as percent of true monoexponential diffusion rate. Random error is denoted by vertical error bars and bias as deviation from the horizontal *dashed line* at 0% error. Two 3 *b* value protocols are compared $b = [0, 400, 800]$ s/mm^2 *(top)* versus $b = [0, 800, 1600]$ s/mm^2 *(bottom* panels) for SNR = 25 *(left)* versus SNR = 50 *(right)* as labeled on each plot. The simulation assumes SNR is measured at $b = 0$ without signal averaging and nonzero *b* values include inherent threefold averaging due to a 3-orthogonal DWI acquisition protocol. *ADC,* Apparent diffusion coefficient; *DWI,* diffusion-weighted imaging; *SNR,* signal-to-noise ratio.

USE OF PHANTOMS FOR QUALITY CONTROL

Performance relevant to DWI includes quantitative accuracy; stability; spatial resolution, distortion, and uniformity; directional artifact (e.g., from eddy currents); and system SNR.[8,33,42,61] Breast DWI QC should also include assessment of fat suppression performance, although for lack of challenging fat-water phantoms, this may have to be subjectively assessed on patient/volunteer DWI (see Fig. 13.6). For simplicity, the following discussion is limited to QC phantoms comprising monoexponential decay materials, thus relevant to breast DWI targeting ADC.

Protocol Compliance

In terms of site certification and periodic QC for inclusion in multicenter clinical trials, adherence to the study-specific protocol is another important consideration, although "performance" in this case may be more a reflection of on-site personnel compliance to responsible protocol creation/curation rather than the MRI system performance. Fortunately, DICOM records many key DWI acquisition parameters that can be polled to assess protocol compliance, although unfortunately some key DWI parameters may be confined to vendor-specific private tags that are subject to change with scanner software version and often inadvertently lost during data anonymization process.

Accuracy Measurement

The term "accuracy" implies measurement relative to known "truth" reference standards. Despite inconvenience of phantom preparation, ice-water based phantoms for temperature control are proven to provide absolute truth in diffusion measurements. A commercially available head-sized DWI phantom (CaliberMRI) was modeled after the QIBA/NIST PVP phantom and allows measurement of ADC bias and linearity (i.e., accuracy) when properly prepared and at thermal equilibrium with ice-water, as shown in Fig. 14.10. The figure summarizes MRI system performance tests established by QIBA using this phantom and a 5 b value protocol. Similar assessment protocol can be implemented with other breast DWI phantoms. The system linearity test is illustrated in Fig. 14.10E, checking that the slope between true and measured ADC is close to 1. Maximum allowed bias threshold may also be established for a given trial (see Fig. 14.10F illustrates the QIBA limit within ±4% established for this protocol).

System Stability

Assessment of system stability and noise of particular relevance for DWI is complicated by the fact that noise is not reliably measured from background ROIs (placed in signal-free air) due to the common practice of image filtration/regularization and parallel imaging reconstruction routines that spatially modulate noise.[62] An alternative QC measure of noise and instability is by intraexamination sequentially repeated DWI scans where all acquisition conditions are held

constant. Then noise (or instability) may be estimated as a spatial mean of pixel-by-pixel temporal standard deviation over the sequential scans.[62] Instability estimation improves with the number of repeated sequential scans, however as a practical balance only four repeated DWI scans were acquired for data shown in Fig. 14.10, as was also used for site certification and periodic QC in ACRIN 6698 and 6702 breast DWI trials (four sequential scans, 3 minutes each scan, for 12 minutes total, Table 14.3).[42,43]

Signal-to-Noise Ratio

Using dedicated DWI QC analysis software, SNR is measured on each b value DWI separately as follows. The temporal mean over sequential scans is denoted as "signal image" and temporal standard deviation denoted as "noise image." Note that temporal mean and standard deviation are performed on a pixel-by-pixel basis. The image analyst next has to define single-slice ROIs (or volumes of interest [VOIs] over multiple slices) in uniform materials on both the signal image and noise image and record the spatial means and standard deviations for each ROI. An estimate of

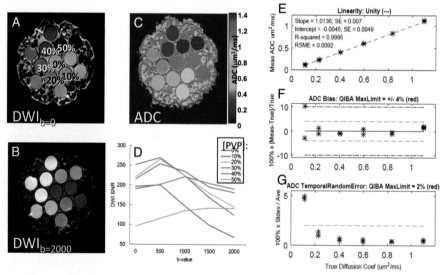

Fig. 14.10 PVP DWI phantom for absolute measure of bias, linearity, and SNR. The PVP phantom DWI at $b = 0$, $b = 2000$ s/mm², and ADC map are shown in (A–C). SNR at b values = 0, 500, 1000, 1500 and 2000 s/mm² is illustrated in (D). Apparent increase in SNR at $b > 1000$ s/mm² for high PVP concentrations is in part due to relatively low ADC and additional directional averaging for nonzero b value acquisitions. Scan system linearity is established through the measured ADC plot (E) versus known phantom ADC values at multiple PVP concentrations. QC plots for bias and random error as a function of ADC (PVP concentration) are shown in (F) and (G), respectively. Phantom temperature at 0°C is controlled by ice-water bath. *ADC*, Apparent diffusion coefficient; *DWI*, diffusion-weighted imaging; *PVP*, polyvinylpyrrolidone; *QC*, quality control; *SNR*, signal-to-noise ratio.

DWI SNR is formed by the ratio of ROI spatial mean of signal image over spatial mean of noise image. Note that although signal decays exponentially with b value, depending on phantom material diffusion rate (see Fig. 14.9), system instability (noise) depends on the number of averages (e.g., three direction for $b > 0$ trace DWI) and is not constant with respect to b value. Therefore plots of DWI SNR versus b value typically do not appear as an exponential decay (see Fig. 14.10D). DWI SNR is a useful QC metric and a minimum acceptable threshold can be established (e.g., QIBA minimum SNR = 45) below which ADC measurement is prone to bias. The 3 T system illustrated in Fig. 14.10 surpasses this minimum SNR performance metric, whereas 1.5 T systems often fall below this minimum SNR for low PVP concentrations at high b values (≥ 1500 s/mm^2, data not shown).

Similar pixel-wise analysis is applied to sequential ADC maps to create temporal mean ("ADC signal image") and temporal standard deviation ("ADC noise image") for estimation of temporal random error in ADC defined as ROI spatial mean (in uniform material) on the ADC noise image divided by ROI spatial mean on ADC signal image, expressed as a percent of true ADC as shown in Fig. 14.10G. Again, a maximum allowed threshold in temporal random error may be established for a QC metric. QIBA limits for ADC bias and random error are indicated in the figure. Note, the temporal random error metric (multiscan SNR) is distinct from the ratio of ROI spatial mean over spatial standard deviation of the ADC signal image because the spatial standard deviation includes static structural artifact in ADC maps (e.g., ringing artifact near high-contrast edges).

Conclusion

Timely clinical translation of promising breast DWI technology requires establishing reproducibility and accuracy of diagnostic results across vendor systems, scan sequences, and data analysis implementations. Protocol optimization and standardization rely on achieving balance in trade-offs between diagnostic yield, complexity, and practicality. Scan time and SNR are driving factors for DWI acquisition optimization. Currently the main limiting aspects for widespread clinical use of breast DWI are questionable added clinical value, reliability, image quality, and protocol complexity. Simplified diffusion scans and parametric models tend to exhibit good repeatability and accuracy for the derived breast diffusion metric. The majority of current clinical trials explore ADC and its histogram derivatives for cancer diagnosis and prediction of therapy response. More advanced multiparametric diffusion models, including IVIM, DTI, and kurtosis, hold potential to provide deeper insights into microstructure of breast pathology but need thorough repeatability and reproducibility studies before utilization as clinical biomarkers. Use of phantom test objects helps evaluate performance and accuracy of emerging scan protocols, correction techniques, and parameter choices to optimize for clinical applications. Ultimately, the benefit of advanced breast DWI protocols has to be established through large-scale multisite clinical trial validation. Standardization of breast DWI protocols is critical for clinical integration to ensure consistent performance and generalizable interpretation guidelines, which is being addressed by international standardization initiatives underway by EUSOBI, QIBA, RSNA, and other cooperative groups.

REFERENCES

1. Baltzer P, et al. Diffusion-weighted imaging of the breast—a consensus and mission statement from the EUSOBI International Breast Diffusion-Weighted Imaging working group. *Eur Radiol.* 2020;30(3):1436–1450.
2. Shukla-Dave A, et al. Quantitative Imaging Biomarkers Alliance (QIBA) recommendations for improved precision of DWI and DCE-MRI derived biomarkers in multicenter oncology trials. *J Magn Reson Imaging.* 2019;49(7):e101–e121.
3. Iima M, Partridge SC, Le Bihan D. Six DWI questions you always wanted to know but were afraid to ask: clinical relevance for breast diffusion MRI. *Eur Radiol.* 2020;30(5):2561–2570.
4. Partridge SC, et al. Diffusion-weighted breast MRI: clinical applications and emerging techniques. *J Magn Reson Imaging.* 2017;45(2):337–355.
5. Aja-Fernandez S, Alberola-Lopez C, Westin CF. Noise and signal estimation in magnitude MRI and Rician distributed images: a LMMSE approach. *IEEE Trans Image Process.* 2008;17(8):1383–1398.
6. Poot DH, et al. Optimal experimental design for diffusion kurtosis imaging. *IEEE Trans Med Imaging.* 2010;29(3):819–829.
7. Malyarenko DI, et al. Retrospective correction of ADC for gradient nonlinearity errors in multicenter breast DWI trials: ACRIN 6698 multiplatform feasibility study. *Tomography.* 2020;6(2):86–92.
8. Newitt DC, et al. Gradient nonlinearity correction to improve apparent diffusion coefficient accuracy and standardization in the American College of Radiology Imaging Network 6698 breast cancer trial. *J Magn Reson Imaging.* 2015;42(4):908–919.
9. Luo J, et al. Diffusion tensor imaging for characterizing tumor microstructure and improving diagnostic performance on breast MRI: a prospective observational study. *Breast Cancer Res.* 2019;21(1):102.

10. Wu D, et al. Characterization of breast tumors using diffusion kurtosis imaging (DKI). *PLoS One*. 2014;9(11). e113240.

11. Malyarenko D, et al. Toward uniform implementation of parametric map Digital Imaging and Communication in Medicine standard in multisite quantitative diffusion imaging studies. *J Med Imaging (Bellingham)*. 2018;5(1):011006.

12. Hu Y, et al. Multishot diffusion-weighted MRI of the breast with multiplexed sensitivity encoding (MUSE) and shot locally low-rank (shot-LLR) reconstructions. *J Magn Reson Imaging*. 2021;53(3):807–817.

13. Otikovs M, et al. Diffusivity in breast malignancies analyzed for $b > 1000$ s/mm^2 at 1 mm in-plane resolutions: insight from Gaussian and non-Gaussian behaviors. *J Magn Reson Imaging*. 2021;53(6):1913–1925.

14. Wisner DJ, et al. High-resolution diffusion-weighted imaging for the separation of benign from malignant BI-RADS 4/5 lesions found on breast MRI at 3 T. *J Magn Reson Imaging*. 2014;40(3):674–681.

15. Keenan KE, et al. Quantitative magnetic resonance imaging phantoms: a review and the need for a system phantom. *Magn Reson Med*. 2018;79(1):48–61.

16. Newitt DC, et al. Multisite concordance of apparent diffusion coefficient measurements across the NCI Quantitative Imaging Network. *J Med Imaging (Bellingham)*. 2018;5(1):011003.

17. Raunig DL, et al. Quantitative imaging biomarkers: a review of statistical methods for technical performance assessment. *Stat Methods Med Res*. 2015;24(1):27–67.

18. Sullivan DC, et al. Metrology standards for quantitative imaging biomarkers. *Radiology*. 2015;277(3):813–825.

19. Dalmis MU, et al. Artificial intelligence-based classification of breast lesions imaged with a multiparametric breast MRI protocol with ultrafast DCE-MRI, T2, and DWI. *Invest Radiol*. 2019;54(6):325–332.

20. Leithner D, et al. Radiomic signatures derived from diffusion-weighted imaging for the assessment of breast cancer receptor status and molecular subtypes. *Mol Imaging Biol*. 2020;22(2):453–461.

21. Zhang L, et al. Automated deep learning method for whole-breast segmentation in diffusion-weighted breast MRI. *J Magn Reson Imaging*. 2020;51(2):635–643.

22. Newitt DC, et al. Repeatability and reproducibility of ADC histogram metrics from the ACRIN 6698 breast cancer therapy response trial. *Tomography*. 2020;6(2):177–185.

23. Newitt DC, et al. Test-retest repeatability and reproducibility of ADC measures by breast DWI: results from the ACRIN 6698 trial. *J Magn Reson Imaging*. 2019;49(6):1617–1628.

24. Iima M, et al. Variability of non-Gaussian diffusion MRI and intravoxel incoherent motion (IVIM) measurements in the breast. *PLoS One*. 2018;13(3):e0193444.

25. Obuchowski NA, et al. Quantitative imaging biomarkers: a review of statistical methods for computer algorithm comparisons. *Stat Methods Med Res*. 2015;24(1):68–106.

26. Spick C, et al. Diffusion-weighted MRI of breast lesions: a prospective clinical investigation of the quantitative imaging biomarker characteristics of reproducibility, repeatability, and diagnostic accuracy. *NMR Biomed*. 2016;29(10):1445–1453.

27. Jensen LR, et al. Diffusion-weighted and dynamic contrast-enhanced MRI in evaluation of early treatment effects during neoadjuvant chemotherapy in breast cancer patients. *J Magn Reson Imaging*. 2011;34(5):1099–1109.

28. Nissan N, et al. Diffusion-tensor MR imaging of the breast: hormonal regulation. *Radiology*. 2014;271(3):672–680.

29. McDonald ES, et al. Mean apparent diffusion coefficient is a sufficient conventional diffusion-weighted MRI metric to improve breast MRI diagnostic performance: results from the ECOG-ACRIN Cancer Research Group A6702 diffusion imaging trial. *Radiology*. 2021;298(1):60–70.

30. Meeus EM, et al. Evaluation of intravoxel incoherent motion fitting methods in low-perfused tissue. *J Magn Reson Imaging*. 2017;45(5):1325–1334.

31. While PT. A comparative simulation study of Bayesian fitting approaches to intravoxel incoherent motion modeling in diffusion-weighted MRI. *Magn Reson Med*. 2017;78(6):2373–2387.

32. Chenevert TL, et al. Diffusion coefficient measurement using a temperature-controlled fluid for quality control in multicenter studies. *J Magn Reson Imaging*. 2011;34(4):983–987.

33. Keenan KE, et al. Variability and bias assessment in breast ADC measurement across multiple systems. *J Magn Reson Imaging*. 2016;44(4):846–855.

34. Malyarenko D, et al. Numerical DWI phantoms to optimize accuracy and precision of quantitative parametric maps for non-Gaussian diffusion. *SPIE Medical Imaging*. 2020;11313.

35. Partridge SC, Amornsiripanitch N. DWI in the assessment of breast lesions. *Top Magn Reson Imaging*. 2017;26(5):201–209.

36. Woodhams R, et al. Diffusion-weighted imaging of the breast: principles and clinical applications. *Radiographics*. 2011;31(4):1059–1084.

37. Onishi N, et al. Impact of MRI protocol adherence on prediction of pathological complete response in the I-SPY 2 neoadjuvant breast cancer trial. *Tomography*. 2020;6(2):77–85.

38. Nogueira L, et al. Breast DWI at 3T: influence of the fat-suppression technique on image quality and diagnostic performance. *Clin Radiol*. 2015;70(3):286–294.

39. Brandao S, et al. Fat suppression techniques (STIR vs. SPAIR) on diffusion-weighted imaging of breast lesions at 3.0T: preliminary experience. *Radiol Med*. 2015;120(8):705–713.

40. Malyarenko D, et al. Multi-system repeatability and reproducibility of apparent diffusion coefficient measurement using an ice-water phantom. *J Magn Reson Imaging*. 2013;37(5):1238–1246.

41. Li W, et al. Predicting breast cancer response to neoadjuvant treatment using multi-feature MRI: results from the I-SPY 2 trial. *NPJ Breast Cancer*. 2020;6(1):63.

42. Partridge SC, et al. Diffusion-weighted MRI findings predict pathologic response in neoadjuvant treatment of breast cancer: the ACRIN 6698 multicenter trial. *Radiology*. 2018;289(3):618–627.

43. Rahbar H, et al. Utility of diffusion-weighted imaging to decrease unnecessary biopsies prompted by breast MRI: a trial of the ECOG-ACRIN Cancer Research Group (A6702). *Clin Cancer Res*. 2019;25(6):1756–1765.

44. Sorace AG, et al. Repeatability, reproducibility, and accuracy of quantitative MRI of the breast in the community radiology setting. *J Magn Reson Imaging*. 2018;48(3):695–707.

45. Tan ET, et al. Denoising and multiple tissue compartment visualization of multi-b valued breast diffusion MRI. *J Magn Reson Imaging*. 2021;53(1):271–282.

46. Keenan KE, et al. Design of a breast phantom for quantitative MRI. *J Magn Reson Imaging*. 2016;44(3):610–619.

47. He Y, et al. 3D-printed breast phantom for multi-purpose and multi-modality imaging. *Quant Imaging Med Surg*. 2019;9(1):63–74.

48. Palacios EM, et al. Toward precision and reproducibility of diffusion tensor imaging: a multicenter diffusion phantom and traveling volunteer study. *AJNR Am J Neuroradiol*. 2017;38(3):537–545.

49. Wagner F, et al. Temperature and concentration calibration of aqueous polyvinylpyrrolidone (PVP) solutions for isotropic diffusion MRI phantoms. *PLoS One.* 2017;12(6):e0179276.

50. Keenan KE, et al. MRI-visible liquid crystal thermometer. *Magn Reson Med.* 2020;84(3):1552–1563.

51. Cho GY, et al. A versatile flow phantom for intravoxel incoherent motion MRI. *Magn Reson Med.* 2012;67(6):1710–1720.

52. Fieremans E, Lee HH. Physical and numerical phantoms for the validation of brain microstructural MRI: a cookbook. *Neuroimage.* 2018;182:39–61.

53. Lee JH, et al. Perfusion assessment using intravoxel incoherent motion-based analysis of diffusion-weighted magnetic resonance imaging: validation through phantom experiments. *Invest Radiol.* 2016;51(8):520–528.

54. Schneider MJ, et al. Assessment of intravoxel incoherent motion MRI with an artificial capillary network: analysis of biexponential and phase-distribution models. *Magn Reson Med.* 2019;82(4):1373–1384.

55. Bickelhaupt S, et al. Radiomics based on adapted diffusion kurtosis imaging helps to clarify most mammographic findings suspicious for cancer. *Radiology.* 2018;287(3):761–770.

56. Sun K, et al. Breast cancer: diffusion kurtosis MR imaging—diagnostic accuracy and correlation with clinical-pathologic factors. *Radiology.* 2015;277(1):46–55.

57. Malyarenko DI, et al. Multicenter repeatability study of a novel quantitative diffusion kurtosis imaging phantom. *Tomography.* 2019;5(1):36–43.

58. Phillips J, Charles-Edwards GD. A simple and robust test object for the assessment of isotropic diffusion kurtosis. *Magn Reson Med.* 2015;73(5):1844–1851.

59. Portakal ZG, et al. Design and characterization of tissue-mimicking gel phantoms for diffusion kurtosis imaging. *Med Phys.* 2018;45(6):2476–2485.

60. Jensen JH, Helpern JA. MRI quantification of non-Gaussian water diffusion by kurtosis analysis. *NMR Biomed.* 2010;23(7):698–710.

61. Delakis I, et al. Developing a quality control protocol for diffusion imaging on a clinical MRI system. *Phys Med Biol.* 2004;49(8):1409–1422.

62. Dietrich O, et al. Measurement of signal-to-noise ratios in MR images: influence of multichannel coils, parallel imaging, and reconstruction filters. *J Magn Reson Imaging.* 2007;26(2):375–385.

Routine and Advanced Breast DWI Techniques and Processing: The Siemens Healthineers Perspective

Gregor Thoermer, PhD, Petra Bildhauer, Thomas Benkert, PhD, Wei Liu, PhD, Robert Grimm and Elisabeth Weiland, PhD

As discussed in detail in earlier chapters of this book, diffusion-weighted imaging (DWI) is a powerful tool in the multiparametric assessment of breast lesions with magnetic reconace imaging (MRI) and can provide decisive information for initial detection and classification of lesions, for treatment selection, and for monitoring the efficacy of treatments and follow-up.[1–5] Whereas dynamic contrast-enhanced MRI studies allow to study tissue vascularity and provide high sensitivity for cancer detection, DWI allows assessing tissue organization at a microscopic level by probing the diffusivity of water molecules in their surroundings.

From a vendor perspective, key objectives in breast DWI are to provide robust diffusion-weighted images with high resolution, to generate few distortions and artifacts in reasonable acquisition times for a seamless integration into daily clinical routine, and to support advanced (clinical and research) applications, such as the assessment of non-Gaussian diffusion or tumor heterogeneity.

Data Acquisition

HARDWARE AND SEQUENCES

Although two decades ago there were no tailored protocols or optimized sequences for DWI of the breast, today every Siemens Healthcare MAGNETOM scanner provides standardized DWI sequences and protocols for imaging of the breast. These protocols have been optimized to make best use of the respective MRI hardware (e.g., gradient slew rate and maximum gradient amplitude) and follow the recommendations of the European Society of Breast Imaging (EUSOBI)

consensus group for breast imaging.[6] As recommended there, the Siemens Healthineers protocols provide coverage of both breasts in axial orientation, an in-plane resolution (acquired, not interpolated) of $\leq 2 \times 2$ mm^2, a typical slice thickness of 4 mm, and two b values: one low $b = 50$ s/mm^2 to minimize the effects of pseudo perfusion (intravoxel incoherent motion [IVIM]), which are observed with b = 0 s/mm^2; and one high b value of 800 s/mm^2, which has been shown to be a sweet spot for reasonable signal-to-noise ratio (SNR) and lesion conspicuity in the breast. To reduce scan time by leveraging higher SNR at low b values, a different number of averages is acquired for the individual b values and can be flexibly adjusted by the user. Up to 15 b values can be acquired within a measurement, and small b value increments for non-Gaussian diffusion models are supported with recent software versions. Furthermore, the user can choose from various diffusion modes (e.g., 3-scan-trace, 3D-diagonal, 4-scan-trace) and between monopolar (single-echo) and bipolar (double-echo) diffusion schemes. To mitigate diffusion anisotropy effects, usually a 3-scan-trace diffusion mode is used, in which acquisitions are performed using three orthogonal diffusion gradient directions sequentially to obtain orientation-averaged apparent diffusion coefficient (ADC)–weighted images, which approximate diffusion tensor imaging (DTI)-orientation-invariant trace-weighted images. With a 4-scan-trace or tetrahedral mode the maximum gradient strength can be applied, facilitating minimal echo times (TEs) and echo-planar imaging (EPI) readouts. Under the assumption that diffusion anisotropy in body oncology applications is neglectable, another highly efficient alternative is the diagonal mode, applying the maximum diffusion gradient strength in all three directions simultaneously and thereby measuring diffusion in a single direction.

Whereas the bipolar diffusion scheme is less sensitive to eddy-current effects (which result in geometrical distortion) and background gradient effects (which might interfere with *b* values), the monopolar scheme has the advantage of shorter TE and repetition time (TR) and provides higher SNR. By applying an image-based dynamic distortion correction algorithm,[7] however, most disadvantages of monopolar acquisition can be compensated, and monopolar is routinely used in the Siemens Healthineers breast DWI protocols. Proper fat saturation is achieved by offering different excitation/fat saturation schemes (e.g., spectral adiabatic inversion recovery [SPAIR], inversion recovery), including the use of gradient reversal for minimizing remaining fat residuals.[8] Typical clinical settings encompass 4-scan-trace, monopolar mode, and SPAIR, whereas for scanning ultra-high *b* values, inversion recovery is recommended.[9] The automated (inline) calculation of ADC maps is a standard feature and is based on a monoexponential diffusion model. In addition, the scanner software enables the inline generation of synthetic (extrapolated) high or ultra-high *b* value images, which have been proposed as a tool to increase lesion conspicuity in DWI by means of better suppression of normal tissue and more pronounced appearance of focal lesions with impaired diffusion.[10] Although clinically reasonable values are in a range of 1500 to 2500 s/mm², the calculation is possible up to a value of 5000 s/mm². However, one should remain cautious that extrapolation from lower *b* value images, assuming diffusion is monoexponential (Gaussian), may result in interpretation errors of some findings (see Chapter 12).

Single-Shot Echo-Planar Imaging

The standard and most widely used sequence for DWI in clinical practice is single-shot echo-planar imaging (ss-EPI), where the measured k-space of an entire 2D plane is filled with one EPI readout following a single radiofrequency (RF)–excitation pulse.

The ss-EPI method has the advantage of speed but suffers from susceptibility artifacts, spatial distortions, and spatial blurring. The choice of imaging parameters significantly impacts artifacts and needs careful optimization. When high spatial resolution is desired,

for example, the matrix size in phase encoding (equal to the EPI factor or echo train length [ETL]) must be increased but consequently more echoes are acquired during the T2* decay of the signal. Furthermore, susceptibility effects are amplified in the images due to a larger echo-spacing (ESP).

Geometrical distortions and susceptibility artifacts ($\Delta d(r)$) in EPI are related to ESP, the field of view (FOV) in phase-encoding direction (FOV_{PH}), the number of interleaves (N_{in}), and the parallel acceleration factor R as follows:

$$\Delta d(r) \sim \frac{ESP\ FOV_{PH}}{N_{in}R}$$

To reduce geometrical distortions, several advanced methods have been developed and introduced that leverage these factors to reduce $\Delta d(r)$.

The achievable minimal ESP is dependent on "fixed" factors, such as the available gradient system of the MRI machine, but can be optimized by adjusting the bandwidth of a specific protocol. Usually high bandwidths in the range of 1200 to 2000 Hz/Px are used in clinical DWI.

The FOV_{PH} can be effectively used in breast MRI to influence $\Delta d(r)$: when acquiring axial slices with phase encoding posterior-anterior, the FOV_{PH} can be substantially reduced, practically only covering both breasts and the axilla but excluding the thorax. Because of the typical geometry of breast coils and the limited sensitivity volume of individual coil elements, the signal picked up from anatomy outside the FOV is moderate, and the advantage of shortened ESP outweighs the risk of foldover artifacts.

Finally, the ability of parallel imaging with multiple coil elements as provided with state-of-the-art breast imaging coils on modern MRI scanners allows to reduce the effective ESP with typical acceleration factors of R = 2.

The preceding optimizations in DWI protocols for breast MRI are implemented in the protocols provided by Siemens Healthineers, and any parameter changes can impact the quality of DWI scans accordingly. Modifications should be performed with care by experienced operators and (if available) with the help of an on-site MRI physicist. It is recommended to keep the defined protocols constant in clinical routine.

Zoomed (Reduced) FOV EPI

The concept of reducing the FOV_{PH}, as introduced earlier, can be further refined by applying specially designed excitation pulses as introduced with the ZOOMit technique.[11] The advantage of this method is to combine short TE and moderate scan time while reducing the risk of foldover artifacts compared to conventional EPI. As illustrated in Fig. 15.1, the reduced FOV method allows to achieve high spatial resolution and SNR, which may help in characterizing tumor heterogeneity and heterogeneity of diffusion characteristics.[12] Although only available initially for 3T systems with parallel transmit technology, this technology is now widely available for both 1.5T and 3T systems as ZOOMit[PRO].

RESOLVE

Another method of improving image quality (at the expense of increased imaging time) is to split the acquisition into several interleaves (N_{in}) with readout-segmented echo-planar diffusion methods (rs-EPI), that is, RESOLVE (readout segmentation of long variable echo trains). Several studies[12–14] have consistently shown that RESOLVE not only provides significantly higher image quality and improved lesion conspicuity by reducing geometrical distortions but also achieves higher diagnostic accuracy for the differentiation of benign and malignant breast lesions compared to conventional ss-EPI. One limitation of RESOLVE, however, is the relatively long acquisition time due to segmented k-space acquisition.

Simultaneous Multislice

To shorten the acquisition time of 2D DWI sequences, simultaneous multislice (SMS) excitation based on the "blipped-CAIPI" (controlled aliasing in parallel imaging) method has been proposed for both ss- and rs-EPI (SMS ss-EPI, SMS rs-EPI) and successfully applied to various scan regions, including breast imaging.[3,15] SMS excites several slices at the same time and uses the spatial sensitivity of multichannel array coils for separating the combined slice images. This allows to reduce the minimum TR for a given number of slices. Thereby the acquisition time can be shortened by up to the slice acceleration factor (typically 2) and/or the spatial resolution can be improved, as shown in Fig. 15.2.

IMAGE QUALITY

In a joint effort with clinical users and based on their feedback, Siemens Healthineers is continuously striving to improve image quality and improve robustness of DWI of the breast. Without going into technical details, the introduction of an external phase correction, dynamic field correction, or sensor network to adjust for frequency drifts in very demanding and enduring EPI scans are some of the measures to achieve this goal. On the postprocessing side, background noise masking has been shown to improve image appearance, in particular when assessing inverted ultra-high b value images in the context of screening (Fig. 15.3).[16]

As a particular topic, DWI of patients with breast implants poses an extra challenge on DWI, as image quality can be impaired by improper fat saturation and N/2 ghosting artifacts and thereby affect assessment. With an optimized frequency selective saturation pulse ("breast SPAIR mode"), both fat and silicone frequencies are well suppressed and high water signal intensity is achieved for routine breast DWI at 3T, as illustrated in Fig. 15.4.

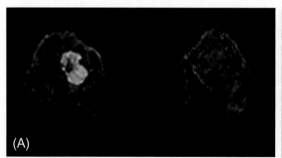 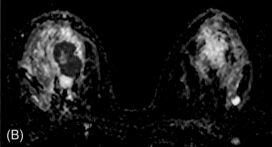

Fig. 15.1 **Case of a histopathologically confirmed invasive ductal carcinoma, nuclear grade 2.** (A) Diffusion-weighted image (b = 1000 s/mm²) and (B) Corresponding apparent diffusion coefficient (ADC) map. The zoomed diffusion-weighted images were acquired at 3T with an (in-plane interpolated) resolution of 0.9 × 0.9 × 3.0 mm³ and were scanned in 3:26 min. (Courtesy Prof. Minseo Bang, Ulsan University Hospital, Republic of Korea.)

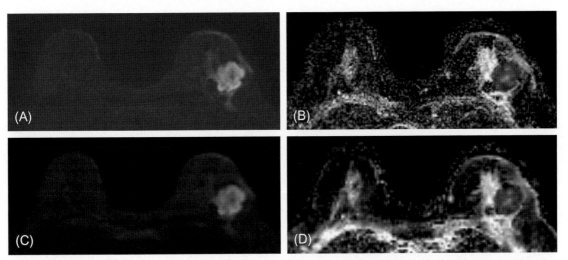

Fig. 15.2 **RESOLVE images of a 64-year-old patient diagnosed with invasive ductal carcinoma (1.5T): (A–B) acquired with simultaneous mul-tislice (SMS) (acquired resolution 1.4 × 1.4 × 5.0 mm³, TA 3:00 min), (C–D) acquired without SMS (acquired resolution 2.1 × 2.1 × 5.0 mm³, TA 3:03 min). (A, C) Diffusion-weighted image (b = 800 s/mm²). (B, D) Corresponding apparent diffusion coefficient (ADC) maps.** (Courtesy Prof. Fuhua Yan, Ruijin Hospital, Shanghai Jiao Tong University School of Medicine, Shanghai, China.)

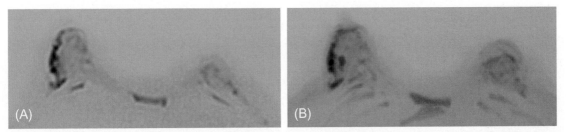

Fig. 15.3 **High *b* value images (b = 2500 s/mm²) of a patient with a moderately differentiated invasive ductal breast cancer and extensive intermediate grade ductal carcinoma in situ (DCIS). Images have an acquired resolution of 2.7 × 2.7 × 4.0 mm³ and were acquired in TA 4:26 min at 3T: (A) single slice (grayscale inverted) and (B) maximum intensity projection (MIP) (grayscale inverted).** (Courtesy Prof. Evelyn Wenkel, University Hospital Erlangen, Friedrich-Alexander-Universität Erlangen-Nürnberg [FAU], Erlangen, Germany.)

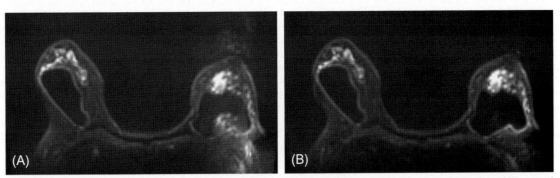

Fig. 15.4 **Diffusion-weighted images of the breast (b = 50 s/mm²) in a volunteer with bilateral silicone implants.** Comparison of (A) conventional SPAIR and (B) optimized SPAIR pulse for the breast shows clear image quality improvement.

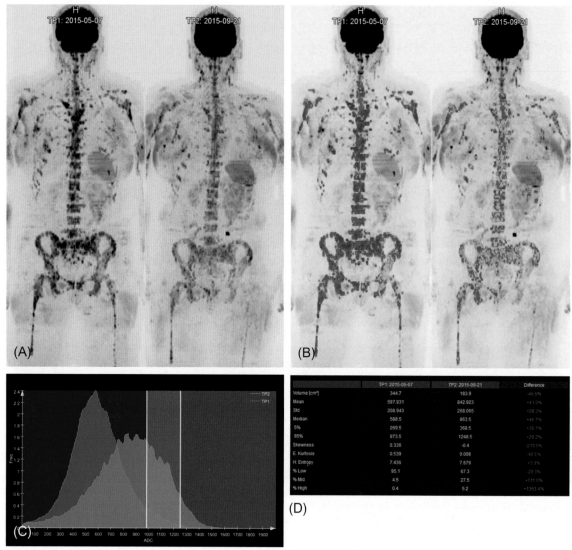

Fig. 15.5 A 50-year-old woman with metastatic invasive breast cancer, estrogen receptor (ER)-positive and human epidermal growth factor receptor 2 (HER-2) neu negative disease was treated with first-line hormonal therapy (exemestane, goserelin) and zoledronic acid. Bone lesions were segmented semiautomatically based on thresholding of the high *b* value maximum intensity projection (MIP) images (A) followed by manual corrections to remove tissue with physiological high diffusion-weighted imaging (DWI) signal intensity such as brain and spleen. The corresponding apparent diffusion coefficient (ADC) ranges are represented as a color-coded overlay, with ADC ranges less than 980 $\mu m^2/s$ that resemble regions of active disease shown in red, 980 to 1250 $\mu m^2/s$ shown in yellow (B). Finally, regions with an ADC greater than 1250 $\mu m^2/s$ are shown in green. On hormone therapy (B, "TP2: 2015-09-21"), a decreased DWI signal intensity is observed on the MIP images, and the ADC histogram shift (C) reflects therapy response in the spine and pelvis with higher ADC values. The histogram parameters (D) indicating response include higher central tendency parameters (mean and median values [units: $\mu m^2/s$]), decreased kurtosis and changes in skewness from positive to negative, and increased dispersion of ADC values (increased standard deviation values and the 5th–95th centile ranges). However, the spatial distribution indicates areas of persistent active disease (red voxels in B) indicating therapy resistance. The patient relapsed with more extensive bone disease on June 06, 2016. (Courtesy Prof. A. R. Padhani, Paul Strickland Scanner Centre, Mount Vernon Cancer Hospital, UK.)

Data Processing and Management

SYNTHESIZED DWI AND ADC

As described before, the scanner software offers inline (automated) calculation of one synthesized high *b* value series and ADC maps as a standard feature. Scanners with software Numaris X offer standard postprocessing tools to generate additional synthesized *b* value images and ADC maps based on a subset of *b* values that can be freely defined by the user.

ADVANCED DISPLAY AND ANALYSIS TOOLS

Siemens Healthineers offers comprehensive reading and reporting software (*syngo*.MR BreVis and *syngo*. MR Breast) that allows an integrative assessment of multiparametric breast MRI cases, for example, by generating maximum intensity projections (MIPs) of high *b* value images, measuring ADC metrics, and fusing/cross-correlating DWI with other contrasts.

To assess diffusion metrics, such as the skewness of the ADC value distribution or changes in the mean and median ADC under therapy, advanced visualization tools may be useful. The postprocessing application *syngo*.via OncoTrend enables in depth evaluation

of diffusion information similar to the clinical example shown in Fig. 15.5.[17]

Works in Progress

ADVANCED ACQUISITION

Key trends driving predevelopment activities in DWI of the breast are the demand for "morphological" spatial resolution and image sharpness in clinically acceptable scan times and the need for more reliable, quantitative metrics for tissue characterization. These developments are seconded by the rise of deep learning techniques in image reconstruction and processing. The long-term vision is to mature DWI to a state where the application of contrast agent may become obsolete for certain clinical questions. Work-in-progress packages allow to transfer emerging scientific approaches and novel methods into clinical testing and validation at collaborating clinical sites.

ADVANCED POSTPROCESSING TOOLS

Similar to scientific collaborations on the acquisition side, *syngo*.via Frontier offers a platform for developing and testing new postprocessing and data analysis

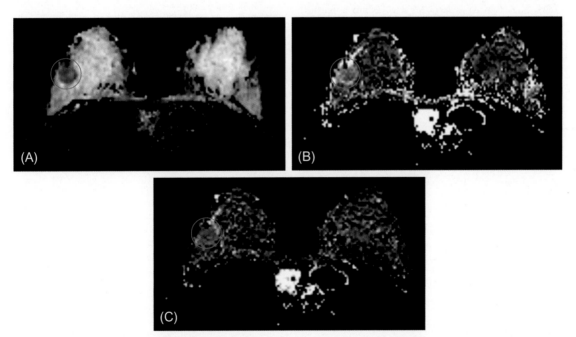

Fig. 15.6   Intravoxel incoherent motion (IVIM) parameter maps for a 40-year-old patient with invasive ductal carcinoma. (A) Diffusion coefficient D, (B) perfusion fraction f$_p$, and (C) pseudodiffusion coefficient D*. (Courtesy Sung Eun Song, Korea University Anam Hospital, Seoul, South Korea.)

prototypes. Researchers can develop and share own algorithms and tools but also may evaluate Siemens Healthineers research applications such as the Body Diffusion Toolbox. This research prototype allows the calculation and assessment of parameter maps based on non-Gaussian diffusion models and enables the export of diffusional kurtosis imaging (DKI) and IVIM results for further investigation (Fig. 15.6).

REFERENCES

1. Ei Khouli RH, Jacobs MA, Mezban SD, et al. Diffusion-weighted imaging improves the diagnostic accuracy of conventional 3.0-T breast MR imaging. *Radiology.* 2010;256(1):64–73.
2. Guo Y, Cai YQ, Cai ZL, et al. Differentiation of clinically benign and malignant breast lesions using diffusion-weighted imaging. *J Magn Reson Imaging.* 2002;16(2):172–178.
3. Ohlmeyer S, Laun FB, Palm T, et al. Simultaneous multislice echo planar imaging for accelerated diffusion-weighted imaging of malignant and benign breast lesions. *Invest Radiology.* 2019;54(8):524–530.
4. Park MJ, Cha ES, Kang BJ, Ihn YK, Baik JH. The role of diffusion-weighted imaging and the apparent diffusion coefficient (ADC) values for breast tumors. *Korean J Radiol.* 2007;8(5):390–396.
5. Sinha S, Lucas-Quesada FA, Sinha U, DeBruhl N, Bassett LW. In vivo diffusion-weighted MRI of the breast: potential for lesion characterization. *J Magn Reson Imaging.* 2002;15(6):693–704.
6. Baltzer P, Mann RM, Iima M, et al. Diffusion-weighted imaging of the breast—a consensus and mission statement from the EUSOBI International Breast Diffusion-Weighted Imaging working group. *Eur Radiol.* 2020;30:1436–1450.
7. Lewis S, Kamath A, Chatterji M, et al. Diffusion-weighted imaging of the liver in patients with chronic liver disease: comparison of monopolar and bipolar diffusion gradients for image quality and lesion detection. *AJR Am J Roentgenol.* 2015;204:59–68.
8. Koh D-M, Blackledge M, Burns S, et al. Combination of chemical suppression techniques for dual suppression of fat and silicone at diffusion-weighted MR imaging in women with breast implants. *Eur Radiol.* 2012;22:2648–2653.
9. Dreher C, Kuder TA, Koenig F, et al. Advanced diffusion-weighted abdominal imaging: qualitative and quantitative comparison of high and ultra-high *b* values for lesion detection and image quality. *Invest Radiol.* 2020;55(5):285–292.
10. Bickel H, Polanec SH, Wengert G, et al. Diffusion-weighted MRI of breast cancer: improved lesion visibility and image quality using synthetic *b* values. *J Magn Reson Imaging.* 2019;50:1754–1761.
11. Park JY, Shin HJ, Shin KC, et al. Comparison of readout segmented echo planar imaging (EPI) and EPI with reduced field-of-view diffusion-weighted imaging at 3 T in patients with breast cancer. *J Magn Reson Imaging.* 2015;42:1679–1688.
12. Bogner W, Pinker-Domenig K, Bickel H, et al. Readout-segmented echo-planar imaging improves the diagnostic performance of diffusion-weighted MR breast examinations at 3.0 T. *Radiology.* 2012;263(1):64–76. https://doi.org/10.1148/radiol.12111494.
13. Kim YJ, Kim SH, Kang BJ, et al. Readout-segmented echo-planar imaging in diffusion-weighted MR imaging in breast cancer: comparison with single-shot echo-planar imaging in image quality. *Korean J Radiol.* 2014;15(4):403–410.
14. Wisner DJ, Nathan R, Deshpande VS. High-resolution diffusion-weighted imaging for the separation of benign from malignant BI-RADS 4/5 lesions found on breast MRI at 3 T. *J Magn Reson Imaging.* 2014;40(3):674–681.
15. Song SE, Woo OH, Cho KR, et al. Simultaneous multislice readout-segmented echo planar imaging for diffusion-weighted MRI in patients with invasive breast cancers. *J Magn Reson Imaging.* 2021;53(4):1108–1115. https://doi.org/10.1002/jmri.27433.
16. Ohlmeyer S, Laun FB, Bickelhaupt S, et al. Ultra-high *b* value DWI-based abbreviated protocols for breast cancer detection. *Invest Radiol.* 2021;56(10). https://doi.org/10.1097/RLI.0000000000000784.
17. Padhani AR, Makris A, Gall P, et al. Therapy monitoring of skeletal metastases with whole-body diffusion MRI. *J Magn Reson Imaging.* 2014;39(5):1049–1078.

Breast Diffusion MRI Acquisition and Processing Techniques: The GE Healthcare Perspective

Ann Shimakawa, MS and Ersin Bayram, PhD

At GE Healthcare, we strive to harness the power of magnetic resonance imaging (MRI) to improve breast care. Breast diffusion-weighted imaging (DWI) exemplifies the potential of MRI, combining morphology of physical structure with functional assessment of disease processes. GE breast MRI products include DWI protocols for all scanner configurations on both our 1.5 T and 3 T platforms, and protocols are compatible with 8-channel HD Breast Array, 16-channel InVivo Sentinelle, 16-channel NeoCoil, and 16-channel Rapid breast arrays, which are all available at both 1.5 T and 3 T. For tomorrow and beyond, our scanners are equipped with expanded research capacity and flexibility, as researchers develop the next generation of state-of-the-art breast MRI. Next we will give a high-level overview of the data acquisition, processing, and reconstruction capabilities on GE MR scanners.

Data Acquisition

To ensure the reliability and quality of breast echo-planar DWI (EP-DWI), system gradient and B_0 fidelity are essential. We provide prospective correction for high-order eddy-current effects (Real Time Field Adjustment [RTFA][1]) and real-time frequency corrections (Real Time Center Frequency [RTCF][2]) to ensure system stability. For object-specific variations, B_0 shimming tools for dual-volume shim prescription and retrospective image distortion correction using reverse polarity gradient approach (PROGRES)[3] are designed to ensure robust image quality for every patient.

Our foundational EP-DWI sequence is the enhanced DWI (eDWI) acquisition. The sequence can be combined with parallel imaging and supports simultaneous-multislice (HyperBand)[4] for increased scan efficiency. HyperBand support is limited to the 16-channel coils due to coil geometry. The eDWI product is designed to provide efficient, flexible, and robust acquisition strategies necessary for diffusion-weighted imaging. For efficiency, the eDWI SmartNEX feature can accommodate multiple b values with different signal averages to ensure that examination time is optimized for each b value. For flexibility, eDWI expands diffusion-direction options to include 3-in-1 and Tetrahedral modes, which use gradient combinations to create diffusion weighting in oblique directions to minimize echo time (TE) and the associated signal loss due to T2 decay. For robust image quality, optional artifact-mitigation strategies include the Dual Echo feature,[5] which combines additional signal refocusing with compensating gradients to correct for eddy-current effects induced by the large gradient waveforms required for DWI. The Optimize TE feature uses intelligent gradient timing to maximize pulse sequence efficiency and reduce TE. For high-performance gradient configurations, the Super G feature allows increased gradient performance for short durations to further reduce TE. Fig. 16.1 shows the user interface for our eDWI sequence, highlighting the variety of tools provided with eDWI.

Our EP-DWI portfolio extends beyond the eDWI sequence to address common challenges posed by breast DWI. For large field-of-view (FOV) applications, multiplexed sensitivity-encoding (MUSE) DWI uses a segmented acquisition to reduce image distortion. MUSE[6] employs an interleaved strategy to

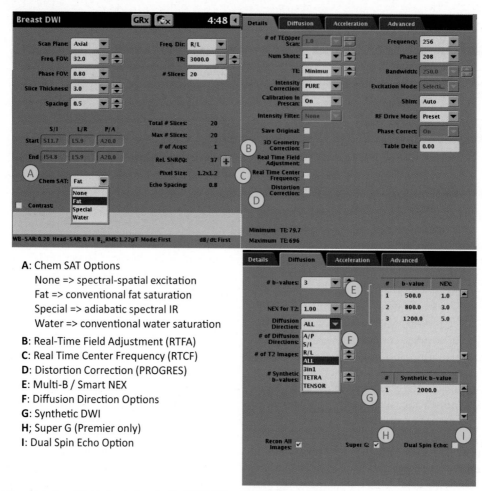

A: Chem SAT Options
  None => spectral-spatial excitation
  Fat => conventional fat saturation
  Special => adiabatic spectral IR
  Water => conventional water saturation
B: Real-Time Field Adjustment (RTFA)
C: Real Time Center Frequency (RTCF)
D: Distortion Correction (PROGRES)
E: Multi-B / Smart NEX
F: Diffusion Direction Options
G: Synthetic DWI
H; Super G (Premier only)
I: Dual Spin Echo Option

Fig. 16.1 eDWI user interface. This interface is shared by the FOCUS DWI and MUSE DWI solutions as well. *DWI*, Diffusion-weighted imaging; *eDWI, enhanced diffusion-weighted imaging; FOCUS*, FOV optimized and constrained undistorted single-shot; *MUSE,* multiplexed sensitivity-encoding.

acquire a subset of the total acquisition, repeated over multiple groupings or "shots." MUSE supports the full array of fat-suppression techniques used in eDWI as well as diffusion-weighting features and parametric image creation options (Fig. 16.2).

For applications that require limited spatial coverage, FOV optimized and constrained undistorted single-shot DWI (FOCUS) reduces image distortion by reducing the total time duration required for the entire acquisition. FOCUS[7] uses a novel radiofrequency (RF) excitation strategy to limit the FOV while simultaneously avoiding aliasing artifacts. In addition, the RF pulses are designed to minimize the fat signal contained in the excited volume, resulting in spatially

and spectrally confined images (Fig. 16.3). FOCUS is available for all platforms and supports the full array of diffusion-weighting features and parametric-image creation options.

Fat suppression is critical for diffusion, in particular in the breast, as residual fat signal can cause artifacts, such as ghosting and chemical shift, and adversely impact the lesion conspicuity. Fat-suppression techniques available for our diffusion sequences include spectral-spatial excitation (SpSp), saturation-based fat suppression (FatSat), short TI inversion recovery fat-nulling (STIR), adiabatic spectral-selective inversion recovery (ASPIR), and slice-select gradient reversal approach (Classic).[8] Multiple techniques can be

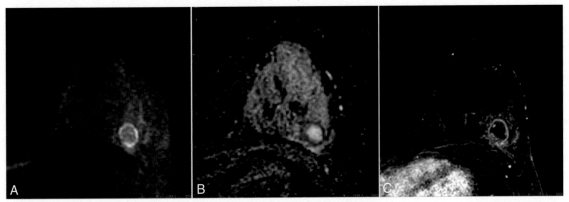

Fig. 16.2 MUSE acquisition of a patient with breast cancer (axial slice, *arrow*). The acquisition pixel size is 1.2 mm × 1.2 mm × 3 mm with T2 ($b = 0$) and $b = 800\,s/mm^2$. The scan time to acquire axial images covering the breast is 6 mins. Note that STIR and spectral-spatial excitation have been combined to provide excellent fat suppression, highlighting the spatial fidelity in the $b = 800\,s/mm^2$ image (A). The ADC map (B) shows a thin ring of tumor denoted by reduced ADC values, corresponding to the area of contrast enhancement on the DCE subtraction (C) image. *ADC*, Apparent diffusion coefficient; *DCE*, dynamic contrast-enhanced; *STIR*, short TI inversion recovery; TI, inversion time. (Data courtesy UCSF Breast Imaging Research Group.)

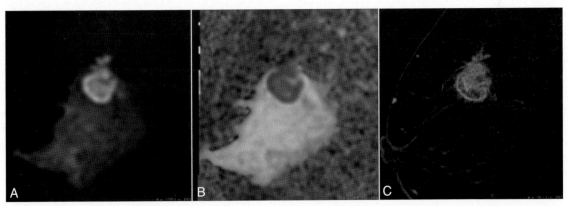

Fig. 16.3 FOCUS acquisition of a patient with breast cancer (sagittal slice, *arrow*). The acquisition pixel size is 1.9 mm × 1.9 mm × 3 mm with $b = 50\,s/mm^2$ and $b = 800\,s/mm^2$. The scan time to acquire sagittal images covering the right breast is 3:37 mins. Note that STIR and FOCUS have been combined to provide excellent fat suppression, highlighting the spatial fidelity in the $b = 800\,s/mm^2$ image (A). The ADC map (B) shows a tumor denoted by reduced ADC values, corresponding to the area of contrast enhancement on the dynamic-contrast-enhanced subtraction (C) image. *ADC*, Apparent diffusion coefficient; *FOCUS*, FOV optimized and constrained undistorted single-shot; *STIR*, short TI inversion recovery; *TI*, inversion time. (Data courtesy Hospital Universitario Quirónsalud Madrid.)

combined (spectral-spatial + STIR or Classic + ASPIR, etc.) for challenging applications such as breast imaging. SpSp provides selective water excitation and enabled by default but imposes a minimum slice thickness requirement. Classic could be enabled if thinner slices are needed than what SpSp could deliver. FatSat, ASPIR, and STIR can be combined with SpSp or Classic as a combo punch for improved fat suppression or can be applied as stand-alone. FatSat is saturation based and thus is quite efficient from a scan-time perspective, but it is both B_0 and B_1 sensitive in that

it is more suitable for use in less challenging scenarios such as 1.5 T, but it should always be combined with SpSp or Classic given the limited FatSat performance. ASPIR is B1 insensitive with an adiabatic inversion but remains B_0 sensitive. It is an excellent choice for fat suppression at 3 T, where B_1 is a bigger concern. Due to inversion pulse, scan efficiency is not as good as FatSat. STIR is spectrally nonselective in that its B_0 insensitive nature provides a robust fat suppression option; however, it comes with a signal-to-noise ratio (SNR) penalty, as water spins are also impacted.

Data Processing and Reconstruction

Parametric image creation can be incorporated into operator workflow with protocol-based options to automatically generate parametric maps such as apparent diffusion coefficient (ADC) and fractional anisotropy (FA) images. Enhanced image-processing tools (READYView) are available to create additional parametric maps, such as synthetic DWI, ADC, eADC, or TRACE, or to perform image segmentation or reformation. Standard DICOM formats are supported for all images. Image reconstruction for diffusion offers a variety of user-selectable options. For multi-*b* value acquisitions, Synthetic DWI (MAGiC DWI)[9] creates mathematical representations of diffusion weighting based on acquired data. Up to four *b* values could be programmed to be automatically synthesized as part of the protocol settings in the range of (100, 2500). By synthesizing higher *b* values instead of acquiring, one can speed up the acquisition significantly and deliver higher SNR because of shorter TE. Retrospective analysis and arbitrary *b* value generation is possible by launching the SyntheticDWI postprocessing application either on the scanner console or on the Advantage Windows Workstation GE Healthcare and using *b* value strength as a slider bar. It is important to note that synthesized *b* values do not contribute to the ADC calculation. Care should be given to minimize potential motion-induced mismatch between *b* values as a confounding factor for synthetic DWI and other parametric map generation, including ADC maps.

GE Healthcare scientists and researchers continue to pioneer transformative technology. Our recent AIR IQ Edition release includes AIR Recon DL (ARDL), which uses a deep convolutional neural network to aid in the reconstruction of raw data to provide high-resolution, low-noise MR images.[10] The supervised learning approach that employed a diverse collection of source images and image augmentations enabled broad generalizability of AIR Recon DL to multiple anatomies, pulse sequences, contrast weightings, and field strengths. In addition to the anatomical imaging, ARDL is now compatible with DWI. We envision using the power behind our ARDL to expand the clinical utility of emerging breast DWI applications. For instance, high *b* value breast DWI may provide unique clinical insights; however, maintaining adequate signal to noise can be challenging for high *b* value acquisitions with conventional reconstruction. AIR Recon DL improves the SNR by removing noise that it does not alter the mean value of the parametric maps but reduces the standard deviation in measurements that it can be used with ADC and other parametric maps as well. Fig. 16.4 demonstrates conventional reconstruction versus AIR Recon DL reconstruction on the same raw data. Noise reduction is evident particularly away from the coil such as in chest wall area in diffusion images. Reduced noise in diffusion images also results

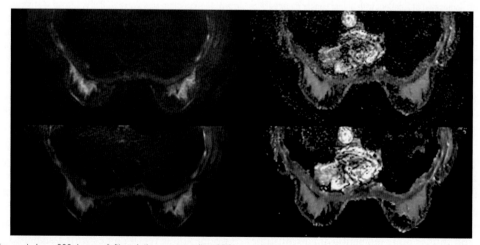

Fig. 16.4 (Top row) $b = 800$ image *(left)* and the corresponding ADC map *(right)*, $b = 0$ image not shown. (Bottom row) Same raw data was processed with AIR Recon DL. $b = 800$ image *(left)* and the corresponding ADC map *(right)*, $b = 0$ image not shown.

in cleaner ADC maps. AIR Recon DL is compatible with MAGiC DWI and the two features could be used synergistically to probe higher diffusion weightings, higher resolution imaging, and/or rapid acquisition.

At GE Healthcare, we are dedicated to improving lives in the moments that matter. Improving breast care continues to challenge us and motivate us as we seek to fully realize the power of breast MRI.

REFERENCES

1. Xu D, Maier JK, King KF, et al. Prospective and retrospective high order eddy current mitigation for diffusion weighted echo planar imaging. *Magn Reson Med.* 2013;70:1293–1305.
2. Fung M, Wu G, Estkowski L, et al. Realtime B_0 inhomogeneity correction in multi-station diffusion imaging [abstract]. In: Proceedings of the 23rd Annual Meeting of the International Society for Magnetic Resonance in Medicine; May 30–June 5, 2015; Toronto, Ontario, Canada. Berkeley (CA): ISMRM; 2015. Abstract #1606.
3. Holland D, Kuperman JM, Dale AM. Efficient correction of inhomogeneous static magnetic field-induced distortion in echo planar imaging. *Neuroimage.* 2010;50(1):175–183.
4. Zhu K, Dougherty RF, Wu H, et al. Hybrid-space SENSE reconstruction for simultaneous multi-slice MRI. *IEEE Trans Med Imaging.* 2016;35(8):1824–1836.
5. Reese TG, Heid O, Weisskoff RM, et al. Reduction of eddy-current induced distortion in diffusion MRI using a twice-refocused spin echo. *Magn Reson Med.* 2003;49:177–182.
6. Blackledge MD, Wilton B, Messiou C, et al. Computed diffusion weighted imaging (CDWI) for improving imaging contrast [abstract]. In: Proceedings of the 17th Annual Meeting of the International Society for Magnetic Resonance in Medicine; April 18–24, 2009; Honolulu, Hawaii, USA. Berkeley (CA): ISMRM; 2009. Abstract #4005.
7. Chen NK, Guidon A, Chang HC, et al. A robust multi-shot scan strategy for high-resolution diffusion weighted MRI enabled by multiplexed sensitivity encoding (MUSE). *Neuroimage.* 2013;72:41–47.
8. Gomori JM, Holland GA, Grossman RI, et al. Fat suppression by section-select gradient reversal on spin-echo MR imaging. Work in progress. *Radiology.* 1998;168(2):493–495.
9. Saritas EU, Cunningham CH, Lee JH, et al. DWI of the spinal cord with reduced FOV single-shot EPI. *Magn Reson Med.* 2008;60:468–473.
10. Lebel RM. Performance characterization of a novel deep learning-based MR image reconstruction pipeline. Preprint. Posted online August 14, 2020. arXiv:200806559.

Chapter 17

Breast DWI Techniques and Processing: The Philips Perspective

Johannes M. Peeters, PhD, Ilse Rubie, Jaladhar Neelavalli, PhD, and Liesbeth Geerts, PhD

Data Acquisition

ESSENTIAL ELEMENTS OF CALIBRATION (B_0 AND B_1)

Most breast diffusion scans are performed with fat suppression and an echo-planar imaging (EPI) readout. Both these elements have optimal performance with uniform B_0 (magnet) and B_1 (radiofrequency) fields. Homogeneity of these fields heavily depends on the patient body habitus and positioning of the breasts with respect to the magnet and the radio frequency (RF) transmit coil, especially at 3 T. At this field strength, patient specific RF shimming[1,2] realizes signal uniformity over both breasts as well as uniform fat suppression. Before the actual scan, a B_1 map is generated to optimize the RF transmission settings to realize a uniform transmit field. A similar strategy is used for image-based B_0 shimming for which a B_0 map is acquired before the diffusion-weighted imaging (DWI) scan. The acquisition of the B_0 map is integrated in the SmartSurvey scan that is the basis for automated, operator-independent planning of the scan geometry. In the B_0 map, segmentation is performed such that shimming is optimized over the breasts and axillae, the clinically relevant areas. This image-based B_0 shimming allows for optimal and reproducible fat suppression in bilateral breast magnetic resonance MRI.[3] In case there is focus on a single breast, a shim volume can be planned to optimize the shimming over the indicated location. The three features of patient body habitus, adaptive B_0 and B_1 shimming, and automated planning of scan geometries are bundled in the SmartExam Breast option, which allows for robust and reproducible B_0 shimming for optimal fat suppression and minimal EPI distortion, optimal B_1 shimming for signal uniformity, and reproducible planning.

Another important aspect for system calibration is the compensation for eddy currents, which arise due to switching gradients and lead to signal loss and distortion. Especially with strong diffusion encoding gradients, these effects can be significant. Eddy current effects are minimized by intrinsic design of the hardware and by preemphasis to compensate upfront for the expected deviations in gradient trajectories. Proper eddy current compensation allows us to use the Stejskal–Tanner type of diffusion encoding without the need for additional sequence compensations, such as twice-refocused diffusion encoding.[4]

ESSENTIAL ELEMENTS OF ACQUISITION AND RECONSTRUCTION

A DWI sequence consists of the following modules: diffusion encoding, fat suppression, readout, and reconstruction. It is possible to perform diffusion imaging without fat suppression, but the use of fat suppression is general practice and recommended in the guidelines.[5] Readout and reconstruction can be regarded as two separate modules, but as these are very much interdependent, we cover them together.

Diffusion Encoding

For the diffusion encoding, the monopolar Stejskal–Tanner encoding scheme is most commonly applied, which is also the default in Philips systems. The diffusion gradient strengths and timings are automatically optimized, considering the parameters in the protocol as set by the echo time (TE), field of view (FOV), and acquisition voxel sizes. With the "specialist option," the user can opt to set diffusion times and gradient timings manually, and to use a twice-refocused or a

A

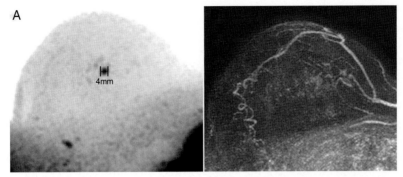

Fig. 17.1 **Examples of screening-detected lesion in a 67-year-old breast cancer screening participant.** (A) DWIBS (b = 1500 s/mm^2) MIP, displayed with black-white inversion, clearly depicts the focal lesion as an area of focal diffusion restriction. (B) First postcontrast subtraction MIP shows an area of subtle enhancement that is partially obscured by generally increased background enhancement. *DWIBS*, Diffusion-weighted whole-body imaging with background body signal suppression; *MIP*, minimum and maximum intensity projections. (Reproduced with permission from Bickelhaupt S, Laun FB, Tesdorff J, et al. Fast and noninvasive characterization of suspicious lesions detected at breast cancer x-ray screening: capability of diffusion-weighted MR imaging with MIPs. *Radiology*. 2016;278(3):689–697.)

more time-efficient asymmetrical non-Stejskal–Tanner encoding scheme. In the latter, dead times in the diffusion encoding module are avoided. This results in a shorter TE but introduces an off-center bias due to concomitant fields.[6]

For DWI, the diffusion encoding gradients are applied in three orthogonal directions, either along the imaging plane axes or via a vector optimized combination of the physical gradient axes independent of the slice orientation, to minimize TE (gradient overplus). An arbitrary number of b values can be chosen with a maximum b value of 25,000 s/mm^2. As the signal-to-noise ratio (SNR) decreases with increasing b value, the number of signal averages (NSA) can be set per b value to allow multiple averages to recover SNR for the higher b values while maintaining a low number of averages for the lower b values to gain efficiency.

For diffusion tensor imaging (DTI),[7,8] predefined schemes are available, as well as the possibility to define any user-defined scheme of b values and orientations of the diffusion encoding gradients.

Fat Suppression

Several fat-suppression techniques are available based on spectral and/or T1 relaxation differences between water and fat protons. Different types of inversion pulses like short tau inversion recovery (STIR), spectral presaturation with inversion recovery (SPIR), and spectral attenuated inversion recovery (SPAIR) exist, as well as slice selective gradient reversal (SSGR)[9] fat suppression, in which the slice encoding and refocusing gradient in a spin-echo acquisition have opposite polarity to avoid refocusing of excited fat protons. STIR exploits slice selective presaturation based on T1 relaxation. The combination of STIR with diffusion encoding, multiple averages, and inversion processing is referred to as DWIBS (Fig. 17.1; see Chapter 11).[10,11] SPIR[12] and SPAIR[5] are spectrally selective presaturation pulses. Looking at these techniques individually, STIR has the best fat suppression performance, but a penalty in SNR is paid, as the water signal will also be partially saturated. From the spectrally selective inversion pulses, SPIR allows time-efficient shorter inversion times and has far less RF power deposition in the body (lower specific absorption rate [SAR]), as the inversion pulse is not of adiabatic nature, and a lower flip angle is used compared with SPAIR pulses. This comes at the cost of sensitivity to B$_1$ nonuniformity. The best fat-suppression performance is realized when the different technologies are combined. The system allows to combine STIR, SPIR or SPAIR, and SSGR. From sequence optimization perspective, SSGR can easily be added to the inversion techniques, as it does not affect optimal sequence timings. On the other hand, combining STIR and SPIR/SPAIR needs careful planning of the inversion and repetition times with respect to steady state such that optimal fat saturation is realized.

Readout and Reconstruction

Single-shot spin-echo EPI is the workhorse for DWI, as it is a very time-efficient readout strategy for the generally long acquisition nature of diffusion scans. The EPI readout train can be reduced with the acceleration techniques SENSE (Sensitivity Encoding)[13] or Compressed SENSE.[14] A shorter readout train is beneficial, as it reduces (1) the TE and thus minimizes T2 shine-through and signal loss due to T2 decay and (2) the distortion related to B_0 inhomogeneity. Of all parallel imaging techniques, SENSE is the most SNR efficient, allowing the use of maximal reduction factor with respect to the geometrical capabilities of the coil. Compressed SENSE adds additional reduction capabilities by using sparsity of the image data to remove g-factor-related noise.[15] Minimizing the EPI train length with these acceleration techniques therefore improves image quality but does not lead to a shorter scan time, as it does not affect the minimally required repetition time (TR). MultiBand SENSE (Fig. 17.2),[16] in which multiple slices are excited simultaneously, is designed to reduce scan time. This reduction is especially useful for long scans with multiple averages, *b* values, and/or directions, such as DTI

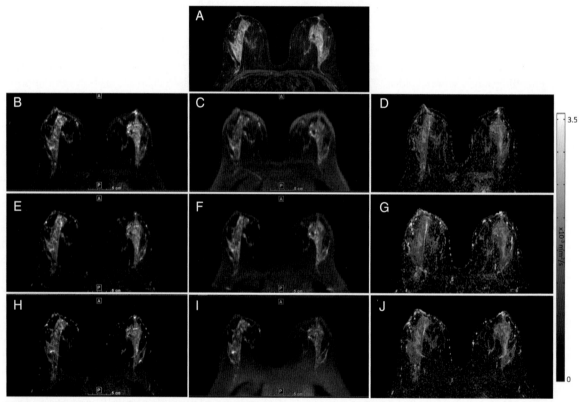

Fig. 17.2 MultiBand breast DW MRI technique implemented to achieve higher spatial resolution. Shown are representative images in a 35-year-old woman undergoing 3T MRI for preoperative staging of recently diagnosed ductal carcinoma in situ (not visualized) comparing standard single-shot EPI DWI with voxel size 1.8 × 1.8 mm and slice thickness of 4 mm, MultiBand single shot EPI DWI with the same voxel size and slice thickness and high resolution MultiBand single shot EPI DWI with voxel size 1.2 × 1.2 mm and slice thickness of 3 mm. (A) reference T2-weighted mDixon TSE; (B) standard DWI, $b = 0$ s/mm²; (C) standard DWI, $b = 800$ s/mm²; (D) standard DWI ADC; (E) MultiBand DWI, $b = 0$ s/mm²; (F) MultiBand DWI, $b = 800$ s/mm²; (G) MultiBand DWI ADC; (H) high-resolution MultiBand DWI, $b = 0$ s/mm²; (I) high-resolution MultiBand DWI, $b = 800$ s/mm²; and (J) high resolution MultiBand DWI ADC. Incorporating MultiBand facilitates increasing spatial resolution and acquiring a greater number of thinner slices (to maintain coverage) versus standard DW MRI without extending scan time. *ADC,* Apparent diffusion coefficient; *DW MRI,* diffusion-weighted MRI; *DWI,* diffusion-weighted imaging; *EPI,* echo-planar imaging; *TSE,* turbo spin echo. (Courtesy Dr. Savannah Partridge, University of Washington, Seattle, WA).

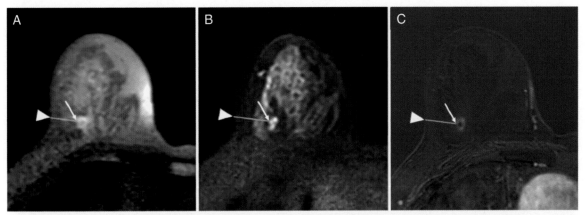

Fig. 17.3 A 60-year-old woman diagnosed with right-invasive ductal carcinoma by lumpectomy. The methods used to evaluate geometrical distortion in TSE-DWI and EPI-DWI. Two matching anatomical sites were used: the site of the lesion closest to the skin *(arrows)* and the site of the skin closest to the lesion *(arrowheads)*. (A) The distance between the sites was calculated as Distance$_{TSE}$ in images of TSE-DWI (b = 850 s/mm^2), (B) Distance$_{EPI}$ in those of EPI-DWI (b = 850 s/mm^2), and (C) Distance$_{DCE-MRI}$ in those of DCE-MR. In this case, Distance$_{TSE}$, Distance$_{EPI}$, and Distance$_{DCE-MRI}$ were 19.1, 25.3, and 19.5 mm, respectively. *DCE-MR*, Dynamic contrast-enhanced magnetic resonance; *EPI-DWI*, echo-planar imaging diffusion-weighted imaging (DWI); *TSE-DWI*, turbo spin echo DWI. (Reproduced with permission from Mori N, Mugikura S, Miyashita M, et al. Turbo spin-echo diffusion-weighted imaging compared with single-shot echo-planar diffusion-weighted imaging: image quality and diagnostic performance when differentiating between ductal carcinoma in situ and invasive ductal carcinoma. *Magn Reson Med Sci.* 2021;20(1):60–68.)

acquisitions and scans used for intravoxel incoherent motion (IVIM) or kurtosis processing. Applicable acceleration factors of SENSE, Compressed SENSE, and MultiBand SENSE increase with the number of receiver elements of the coil being used. Depending on the type of scanner, 2-, 4-, 7-, or 16-channel breast coils are available.

One of the downsides of EPI is the sensitivity for B$_0$-related distortion, which can be completely overcome with a turbo spin-echo (TSE) readout (Fig. 17.3).[17] In TSE DWI, SENSE or Compressed SENSE are used to realize complete coverage of the breast with a decent resolution. For higher resolutions, MultiVane XD facilitates the use of a multishot approach, in which the blade orientation of each TSE shot is rotated to provide motion robustness. The phase interleaved multishot EPI approach, image reconstruction using image-space sampling functions (IRIS),[18,19] is a good compromise between the scan time efficiency of single-shot EPI and the distortion-free properties of a TSE readout. In such a phase-interleaved approach, as the EPI train length decreases proportionally with an increasing number of shots, distortion too is reduced to

the same extent. When distortion is not a limiting factor, IRIS can be used to enhance the resolution, as illustrated in Fig. 17.4. Partial Fourier in phase-encoding direction (Halfscan) can be applied to the EPI and TSE readout types to reduce TE or the TSE train length.

USER INTERFACE

In the user interface, the user can provide the intended TE and geometrical properties like FOV, orientation and acquisition, and reconstruction voxel size. Next to numerical values, the TE can also be set to shortest, by which the system automatically generates the minimal echo time achievable given the geometrical input (FOV, slice orientation, etc.), hardware capabilities, and physiological limitations such as peripheral nerve stimulation limits. In the sequence information page, the resulting TE is provided. This allows for easy sequence optimization, for instance when geometrical updates are required for adapting to patient specific body habitus.

For EPI readouts, reconstruction contains automatic corrections to eliminate EPI ghosting due to gradient delays. Reconstruction also has the optional low

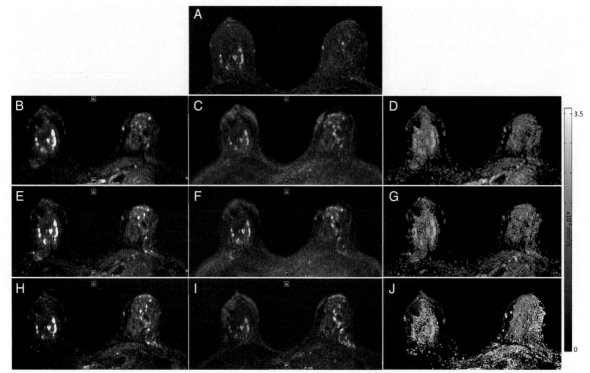

Fig. 17.4 **IRIS phase interleaved multishot EPI breast DWI to achieve higher spatial resolution with low distortion.** Shown are representative images in a 52-year-old woman undergoing 3 T MRI for high-risk screening, including standard single-shot EPI DWI with voxel size 1.8 × 1.8 mm, high-resolution single-shot EPI DWI with voxel size 1.2 × 1.2 × 4 mm, and dual shot IRIS DWI with voxel size 1.2 × 1.2 mm. All have a slice thickness of 4 mm. (A) reference T2-weighted mDixon TSE; (B) standard single-shot DWI, b = 0 s/mm²; (C) standard single-shot DWI, b = 800 s/mm²; (D) standard single-shot DWI ADC; (E) high-resolution single-shot DWI, b = 0 s/mm²; (F) high-resolution single-shot DWI, b = 800 s/mm²; (G) high-resolution single-shot DWI ADC; (H) IRIS, b = 0 s/mm²; (I) IRIS, b = 800 s/mm²; and (J) IRIS ADC. *ADC*, Apparent diffusion coefficient; *DWI*, diffusion-weighted imaging; *EPI*, echo-planar imaging; *IRIS*, image reconstruction using image-space sampling functions. (Courtesy Dr. Savannah Partridge, University of Washington, Seattle, WA.)

variance apparent diffusion coefficient (ADC) functionality, a pixel-wise intensity correction[20] to remove off-center biases in ADC maps due to gradient nonlinearity.

Essential Elements of Postprocessing

The postprocessing of diffusion data can serve two different goals: enhanced lesion visualization and extraction of quantitative information.

ENHANCED VISUALIZATION

Basic inline processing steps like subtraction, multiplanar reformat (MPR), volume renderings, minimum and maximum intensity projections, and

inversion, can be performed. Visualization using the combination of subtraction and inversion has proven to be useful for diffusion-weighted whole-body imaging with background body signal suppression (DWIBS).[21] Also, the computation of enhanced apparent diffusion coefficient (eADC), computed DWI (cDWI),[22,23] and fibertracking options are available. eADC allows to generate diffusion images of the acquired *b* value, in which the T2-decay and proton density weighting are removed, to create a purely diffusion-weighted image contrast. cDWI (Fig. 17.5) allows to generate synthetic high *b* value diffusion-weighted images from acquired low *b* value data. For DTI acquisitions, fibertracking can

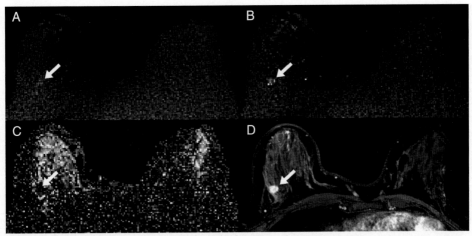

Fig. 17.5 Axial DWIs of a 45-year-old woman with IDC (1 cm and histological grade I) for (A) an acquired *b* value of 1500 s/mm^2 (A-b-1500) and (B) a cDWI *b* value of 1500 s/mm^2 (C-b-1500). Note the IDC lesion *(arrow)* in her right breast, which was missed by all three readers in A-b-1500, but was well seen in C-b-1500. All readers rated this as 4 in C-b-1500. (C) ADC map showed a mass with low ADC value. (D) Axial DCE image showed an irregular enhancing mass in the right breast in correlating area. *ADC,* Apparent diffusion coefficient; *cDWI,* computed diffusion-weighted imaging; *DCE,* dynamic contrast-enhanced; *DWI,* diffusion-weighted imaging; *IDC,* invasive ductal carcinoma. (Reproduced with permission from Park JH, Yun B, Jang M, et al. Comparison of the diagnostic performance of synthetic versus acquired high b value (1500 s/mm^2) diffusion-weighted MRI in women with breast cancers. *J Magn Reson Imaging.* 2019;49(3):857–863.)

be used to visualize the dominant diffusion directions. eADC, cDWI, and fibertracking are assuming monoexponential signal decay under diffusion encoding. Hence one should keep in mind that the presence of non-Gaussian diffusion will not be reflected in the eADC or cDWI maps, which may result in interpretation differences (see Chapter 12).

QUANTITATIVE INFORMATION

ADC is the best-known quantitative diffusion parameter and is derived via pixel-wise fitting of a monoexponential decay. With the inline DWI processing package, a retrospective selection of *b* values to be included in the fit can be made, such that low or high *b* values can be excluded, to only fit in the Gaussian diffusion regime. Background segmentation can be enabled to avoid overwhelming intensities in the ADC maps.

Alternative models to the monoexponential model, like biexponential, simplified IVIM, kurtosis, and combinations of these, are available in the advanced diffusion analysis (ADA) package. These models provide perfusion fraction (f), pseudo diffusivity (D*), diffusivity (D), and kurtosis maps.

Depending on the input *b* values, an applicable model can be chosen and a "goodness of fit" map indicates the fitting quality of the selected model. An example of monoexponential plus kurtosis fitting is provided in Fig. 17.6.

On top of the already mentioned parametric maps, the DTI processing packages can provide fractional anisotropy, color direction, axial diffusivity, and radial diffusivity maps.

Future Aspects

Over the last few decades, DWI has undergone major steps as a result of increasing field strength, the introduction of multichannel receiver coils, parallel imaging acquisition and reconstruction, improved gradient performance and calibration, and shimming capabilities. With ever-increasing gradient performance, more advanced diffusion encoding strategies will become feasible. Deep learning may be integrated in the multichannel reconstruction framework to allow for a higher acceleration factor to shorten scan times, reduce distortion, and improve quantitative analysis by minimizing the impact of image noise.

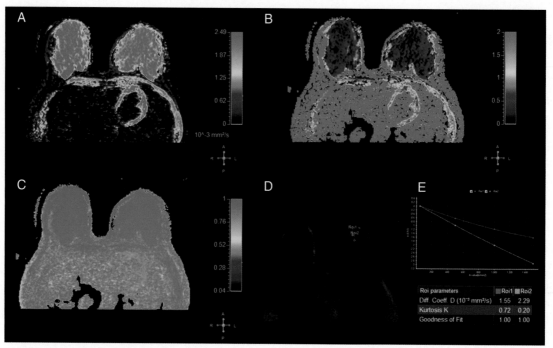

Fig. 17.6 **Example of monoexponential plus kurtosis fitting with the advance diffusion analysis package.** (A) Diffusion coefficient map, (B) kurtosis map, (C) goodness-of-fit map, (D) b = 1500 s/mm^2 DWI image, and (E) fitting curves for regions of interest (ROIs) in (D) with respective diffusion coefficient, kurtosis, and goodness-of-fit values for these ROIs. (Courtesy Dr. Nora Voormolen, Leiden University Medical Center, Leiden, The Netherlands.)

REFERENCES

1. Rahbar H, Partridge SC, Demartini WB, et al. Improved B$_1$ homogeneity of 3 tesla breast MRI using dual-source parallel radiofrequency excitation. *J Magn Reson Imaging.* 2012;35(5):1222–1226.
2. Trop I, Gilbert G, Ivancevic MK, et al. Breast MR imaging at 3 T with dual-source radiofrequency transmission offers superior B$_1$ homogeneity: an intraindividual comparison with breast MR imaging at 1.5 T. *Radiology.* 2013;267(2):602–608.
3. Ishizaka K, Kato F, Terae S, et al. Bilateral breast MRI by use of dual-source parallel radiofrequency excitation and image-based shimming at 3 tesla: improvement in homogeneity on fat-suppression imaging. *Radiol Phys Technol.* 2015;8(1):4–12.
4. Geerts L, Lippe R, Nijenhuis M. How to minimize eddy current related distortion in DTI? *Proceedings of OHBM.* 2015:1755.
5. Baltzer P, Mann RM, Iima M, et al; EUSOBI international Breast Diffusion-Weighted Imaging Working Group. Diffusion-weighted imaging of the breast: a consensus and mission statement from the EUSOBI International Breast Diffusion-Weighted Imaging Working Group. *Eur Radiol.* 2020;30(3):1436–1450.
6. Szczepankiewicz F, Westin CF, Nilsson M. Maxwell-compensated design of asymmetric gradient waveforms for tensor-valued diffusion encoding. *Magn Reson Med.* 2019;82(4):1424–1437.
7. Furman-Haran E, Nissan N, Ricart-Selma V, et al. Quantitative evaluation of breast cancer response to neoadjuvant chemotherapy by diffusion tensor imaging: initial results. *J Magn Reson Imaging.* 2018;47(4):1080–1090.
8. Luo J, Hippe DS, Rahbar H, et al. Diffusion tensor imaging for characterizing tumor microstructure and improving diagnostic performance on breast MRI: a prospective observational study. *Breast Cancer Res.* 2019;21(1):102.
9. Kwee TC, Takahara T, Vermoolen MA, et al. Whole-body diffusion-weighted imaging for staging malignant lymphoma in children. *Pediatr Radiol.* 2010;40(10):1592–1602.
10. Takahara T, Imai Y, Yamashita T, et al. Diffusion weighted whole body imaging with background body signal suppression (DWIBS): technical improvement using free breathing, STIR and high resolution 3D display. *Radiat Med.* 2004;22(4):275–282.
11. Stadlbauer A, Bernt R, Gruber S, et al. Diffusion-weighted MR imaging with background body signal suppression (DWIBS) for the diagnosis of malignant and benign breast lesions. *Eur Radiol.* 2009;19(10):2349–2356.
12. Merchant TE, Thelissen GR, Kievit HC, et al. Breast disease evaluation with fat-suppressed magnetic resonance imaging. *Magn Reson Imaging.* 1992;10(3):335–340.
13. Bammer R, Keeling SL, Augustin M, et al. Improved diffusion-weighted single-shot echo-planar imaging (EPI) in stroke using sensitivity encoding (SENSE). *Magn Reson Med.* 2001;46(3):548–554.
14. Sprenger P, Morita K, Nakaura T, et al. Body diffusion MR imaging with compressed SENSE based on single-shot EPI at 3 T and 1.5 T: technical feasibility and initial clinical experience. *Proceedings of ISMRM.* 2020:2611.

15. Pruessmann KP, Weiger M, Scheidegger MB, Boesiger P. SENSE: sensitivity encoding for fast MRI. *Magn Reson Med.* 1999 Nov;42(5):952-62. PMID: 10542355.

16. DelPriore MR, Biswas D, Hippe DS, et al. Breast cancer conspicuity on computed versus acquired high *b* value diffusion-weighted MRI. *Acad Radiol.* 2021;28(8):1108–1117.

17. Mori N, Mugikura S, Miyashita M, et al. Turbo spin-echo diffusion-weighted imaging compared with single-shot echo-planar diffusion-weighted imaging: image quality and diagnostic performance when differentiating between ductal carcinoma in situ and invasive ductal carcinoma. *Magn Reson Med Sci.* 2021;20(1):60–68.

18. Jeong HK, Gore JC, Anderson AW. High-resolution human diffusion tensor imaging using 2-D navigated multishot SENSE EPI at 7 T. *Magn Reson Med.* 2013;69(3):793–802.

19. Rahbar H, Kitch AE, Peeters H, et al. High resolution breast diffusion weighted imaging using 2-D navigated multi-shot SENSE EPI with image reconstruction using image-space sampling function (IRIS) at 3T. *Proceedings of ISMRM.* 2017:4923.

20. Malyarenko DI, Newitt DC, Amouzandeh G, et al. Retrospective correction of ADC for gradient nonlinearity errors in multi-center breast DWI trials: ACRIN6698 Multiplatform Feasibility Study. *Tomography.* 2020;6(2):86–92.

21. Bickelhaupt S, Laun FB, Tesdorff J, et al. Fast and noninvasive characterization of suspicious lesions detected at breast cancer x-ray screening: capability of diffusion-weighted MR imaging with MIPs. *Radiology.* 2016;278(3):689–697.

22. Park JH, Yun B, Jang M, et al. Comparison of the diagnostic performance of synthetic versus acquired high *b* value (1500 s/mm^2) diffusion-weighted MRI in women with breast cancers. *J Magn Reson Imaging.* 2019;49(3):857–863.

23. Tamura T, Takasu M, Higaki T, et al. How to improve the conspicuity of breast tumors on computed high *b* value diffusion-weighted imaging. *Magn Reson Med Sci.* 2019;18(2):119–125.

Diffusion-Weighted Imaging (DWI) for Breast Lesion Characterization: The Olea Medical Perspective and the Utilization of Olea Sphere Software

Margarita Arango-Lievano, PhD, Timothé Boutelier, PhD, Lucile Brun, Ms, Brianna Bucciarelli, MSc, Sophie Campana, PhD, Adam J. Davis, MD, Florence Feret, MRT, Aurélia Hermoso, and Anca Mitulescu, PhD

The Importance of Postprocessing and Data Analysis for Breast Diffusion Weighted Imaging

The role of magnetic resonance imaging (MRI) in breast cancer diagnosis and management is evolving as a supplemental screening tool for high-risk populations.[1] Nowadays, a myriad of magnetic resonance (MR) sequences is applicable to breast imaging, with common protocol consisting in T1-weighted contrast-enhanced and T2-weighted imaging. Dynamic contrast-enhanced (DCE) MRI is highly sensitive, improving detection compared with mammography alone[1] and approaching, with automation techniques, a sensitivity of 89% for all breast cancers.[2] However, specificity remains an issue. Though not yet generalized in the clinical practice, diffusion-weighted imaging (DWI) could improve the diagnostic specificity of DCE (i.e., decrease the false positive rate and consequently reduce the number of unnecessary biopsies). If different MRI sequences offer specific information on lesion morphology and physiology, they could, when combined, guide the operator toward improved lesion identification and characterization. However, the widespread use of breast DWI is limited by its high sensitivity factors that diminish image quality (e.g., residual eddy-currents- and susceptibility-induced distortions). Newer DWI sequences are emerging in complement of standard spin-echo echo-planar DWI, such as readout segmented (RS), multishot, simultaneous multislice (SMS), and zoomed two-dimensional spatially selective radiofrequency (2D RF) excitation pulses, to reduce those effects.[3,4] Yet, there is very little agreement on the optimal protocol to acquire data and even less on the analysis method to characterize the malignant nature of a breast lesion, tumor aggressiveness, or grade.[5,6]

This lack of consensus in the clinical community leaves the vendor uncertain as to what characteristics in their software product would be the most applicable for the market. In an effort to address these discrepancies that affect clinicians and vendors alike, the European Society of Breast Imaging (EUSOBI) recently published the first guidelines regarding DWI breast parameters from the consensus of an international group of experts. They include specifications for data acquisition: axial acquisition with at least two b values of 0 and 800 s/mm^2, fat saturation, and a minimal spatial resolution of 2 × 2 mm. Guidelines also recommend to compute standard apparent diffusion coefficient (ADC) maps from these raw diffusion images. Yet there is little information on data analysis besides region-of-interest (ROI) positioning. The determination of the possible malignant nature of a specific lesion based on DWI relies on a combination of observations and metrics based on b-800, ADC maps, and a range of ADC values of the ROI.[7]

Diffusion imaging covers a broad spectrum of techniques, from the mapping of apparent diffusion coefficient (ADC) values using the mono-exponential model to advanced diffusion models such as Intravoxel incoherent motion (IVIM) and Diffusion Kurtosis imaging (DKI) (see Chapters 1 and 8) or diffusion tensor imaging (DTI) (see Chapter 9)

In this chapter, we describe the technical options currently available in the Olea Medical portfolio for the advanced postprocessing of diffusion imaging, compatible with clinical practice expectations in terms of time-effectiveness and clinical impact, in breast lesion assessment.

Breast Diffusion Image Pre- and Postprocessing in Olea Sphere

PREPROCESSING

Background Extraction

In an effort to optimize calculation time and reduce background noise, Olea Sphere automatically applies a background segmentation based on a histogram analysis of the raw diffusion images. The user can manually adjust the thresholds and visualize the filtering process on the displayed series.

Noise Reduction

If several acquisitions of the same b value are made in several orientations, Olea Sphere averages the data using the geometrical mean. This operation improves the signal-to-noise ratio (SNR) for isotropic acquisitions.

Motion Correction

To cancel moderate patient motion during image acquisition, Olea Sphere includes a 2D motion correction algorithm that achieves in-plane rigid coregistration of all raw images (b values) of a given slice to the first acquired image, usually the b0 acquisition. The coregistration minimizes the sum of squares differences between the reference and the target images.

Geometrical Distortion Correction on DTI Series

Due to the high gradient amplitudes and short echo time (TE) used during acquisition, DTI imaging is particularly prone to eddy-currents distortions. Motion artifacts due to the patient's movement during the examination can also affect estimation of diffusion parameters. Although most of these artifacts have been reduced by manufacturers with active shielding of the gradient coils and adjustments on the acquisition protocols, diffusion postprocessing software must reduce the remnant artifacts. In Olea Sphere, all diffusion volumes are aligned to the b0 volume using a 12-degrees-of-freedom affine transformation. The algorithm takes into account translation, rotation, and scaling due to movements as well as shearing due to eddy currents.

MODEL PARAMETER ESTIMATES

Spectrum of Techniques

Diffusion imaging covers a broad spectrum of techniques implemented within Olea Sphere (Fig. 18.1), from the mapping of ADC values using the monoexponential model (see Chapter 1) to advanced diffusion models such as IVIM, DKI (see Chapter 8), and DTI (see Chapter 9), along with the capability of generating computed b values if needed.

DWI is quantified by computing the ADC (Fig. 18.2A). Previous studies have shown that ADC values vary between malignant and benign breast lesions.[8,9] However, an overlap may occur, as benign breast changes can occasionally mimic malignancy. Suspicious lesions are typically hyperintense on DWI images with corresponding low ADC values, indicating restricted diffusion and hypercellularity (Fig. 18.3).

Although a simplistic ADC model may be sufficient for some clinical purposes, emerging data suggest that some clinically relevant findings may be found in more complex models. In particular, two advanced models are more adapted to describe the non-Gaussian diffusivity in the tissue: IVIM[10,11] and DKI.[12]

IVIM (Fig. 18.2B) provides separate quantitative measures of D (tissue diffusion coefficient) for cellularity, f (perfusion fraction) and D* (tissue perfusion related coefficient) for vascularity, which are helpful biomarkers for differentiating benign from malignant breast lesions (see Fig. 18.3).[13] However, the acquisition is longer than for conventional DWI because at least four b values are required for postprocessing in Olea Sphere, including at least two b values between 0 and $200\,s/mm^2$ and one higher than $200\,s/mm^2$.

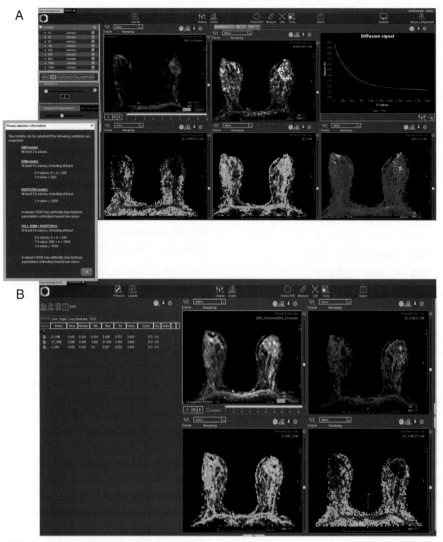

Fig. 18.1 Diffusion postprocessing in Olea Sphere. (A) In the left panel, all available *b* values are displayed with the diffusion models that can be applied *(blue rectangle)*; information is provided on *b* values required for each model *(blue rectangle inset)*. Background segmentation can be manually adjusted *(pink rectangle)*. The top left panel displays the preprocessed diffusion images, where each phase corresponds to a *b* value. The top middle panel can be adjusted to display any computed or raw image - here a SNR map. Finally, the top right panel displays the raw *(blue)* and fitted *(red)* diffusion signal over all *b* values. The bottom panels display rainbow parametric maps corresponding to D*, f, and D metrics, respectively from left to right. (B) The picture shows an example of quantitative measures performed on diffusion parametric maps in Olea Sphere. VOIs can be selected on any image series and propagated to all maps *(pink VOI)*. On the left panel are displayed the mean, median, min, max, SD, and volume of the VOI for each parametric map – D, D*, and f in this case. *SD*, Standard deviation; *SNR*, signal-to-noise ratio; *VOI*, volume of interest.

DKI is a clinically feasible process that requires minor changes in data acquisition compared with conventional monoexponential DWI. This model is based on the acquisition of *b* values higher than 1000 s/mm² to observe the restricted diffusion in the tissue. To obtain a mean kurtosis value, a fast DKI acquisition (1–2 minutes) can be performed.[14] The D parameter representing the Gaussian diffusion and the K kurtosis representing the non-Gaussian diffusion can be both estimated with the model (Fig. 18.2C). DKI has been demonstrated

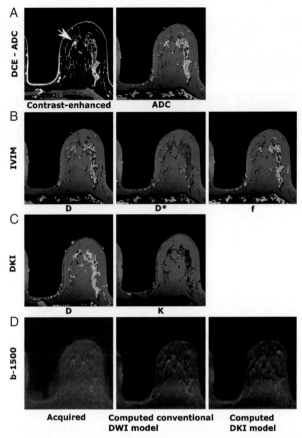

Fig. 18.2 Example of breast diffusion maps and computed *b* values generated by Olea Sphere. Diffusion maps are overlaid on T2-w images. (A) Breast lesion visible on contrast-enhanced imaging (white arrow) and ADC. (B) D, D*, and f maps generated with the IVIM model. (C) D and K maps generated with the DKI model. (D) Example of native *b*-1500 and computed *b*-1500 with both conventional DWI and DKI models. Computed *b* values display better image quality, with higher resolution and lower noise. *ADC*, Apparent diffusion coefficient; *DKI*, diffusion kurtosis imaging; *DWI*, diffusion-weighted imaging; *IVIM*, intravoxel incoherent motion. (Courtesy Dr. Virgil Ionescu, Monza Metropolitan Hospital, Romania.)

as an efficient method to discriminate and characterize breast lesions in several studies (see Fig. 18.3).[15–17]

DTI requires measuring diffusion along at least six different directions, with measurements achieved for each nonzero *b* value. In Olea Sphere, different metrics such as mean diffusivity (MD), axial and radial diffusivities (AD and RD), and fractional anisotropy (FA) can be derived. DTI models have been optimized for brain imaging, but their application to breast imaging is still in progress.

High *b* values, either acquired or calculated, are furthermore of interest for breast lesion characterization,[18] and Olea Sphere "multi-b" capability offers the possibility of computing images with new *b* values to facilitate the visualization of breast lesions (Fig. 18.2D).

The Bayesian Method in Diffusion Imaging: Technical Overview

A noteworthy implementation within Olea Medical software is the use of a Bayesian method to estimate the diffusion coefficients, ameliorating their high sensitivity to noise and sampling. Unlike the least-squares algorithm, the Bayesian approach yields more robust parameter estimates (i.e., calculated values that are more stable and more accurate). Rather than minimizing a residual error, the Bayesian method estimates the uncertainty of each parameter separately, with a narrow probability density function indicating a well-resolved value.[19] The Bayesian method relies on the computation of the joint posterior probability of the values of the parameters to be estimated (e.g., ADC,

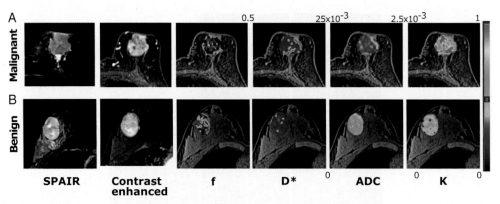

Fig. 18.3 Example of diffusion maps of malignant and benign breast lesions generated by Olea Sphere. Maps are overlaid on T1-w images. (A) A 81-year-old woman, breast cancer (luminal B type) with noncircumscribed mass in the breast, showing relatively low f and ADC values and high K kurtosis. (B) A 22-year-old woman, fibroadenoma. The f value is high, mainly on the periphery of the tumor. Tumoral tissue is associated with high ADC and low K. All analyses were performed with the DKI model. Color bars are rainbow, with max/min values displayed and same scale for both cases. *ADC,* Apparent diffusion coefficient; *DKI,* diffusion kurtosis imaging. (Courtesy Dr. Mami Iima, Kyoto University, Japan.)

D*, f or K; see Chapter 8) from the noisy data, assuming general prior knowledge about the parameters statistics in the organ under study. The accuracy on the parameters depends on the noise of the images but also on the tuning of the computation algorithm (number of sampling points, ranges for the estimated parameters).

The ranges and the number of sampling points can be configured by the user. In Olea Sphere, default values have been chosen to find the best compromise between precision and computation time.

Comparison of the Bayesian Method With Conventional Methods

Numerical simulation was used to validate the Bayesian estimation method and compare its performance to the classical nonlinear least-squares estimation method. Simulated data sets with different b values and noise levels were considered. The simulated signal was then embedded into DICOM files to be analyzed with Olea Sphere. Next, the estimated parameter maps were compared with the ground truth used to generate the numerical phantoms. This analysis allowed to compute the precision and accuracy of a given estimation method and to define the acquisition requirement in terms of number and repartition of b values, as well as noise to ensure reliable parameter estimation.

The phantom used to validate our algorithm was generated with D = (0.5, 1.0, 1.5, 2.0, 2.5) $\times$ 10^{-3}

mm²/s; D* = (10, 15, 20, 25, 30) $\times$ 10^{-3} mm²/s; f = (0, 5, 10, 15, 20)%; and K = (0, 0.25, 0.50, 0.75, 1.0, 1.25, 1.50). The signal was generated for b value = (0, 150, 800, 1000, 1500, 2000) s/mm² and an SNR of 25, 50, 100 and 200. The analysis of the phantom results demonstrated the good performance of the Bayesian method compared with the classical nonlinear least-squares method, with an improved accuracy and precision, even at low SNR (Fig. 18.4).

In a clinical context, comparison of conventional and Bayesian method for ADC calculation from the same acquisitions (b value = [0, 150, 800, 1000, 1500, 2000] s/mm²) shows a sharper estimation within the range of ADC values with the Bayesian method (see Fig. 18.4). Furthermore, a recent study demonstrated higher accuracy of IVIM parameter estimation with the Bayesian method, leading to an improved breast cancer lesion classification.[20]

Future Directions

Relatively recent studies suggested that the mammary ductal network, along with surrounding stroma, could result in diffusion anisotropy in healthy fibroglandular tissue, and this organization may be disrupted by neoplastic tissue.[21,22] Therefore DTI may be an interesting and promising option in breast lesion characterization, offering the possibility to collect quantitative information on the directional diffusivity of water molecules in biological tissues.[23]

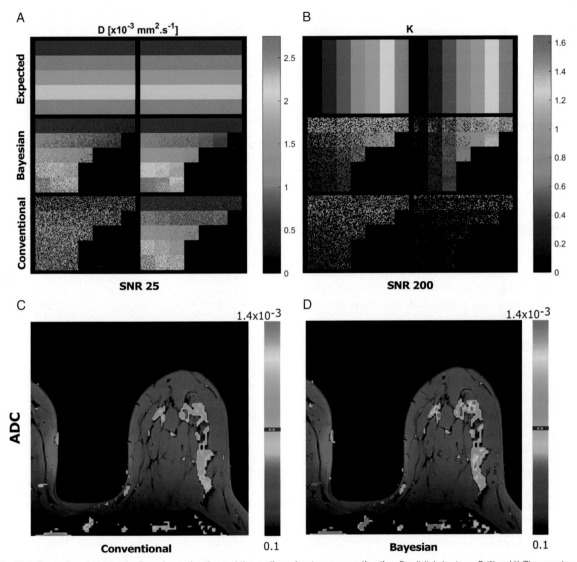

Fig. 18.4 **Comparison between the Bayesian estimation and the nonlinear least-squares estimation.** For digital phantoms, D (A) and K (B) parameters, at SNR = 25 and SNR = 200. The top row is the expected parameter map, the middle row is the estimated parameter map with the Bayesian method, and the bottom row is the estimated parameter map with the conventional estimation method. The phantom was generated with D = (0.5, 1.0, 1.5, 2.0, 2.5) × 10⁻³ mm²/s and K = (0, 0.25, 0.50, 0.75, 1.0, 1.25, 1.50). The signal was generated for b value = (0, 150, 800, 1000, 1500, 2000) s/mm² and an SNR of 25 and 200. ADC estimation with conventional (C) and Bayesian (D) methods on breast examinations. Color bars represent ADC values expressed in mm²/s. A sharper estimation within the range of the ADC values can be observed with the Bayesian method. *ADC,* Apparent diffusion coefficient; *SNR,* signal-to-noise ratio.

Olea Medical provides vendor-neutral advanced solutions for the postprocessing of MR images within Olea Sphere software. breastscape is a dedicated solution for breast MRI that includes modules to assist diagnosis, follow-up, and interventional planning. breastscape provides multiparametric maps, subtraction, lesion segmentation, and classification using the last edition of the Breast Imaging Reporting and Data System (BI-RADS) lexicon from the American College of Radiology, assisting radiologists with dedicated review steps, including follow-up examinations.

breastscape, combined with diffusion and permeability, relaxometry, and texture plug-ins, offers a large spectrum of metrics for breast lesion characterization and/or grading for basic and advanced assessment. However, until clinical consensus has been reached regarding the relevance of these metrics for fast and reliable diagnosis, vendors can only support the clinicians by offering access to multiparametric analysis. It is in the hands of the medical community to create consensus—or at least uniformity. Commercial postprocessing products such as Olea Sphere and breastscape can markedly facilitate the standardization process of acquisition protocols and workflows in breast imaging for the benefit of the physician and, most importantly, the patient.

Acknowledgments

The authors wish to thank Dr. Mami Iima, MD, PhD, Kyoto University, Japan, and Dr. Virgil Ionescu, MD, PhD, Monza Metropolitan Hospital, Romania, for their support with image acquisition, advanced postprocessing, and clinical expertise.

REFERENCES

1. Warner E, Messersmith H, Causer P, Eisen A, Shumak R, Plewes D. Systematic review: using magnetic resonance imaging to screen women at high risk for breast cancer. *Ann Intern Med.* 2008;148(9):671–679.
2. Gubern-Mérida A, Martí R, Melendez J, et al. Automated localization of breast cancer in DCE-MRI. *Med Image Anal.* 2015;20(1):265–274.
3. Partridge SC, Nissan N, Rahbar H, Kitsch AE, Sigmund EE. Diffusion-weighted breast MRI: clinical applications and emerging techniques. *J Magn Reson Imaging.* 2017;45(2):337–355.
4. McKay JA, Church AL, Rubin N, et al. A comparison of methods for high-spatial-resolution diffusion-weighted imaging in breast MRI. *Radiology.* 2020;297(2):304–312.
5. Clauser P, Mann R, Athanasiou A, et al. A survey by the European Society of Breast Imaging on the utilisation of breast MRI in clinical practice. *Eur Radiol.* 2018;28(5):1909–1918.
6. Romeo V, Cuocolo R, Liuzzi R, et al. Preliminary results of a simplified breast MRI protocol to characterize breast lesions: comparison with a full diagnostic protocol and a review of the current literature. *Acad Radiol.* 2017;24(11):1387–1394.
7. Baltzer P, Mann RM, Iima M, et al. Diffusion-weighted imaging of the breast—a consensus and mission statement from the EUSOBI International Breast Diffusion-Weighted Imaging working group. *Eur Radiol.* 2020;30(3):1436–1450.
8. Chen X, Li WL, Zhang YL, Wu Q, Guo YM, Bai ZL. Meta-analysis of quantitative diffusion-weighted MR imaging in the differential diagnosis of breast lesions. *BMC Cancer.* 2010;10:693.
9. Shi R-Y, Yao Q-Y, Wu L-M, Xu J-R. Breast lesions: diagnosis using diffusion weighted imaging at 1.5T and 3.0T—systematic review and meta-analysis. *Clin Breast Cancer.* 2018;18(3):e305–e320.
10. Yablonskiy DA, Sukstanskii AL. Theoretical models of the diffusion weighted MR signal. *NMR Biomed.* 2010;23(7):661–681.
11. Niendorf T, Dijkhuizen RM, Norris DG, Van Lookeren Campagne M, Nicolay K. Biexponential diffusion attenuation in various states of brain tissue: implications for diffusion-weighted imaging. *Magn Reson Med.* 1996;36(6):847–857.
12. Jensen JH, Helpern JA. MRI quantification of non-Gaussian water diffusion by kurtosis analysis. *NMR Biomed.* 2010;23(7):698–710.
13. de Bazelaire C, Calmon R, Thomassin I, et al. Accuracy of perfusion MRI with high spatial but low temporal resolution to assess invasive breast cancer response to neoadjuvant chemotherapy: a retrospective study. *BMC Cancer.* 2011;11:361.
14. Hansen B, Lund TE, Sangill R, Jespersen SN. Experimentally and computationally fast method for estimation of a mean kurtosis. *Magn Reson Med.* 2013;69(6):1754–1760.
15. Christou A, Ghiatas A, Priovolos D, Veliou K, Bougias H. Accuracy of diffusion kurtosis imaging in characterization of breast lesions. *Br J Radiol.* 2017;90(1073):20160873.
16. Sun K, Chen X, Chai W, et al. Breast cancer: diffusion kurtosis MR imaging-diagnostic accuracy and correlation with clinical-pathologic factors. *Radiology.* 2015;277(1):46–55.
17. Huang Y, Lin Y, Hu W, et al. Diffusion kurtosis at 3.0T as an in vivo imaging marker for breast cancer characterization: correlation with prognostic factors. *J Magn Reson Imaging.* 2019;49(3):845–856.
18. Choi BH, Baek HJ, Ha JY, et al. Feasibility study of synthetic diffusion-weighted MRI in patients with breast cancer in comparison with conventional diffusion-weighted MRI. *Korean J Radiol.* 2020;21(9):1036–1044.
19. Dyvorne HA, Galea N, Nevers T, et al. Diffusion-weighted imaging of the liver with multiple b values: effect of diffusion gradient polarity and breathing acquisition on image quality and intravoxel incoherent motion parameters: a pilot study. *Radiology.* 2013;266(3):920–929.
20. Vidić I, Jerome NP, Bathen TF, Goa PE, While PT. Accuracy of breast cancer lesion classification using intravoxel incoherent motion diffusion-weighted imaging is improved by the inclusion of global or local prior knowledge with bayesian methods. *J Magn Reson Imaging.* 2019;50(5):1478–1488.
21. Furman-Haran E, Grobgeld D, Nissan N, Shapiro-Feinberg M, Degani H. Can diffusion tensor anisotropy indices assist in breast cancer detection? *J Magn Reson Imaging.* 2016;44(6):1624–1632.
22. Luo J, Hippe DS, Rahbar H, Parsian S, Rendi MH, Partridge SC. Diffusion tensor imaging for characterizing tumor microstructure and improving diagnostic performance on breast MRI: a prospective observational study. *Breast Cancer Res.* 2019;21(1):102.
23. Iima M. IVIM and non-Gaussian diffusion MRI of the breast: clinical application of ultrafast DCE-MRI in breast cancer. JSMRM-KSMRM Joint Symposium SY12-01. March 28–30, 2019:1–7.

Index

Note: Page numbers followed by '*f*' indicate figures those followed by '*t*' indicate tables.

A

ADC. *See* Apparent diffusion coefficient (ADC)
Adiabatic spectral-selective inversion recovery (ASPIR), 252–253
AIR Recon DL (ARDL), 254–255
American College of Radiology Imaging Network (ACRIN), 76–77, 222*t*
American Joint Committee on Cancer's (AJCC) TNM staging classification, 49
Anisotropic diffusion, 11
Anisotropy indices, 145
Apparent diffusion coefficient (ADC), 50, 108–109, 116, 186
  basic model, 4
  biological tissue, 4–5
  diffusion times, 45
  diffusion weighting, 45
  Einstein's equation, 4
  fat suppression techniques, 45
  image quality, 46
  metrics, 210
  multicenter trials, 82
  neoadjuvant chemotherapy (NAC) monitoring, 72*f*
    ADC changes, 75–76
    advanced DWI modeling approaches, 78–79
    histograms, 77–79, 77*f*
    intravoxel incoherent motion (IVIM), 78–79
    MRI time point selection, 76
    multicenter clinical trials, 76–77
    pretreatment determination, 75
    texture-based DWI parameters, 77–78
  noise effect, 15*f*
  quantitative assessment
    ADC threshold, 43–44
    categorization proposal, 44, 45*t*
    clinical practice, 43*f*
    cutoff value, 43–44
    region of interest (ROI), 42–43
    subtype dependency, 81–82
    test-retest repeatability, 224, 225*f*
    T2-signal, 46
    variability of postprocessing, 45–46
Artifacts
  echo-planar imaging, 212–213
  gradient, 211–212
  metal, 216
Artificial intelligence approaches, 132–134
Artificial intelligence (AI)-enhanced breast magnetic resonance imaging (MRI)
  breast cancer risk prediction, 171–172
  cancer recurrence scores, 171
  challenges, 172
  current studies, 166*t*
  detection
    breast biopsies, 167–168
    convolutional neural networks (CNNs), 166–167
    DCE MRI radiomics, 167
    DWI with background suppression (DWIBS), 167
    multiparametric MRI protocol, 167
    subcentimeter enhancing lesions, 167–168
    unenhanced, abbreviated DWI (ueMRI), 167
  molecular subtyping
    DCE MRI radiomic signatures, 168–169
    gene-expression profiling, 168
    HER2-enriched tumors, 168
    Ki-67 proliferation index, 169–170
    luminal A cancer, 169, 169*f*
    luminal B subtype, 168
  treatment response prediction and assessment, 170–171
  use cases, 166–172
Axially reformatted simultaneous multi-slice (AR-SMS) approach, 197
Axillary lymph node metastasis, 65–66

B

Background parenchymal enhancement (BPE), 22, 108
Background parenchymal signal (BPS), 97–98
Ballistic regime, 118–119
Bayesian estimation
  vs. nonlinear least-squares estimation, 269*f*
  numerical simulation, 268
  parameter uncertainty, 267–268
  phantom results, 268
Bayesian shrinkage prior, 132
Bias analysis and correction guidelines, 224–227
Biexponential IVIM model, 131–132
Biexponential model, 118
Bilateral silicone implants, 247*f*
Biomarkers
  diffusion-weighted imaging
    KI-67, 64
    lymphovascular invasion (LVI), 64
    peritumoral tissue, 64–65
    tumor grade, 61–64
    tumor infiltrating lymphocytes (TILs), 64
  DNA microarrays, 50–51
  estrogen receptor (ER) biology, 51
  non-Gaussian DWI, 128–129, 128*f*
Bipolar diffusion scheme, 245
Breast cancer
  BRCA1/2 mutation carriers, 49–50
  classification, 50–61
  death rate, 49
  diffusion-weighted imaging (DWI), 50
  genomic expression pattern analysis, 50–51
  intravoxel incoherent motion (IVIM), 8*f*
  molecular subtypes, 51, 52*t*
    human epidermal growth factor receptor 2 (HER2), 54–60
    luminal tumors, 51–54

Breast cancer (*Continued*)
triple negative breast cancers
(TNBCs), 60–61
noninvasive (in situ) breast cancer,
49
treatment choices, 50–61
Breast diffusion-weighted imaging
(DWI). *See also* Diffusion-
weighted (DW) magnetic
resonance imaging (DW MRI)
goals of, 118
image acquisition schemes, 129–131
postprocessing and data analysis,
264–265
techniques and processing
GE Healthcare perspective. *See* GE
Healthcare perspective
Philips perspective. *See* Philips
perspective
test objects and quality control,
233–241
Breast ice-water DWI phantom, 236f
Breast imaging
diffusion-weighted imaging (DWI),
36–37
image-guided biopsy
cytological procedures, 23
histological sampling, 24, 24f
magnetic resonance imaging
guidance, 24–25, 25f
tissue sampling, 23
vacuum-assisted biopsy, 24
magnetic resonance imaging (MRI)
background parenchymal
enhancement (BPE), 22
Breast Imaging Reporting and Data
System (BI-RADS) lexicon, 40
central necrosis, 22–23
contrast-enhanced, 21
contrast-enhanced T1-weighted
imaging, 21–22
cost-effectiveness, 29
dynamic contrast-enhanced
magnetic resonance imaging
(DCE-MRI), 40
family history, 28
fat suppression, 22
gadolinium-based contrast agents,
21
lesion physiological enhancement
behavior, 22
with mammography, 28, 29f

masses and foci, 22
neovascularization, 21
nonmass enhancement, 22
subtraction, 22
T2-weighted acquisitions, 22–23
mammography, 18–20
ultrasound
BI-RADS lexicon, 20–21
elastography, 21
high-frequency transducers and
probes, 20
lesion classification, 21
ultrasonic waves, 20
Breast Imaging Reporting and Data
System (BI-RADS), 19
classification, 116
lexicon, 40, 269
scores, 25–26, 26t
Breast lesion characterization
breastscape, 269–270
DTI, 268
Olea Sphere. *See* Olea Sphere
Breast physiology status
involution, 110–111
menopause, 111–113
menstrual cycle, 108–109
pregnancy and lactation, 109–110
Breastscape, 269–270
Brownian motion, 1

C

Centralized image analysis (Cis), 232
Chemically selective saturation
(CHESS), 189–190
Chemical shift selective method,
177–179
Clinical interpretation
clinical sequences, 204–205
lesion classification, 205–206, 206f
lymph node detection, 208
morphological assessment, 206–207
picture archiving and
communication system (PACS),
204–205
problem-solving, 207–208
recommended image review process,
205t
treatment response, 208–209
unenhanced screening, 208
Complicated/proteinaceous cysts, 92, 92f
Computed diffusion-weighted imaging
(cDWI), 260–261

Constrained values, non-Gaussian
DWI, 134–135
Contrast-to-noise ratio (CNR),
179–180, 179f, 186
Conventional breast imaging
asymptomatic women screening
breast cancer–specific survival,
26
false positives detection, 27
mammographic screening, 26–27
MRI, 28–29
overdiagnosis, 27
tomosynthesis, 27
ultrasound, 27–28
underdiagnosis, 27
Wilson and Junger's criteria, 26t
Breast Imaging Reporting and Data
System (BI-RADS) scores,
25–26, 26t
breast symptoms
breast pain, 31
cysts, ultrasound, 30, 30f
DCIS, 31
fibroadenoma, 30
mammography, 29–30
MRI limitations, 31
nipple discharge, 31
papilloma, 31
spontaneous nipple retraction,
31
ultrasound, 31
clinical scenario, 25
proven breast cancer
axillary lymph node assessment,
35–36
histological types, 34
human epidermal growth factor
receptor 2 (HER2)-positive
cancers, 34
magnetic resonance imaging,
34–35, 36f
molecular subtypes, 34
neoadjuvant surgery, 34–35
preoperative staging, 34
spatial heterogeneity, 34
TNM staging, 32, 33t
tumor size, 32
Convolutional neural networks
(CNNs), 164
Cooper ligaments, 31
Covariance, 134
Cumulant expansion, 119

D

Data acquisition
GE Healthcare perspective
fat suppression, 252–253
FOCUS acquisition, 252, 253f
MUSE acquisition, 251–252, 253f
Philips perspective, 256–260
Siemens Healthineers perspective
hardware and sequences, 244–246
image quality, 246
RESOLVE, 246
simultaneous multislice (SMS) excitation, 246
single-shot EPI, 245
zoomed (Reduced) FOV EPI, 246
Data-driven MUSe variants, 195–196, 196f
DBT. See Digital breast tomosynthesis (DBT)
Deep learning (DL)
feature extraction and classification, 163–164
in medical imaging, 164
neural networks, 163–164
validation steps, 164
DICOM. See Digital Image and Communications in Medicine (DICOM)
Difference method approach, 215
Diffusion coefficient, 1
Diffusion encoding
Philips perspective, 256–257
principles, 3f
Diffusion in tissue, 117–118
Diffusion kurtosis imaging (DKI), 83, 119–120
phantoms, 237–238, 238f
Diffusion magnetic resonance imaging (MRI)
advanced, 5–11
apparent diffusion coefficient (ADC), 4–5
degree of sensitivity, 3–4
diffusion coefficient, 1
diffusion encoding, 3f
diffusion signal attenuation, 5f
diffusion tensor imaging (DTI), 10–11
free vs. hindered diffusion, 2f
incorrect fat suppression, 12
kurtosis model, 8–9
noise, 14–15

non-Gaussian diffusion effects, 8–10
relaxation times, 1–3
signal attenuation, 1–3
space and time, tissues, 8
spin-echo sequence, 3–4
very low b values, 6–8
water diffusion, 1
water diffusion-driven displacement distributions, 1
Diffusion propagator, 117–118, 117f
Diffusion signal attenuation, 5f
Diffusion tensor distribution (DTD), 158
Diffusion tensor imaging (DTI), 10–11, 78–79
anisotropy, 144
anisotropy indices, 145
average diffusivity, 145
benign vs. malignant lesions, 153–154
biological stratification, 144
breast cancer invasiveness diagnosis, 154
clinical decision-making, 157
differential diagnosis, 153–154
diffusion tensor distribution (DTD), 158
diffusion time, 157
ductal tree
anisotropy, 152
brain white matter tracking, 152
b value, 152–153
tractography, 152–153
water diffusion, 152
eigenvalue repulsion, 146
fibroglandular tissue (FGT), 144–153
fractional anisotropy (FA), 145
glandular microstructure, 144–145
histological properties, 154–156
invasive vs. ductal carcinoma in situ, 154, 155t
lactating breast, 150–151
lactating volunteers, 109–110, 110f
malignant lesions, 145–146
malignant transformation, 144–145
mammary ductal network, 144–145
metrics, 144–146, 154–156
model-based denoising method, 158–159
pitfalls, 144–146
postmenopausal breast, 150

pregnancy-associated breast cancer (PABC), 111
premenopausal and postmenopausal volunteers, 151t
principal diffusion directions, 145
restriction spectrum imaging (RSI), 157–158, 158f
standardization. See Standardization
treatment response monitoring, 156–157
Diffusion time dependence, 120–121
Diffusion-weighted (DW) magnetic resonance imaging (DW MRI), 3–4
acquired vs. synthesized, 13–14, 13f
acquisition challenges, 213–216
b value choice, 214
fat suppression, 215
minimum requirements, 213t
shimming, 215–216
SNR, 214–215, 214f
acute cerebral infarction, 176
advantages, 82
apparent diffusion coefficient (ADC), 40–41, 203–204
categorization proposal, 44, 45t
clinical practice, 43f
cutoff value, 43–44
diffusion times, 45
diffusion weighting, 45
fat suppression techniques, 45
image quality, 46
region of interest (ROI), 42–43
threshold, 43–44
T2-signal, 46
variability of postprocessing, 45–46
artifacts, 211–213
breast imaging, 36–37
b values, 40–41, 186, 203
clinical interpretation, 204–209
diffusion gradients, 186
diffusive motion, 186
disease and treatment monitoring. See Disease and treatment monitoring
errors and pitfalls, 210–211, 211f
extrapolated, 13–14
high-resolution. See High-resolution diffusion-weighted breast MRI acquisition

Diffusion-weighted (DW) magnetic
 resonance imaging (DW MRI)
 (Continued)
 human epidermal growth factor
  receptor 2 (HER2)-enriched
  tumors, 58–60, 59*f*
 image interpretation
  algorithms, 98*f*
  background parenchymal signal,
   97–98
  image quality, 94–97
 invasive breast cancer detection, 86*f*
 limitation, 176
 luminal tumors
  Dp kurtosis, 53–54
  hormone receptor status, 53–54
  imaging parameters, 53, 56*t*–58*t*
  intravoxel incoherent motion
   (IVIM) analysis, 53–54
  luminal A, 54*f*
  palpable mass, 55*f*
 minimum requirements, 213*t*
 multiparametric breast MRI protocol,
  42*f*
  acquisition parameters, 41–42
  spectrally adiabatic inversion
   recovery (SPAIR) technique,
   41–42
  T2-weighted acquisitions, 41–42
 patient factors, 216
 physical principle, 40–41
 protocol, 10*f*
 pseudoincoherent motion, 40–41
 qualitative assessment, 42, 99
 region of interest (ROI) assessment,
  209–210
 routine and advanced, Siemens
  Healthcare. *See* Siemens
  Healthineers Perspective
 sensitivity, 203
 signal attenuation, 203
 stand-alone modality. *See* Stand-
  alone unenhanced breast
  magnetic resonance imaging
 standardized parameters, 93*t*
 synthesized, 14
 tissue cellularity, 71
 treatment monitoring
  acquisition and ADC mapping,
   72–73
  advanced DWI modeling
   approaches, 78–79
 apparent diffusion coefficient
  (ADC). *See* Apparent diffusion
  coefficient (ADC)
 combined DCE and DWI
  approaches, 79–81
 image analysis, 73–74
 neoadjuvant chemotherapy
  (NAC), 71–72, 72*f*
 triple negative breast cancers
  (TNBCs), 61
 tumor aggressiveness
  ductal carcinoma in situ (DCIS),
   61
  KI-67, 64
  lymphovascular invasion (LVI),
   64
  peritumoral tissue, 64–65
  tumor grade, 61–64
  tumor infiltrating lymphocytes
   (TILs), 64
 tumor staging and surgical planning
  axillary lymph node metastasis,
   65–66
  multifocality, 65
 unenhanced screening modality,
  92–94
 water diffusion, 203
Diffusion-weighted (DW) magnetic
 resonance imaging Breast
 Cancer Screening (DWIST),
 103–104, 103*t*
Diffusion-weighted whole-body
 imaging with background body
 signal suppression (DWIBS)
 breast cancer detection
  contrast-enhanced (CE)-MRI,
   180–181
  dynamic contrast-enhanced (DCE)
   MRI, 181
  gadolinium-based contrast agents
   (GBCAs), 181
  HER2-positive breast cancer, 182*f*
  typical sequence parameters, 183*t*
  unenhanced (UE)-MRI, 180–181
 echo-planar imaging (EPI), 176–177
 EGFR mutation–positive lung
  adenocarcinoma, 177, 178*f*
 false positive findings, 182, 183*f*
 fat-suppression effect
  fat and mammary fibroglandular
   tissue signal, 179*f*
  pseudotransparent effect, 179*f*
 slice selective gradient reversal
  (SSGR), 179
 SNR and contrast-to-noise ratio
  (CNR), 179–180, 179*f*
 spectral attenuated inversion
  recovery (SPAIR), 177
 STIR method, 177–179
 tumor/background contrast, 180,
  180*f*
 tumor visibility, 181*f*
 2D images, 177
 free breathing scanning, 176–177
 image quality adjustment, 182,
  184*f*
 limitations, 182–184
 maximum intensity projections
  (MIPs) images, 176–177
 multiple signal acquisitions,
  176–177
Diffusivity, 186
Digital breast tomosynthesis (DBT),
 19, 27
Digital Image and Communications in
 Medicine (DICOM), 221–222
Disease and treatment monitoring
 diffusion-weighted imaging (DWI)
  acquisition and ADC mapping,
   72–73
  advanced DWI modeling
   approaches, 78–79
  apparent diffusion coefficient
   (ADC). *See* Apparent diffusion
   coefficient (ADC)
  combined DCE and DWI
   approaches, 79–81
  image analysis, 73–74
  neoadjuvant chemotherapy
   (NAC), 71–72, 72*f*
 image analysis, 73–74
  longitudinal trials, 74
  "pseudo-3D" regions, 74
  region of interest (ROI)
   complexity, 73–74, 73*f*
  tumor localization and
   delineation, 73
 neoadjuvant chemotherapy (NAC),
  71–72, 72*f*
 statistical analysis, response
  prediction
  pCR predictive ability, 74–75
  tumor mean ADC, 75–77
Dixon-based approach, 22

DKI. *See* Diffusion kurtosis imaging (DKI)

Double-echo steady state (DESS) DWI, 131, 198

DTI. *See* Diffusion tensor imaging (DTI)

Ductal carcinoma in situ (DCIS), 31, 61
  false-negative lesions, 87–92

Ductal tree
  diffusion tensor imaging (DTI)
    anisotropy, 152
    brain white matter tracking, 152
    b value, 152–153
    tractography, 152–153
    water diffusion, 152
  ductography, 151–152
  in vivo 3D tracking, 152, 153*f*

DWIBS. *See* Diffusion-weighted whole-body imaging with background body signal suppression (DWIBS)

DW MRI. *See* Diffusion-weighted (DW) magnetic resonance imaging (DW MRI)

Dynamic contrast-enhanced magnetic resonance imaging (DCE MRI), 86–87, 117
  and diffusion-weighted imaging (DWI), outcome prediction
    apparent diffusion coefficient (ADC) measure, 81
    kinetic parameters, 79
    logistic regression modeling, 79
    multicenter ACRIN 6698 study, 79
    pathological and survival outcome variables, 79
  gadolinium-based contrast agent injection, 165
  pregnancy-associated breast cancer (PABC), 111
  tumor conspicuity, 111

E

Eastern Cooperative Oncology Group (ECOG) ACRIN, 222–223

Echo-planar diffusion-weighted imaging (EP-DWI), 176–177
  eddy currents, 12*f*
  GE Healthcare perspective
    data acquisition, 251–253
    enhanced DWI (eDWI) acquisition, 251, 252*f*

geometrical distortion, 11, 12*f*
magnetic interfaces, 11
parallel acquisitions, 11
segmented acquisitions, 11
single-shot, 11
switching gradient pulses, 11
2D imaging, 131

Eddy currents, 12*f*, 211, 256

Eigenvalue repulsion, 146

Eigenvectors, 11

Einstein's equation, 4

Elastography, 21

Enhanced apparent diffusion coefficient (eADC), 260–261

Enhanced DWI (eDWI) acquisition, 251, 252*f*

Erb-B2 oncogene overexpression, 54–55

Estrogen receptor (ER) biology, 51

European Society of Breast Imaging (EUSOBI) organization, 45, 222*t*, 223

F

Fat-suppression methods
  chemically selective, 189–190
  diffusion-weighted whole-body imaging with background body signal suppression (DWIBS)
    fat and mammary fibroglandular tissue signal, 179*f*
    pseudotransparent effect, 179*f*
    slice selective gradient reversal (SSGR), 179
    SNR and contrast-to-noise ratio (CNR), 179–180, 179*f*
    spectral attenuated inversion recovery (SPAIR), 177
    STIR method, 177–179
    tumor/background contrast, 180, 180*f*
    tumor visibility, 181*f*
    2D images, 177
  GE Healthcare perspective, 252–253
  Philips perspective, 257
  shimming approaches, 190
  short TI inversion recovery (STIR), 190, 215
  spectral attenuated inversion recovery (SPAIR), 215
  spectral presaturation with inversion recovery (SPIR), 215

water-only excitation, 190

Fibroadenoma, 30

Fibroglandular tissue (FGT) diffusion tensor imaging
  ductal tree, 151–153
  lactating breast, 150–151
  normal breast tissue
    axial and radial diffusivity parametric maps, 148*f*
    b value, 146
    diffusion parameters, 146, 147*t*
    DTI parameters distribution, 148–149
    ellipsoids and parametric DTI maps, 149, 149*f*
    radial diffusion, 146–148
    stimulated-echo approach, 146–148
    water diffusion, 146–148
    2D histogram analysis, 148–149
  postmenopausal breast, 150, 151*t*
  pregnancy, 151

Field-of-view optimized and constrained undistorted single-shot DWI (FOCUS), 252, 253*f*

Fitting algorithm, non-Gaussian DWI, 135

Fractional anisotropy (FA), 145

Free diffusion, 2*f*

G

Gaussian diffusion, 117–118
  diffusion coefficient, 117–118
  displacement, 117–118
  propagators, 117–118

Gaussian diffusion model, 186

GE Healthcare perspective
  data acquisition
    fat suppression, 252–253
    FOCUS acquisition, 252, 253*f*
    MUSE acquisition, 251–252, 253*f*
  data processing and reconstruction, 254–255
  MRI products, 251

Generalized diffusion signal decay curve, 116*f*

Gradient artifacts, 211–212

Gradient nonlinearity correction (GNC), 233

Gradient system-dependent ADC bias, 226*f*

H

Handcrafted radiomics methodology, 163
High-resolution diffusion-weighted
　　breast MRI acquisition
　cones DESS sequence, 199*f*
　contrast-to-noise ratio (CNR), 186
　deep learning, 199–200
　diffusion-prepared single-shot spin-
　　echo-train-imaging, 198–199
　echo-planar imaging (EPI)
　　distortion and blurring reduction,
　　　190–197
　　fat-suppression methods, 189–190
　　interleaved multishot, 194–195
　　multishot EPI methods, 193–196
　　readout-segmented, 195
　　single-shot, 187–189
　magnetic resonance fingerprinting,
　　199–200
　MUlteplexed SEnsitivity encoding
　　(MUSE), 195
　PROPELLER blades, 199
　relaxometry methods, 199–200
　self-navigated interleaved spirals
　　(SNAILS), 199
　short-axis PROPELLER (SAP), 199
　simultaneous multislice (SMS)
　　imaging, 196–197
　spatiotemporal encoding (SPEN), 197
　steady-state gradient-echo DWI, 198
Hindered diffusion, 2*f*
Histograms, 77–79, 77*f*
Human epidermal growth factor
　　receptor 2 (HER2)-enriched
　　tumors
　aggressive tumor growth, 58
　anti-HER2 therapy, 54–55
　diffusion-weighted imaging, 58–60
　Erb-B2 oncogene overexpression,
　　54–55
　Ki-67 overexpression, 54–55
　mammography, 55
　ultrasound, 55
Human epidermal growth factor
　　receptor 2 (HER2)-positive
　　cancers, 34

I

Image quality
　apparent diffusion coefficient
　　(ADC), 46

diffusion-weighted whole-body
　　imaging with background body
　　signal suppression (DWIBS),
　　182, 184*f*
　Siemens Healthineers perspective,
　　246
Interleaved multishot echo-planar
　　imaging (ss-EPI), 194–195
Intravoxel incoherent motion (IVIM),
　　53–54, 78–79, 116–117
　acquisition parameters, 130*t*
　benefit, 117
　biexponential model, 118
　biophysical complexity, 137–138
　biophysical model, 118
　breast cancer treatment response,
　　127
　cancer imaging, 7–8, 8*f*
　clinical application, 122–129
　clinical research, 117
　data analysis
　　artificial intelligence approaches,
　　　132–134
　　Bayesian approaches, 132, 133*f*
　　biexponential IVIM model,
　　　131–132
　　b value, 133–134
　　curve-stripping, 132
　　fitting algorithm, 133–134
　　individual voxels, 132
　　multiexponential fitting proble,
　　　132
　　perfusion fraction, 134
　　spatial priors, 132
　direct estimation, 137
　histogram analysis, 123
　lactating breast, 109–110
　lactation, 127–128, 128*f*
　malignant and benign tumors
　　differentiation, 122–123, 122*f*
　metrics, literature survey, 123*f*
　molecular prognostic factors, 123
　multiparametric breast MRI, 123–127
　parameters, 118, 124*t*–125*t*
　perfusion phantoms, 237
　practical clinical benefit, 137–138
　pseudodiffusion, 6–7
　pseudodiffusive behavior, 118–119
　subtypes, 123
　tumor characterization, 123
　very low *b* values, 7

Invasive breast cancer
　detection, 86*f*
　neoadjuvant chemotherapy (NAC)
　　treatment plan, 71*f*
Invasive ductal carcinoma (IDC),
　　112–113
　IVIM parameter maps, 249*f*
　lumpectomy, 259*f*
　moderately differentiated, *b* value
　　images, 247*f*
　nuclear grade 2, 246*f*
　RESOLVE images, 247*f*
Invasive ductal carcinoma of no special
　　type (IDC-NST), 34
Invasive lobular carcinoma (ILC), 34
Involution, 110–111
IVIM. *See* Intravoxel incoherent motion
　　(IVIM)

K

KI-67, 64
Ki-67 proliferation index, 169–170
Kurtosis, 1

L

Lactating breast, diffusion tensor
　　imaging (DTI), 150–151
Lactation, intravoxel incoherent motion
　　(IVIM) model, 127–128. *See also*
　　Pregnancy and lactation
Lactogenesis, 109
Lesion classification, 205–206, 205*f*, 206*f*
Local spatial prior, 132
Logistic regression models, 79, 80*f*
Luminal tumors
　diffusion-weighted imaging, 53–54
　luminal A tumors, 51–53
　luminal B tumors, 53
　mammography, 53
　MRI features, 53
　ultrasound, 53
Lymph node detection, 208
Lymphovascular invasion (LVI), 64

M

Machine learning, 66
MAGiC DWI, 254–255
Mammary gland
　diffusivity and microstructural
　　changes, 110–111
　involution, 110

Mammography
  axillary view, 18
  calcifications, 19–20
  case-control studies, 26–27
  cleavage view, 18
  compression mechanism, 18
  craniocaudal (CC) view, 18
  density categories, 19, 19f
  digital breast tomosynthesis (DBT), 19
  Eklund view, 18
  false positives detection, 27
  human epidermal growth factor receptor 2 (HER2)-enriched tumors, 55
  mediolateral oblique (MLO) view, 18, 19f
  nipple views, 18
  overdiagnosis, 27
  randomized controlled trials, 26–27
  standard mammogram, 18
  underdiagnosis, 27
  x-ray tube and detector, 18
Maximum intensity projections (MIPs) images, 176–177
Menopause
  breast changes, 112
  diffusion MRI, 112–113
  diffusion tensor imaging (DTI), 112–113
  hormonal replacement therapy (HRT), 111–112
Menstrual cycle
  background parenchymal enhancement (BPE), 108
  breast diffusion tensor imaging (DTI), 108–109
  diffusion MRI, 108–109
  fibroglandular tissue variation, 108
  follicular and luteal phases, 108
Metal artifacts, 216
Microinvasive ductal carcinoma, 90f
Model-based denoising method, 158–159
Molecular diffusion, 1, 118
Molecular tumor characterization, 162
Mono-exponential/Gaussian diffusion phantoms, 235–236
Monoexponential plus kurtosis fitting, 262f
Monopolar scheme, 245

Morphological assessment, 206–207
Mucinous carcinoma, 87–92, 91f
  false positive and false negative findings, 207
MUlteplexed SEnsitivity encoding (MUSE), 131, 195
  GE Healthcare perspective, 251–252, 253f
MultiBand breast DW MRI technique, 258f
Multifocality, 65
Multiple acquisition methods, 214
Multishot echo-planar imaging, 131
  data-driven MUSe variants, 195–196
  interleaved, 194–195
  MUlteplexed SEnsitivity encoding (MUSE), 195
  readout-segmented EPI, 195
  reduced k-space, 193–194
  simultaneous multislice (SMS), 196–197
  vs. single-shot EPI, 194f

N

National Cancer Institute (NCI), 222–223
National Comprehensive Cancer Network (NCCN), 222t
National Institute of Standards and Technology (NIST), 222t
NCI National Clinical Trial Network (NCTN), 222t
Neoadjuvant chemotherapy (NAC) response monitoring
  artificial intelligence (AI)-enhanced breast MRI, 170–171
  intravoxel incoherent motion (IVIM) model, 127
  treatment plan, 71, 71f
Nipple retraction, 36f
Noise effect, DWI-derived metrics, 135–136, 135f
Non-Gaussian descriptors, 116–117
Non-Gaussian diffusion index (NGD), 10
Non-Gaussian diffusion phantoms, 236–238
Non-Gaussian diffusion-weighted imaging, 116–117
  ancillary clinical benefits, 129
  benefit, 117

biomarkers, malignancy determination, 128–129
biophysical complexity, 137–138
clinical application, 122–129
constrained values, 134–135
covariance, 134
direct estimation, 137
empirical perspective, 119
fitting algorithm, 135
fixed values, 134
initialization, 134
microscopic heterogeneity, 120
model fitting, 134–135
model parameters, 119f
noise handling, 135–136, 135f
non-Gaussianity
  bi- and triexponentials, 120
  diffusion kurtosis imaging (DKI), 119–120
  diffusion time dependence, 120–121, 121f
  spatial scale, 119–120
  stretched exponential, 120
practical clinical benefit, 137–138
representation performance, 136–137
sample non-Gaussianity, 119
time-dependent diffusion, 129
Non-Gaussian intravoxel incoherent motion (NG-IVIM)
  restriction spectrum imaging (RSI), 121
  sampling, 121
  vascular, extracellular, and restricted diffusion for cytometry in tumors (VERDICT) model, 121
Nonmass enhancement (NME), 206–207
  lesions, 206–207

O

Olea Sphere
  background extraction, 265
  breast diffusion image preprocessing, 265
  diffusion postprocessing, 266f
  model parameter estimates
    Bayesian method, 267–268
    diffusion maps and computed b values, 265, 267f

Olea Sphere (*Continued*)
  diffusion tensor imaging (DTI), 267
  DKI, 266–267
  high *b* values, 267
  intravoxel incoherent motion
    (IVIM), 265
  motion correction, 265
  noise reduction, 265
Oncotype DX recurrence score, 171
Oscillating gradient spin echo (OGSE)
    sequence, 3–4, 129

P

Papillomas, 31
Parametric response map (PRM)
    technique, 76
Patient motion, 216
Perfusion fraction (f), 110–111
Periodically rotated overlapping
    parallel lines with enhanced
    reconstruction (PROPELLER),
    131
Peritumoral tissue, 64–65
Personalized medicine, 162
Phantoms
  advanced system phantoms (NIST),
    234
  commercial, 234
  DKI, 237–238
  IVIM perfusion, 237
  mono-exponential/Gaussian diffusion
    phantoms, 235–236
  morphology, 234
  MRI breast, 234
  non-Gaussian diffusion phantoms,
    236–238
  physical, 233
  polyvinylpyrrolidone (PVP)-based,
    235–236
  quality control
    accuracy measurement, 239–240
    protocol compliance, 239
    signal-to-noise (SNR) ratio,
      240–241
    system stability, 240
  specifically designed, 235–239
  water-fat, 234–235
Philips perspective
  data acquisition
    calibration (B0 and B1) elements,
      256
    diffusion encoding, 256–257

eddy currents, 256
fat-suppression, 257
readout and reconstruction,
    258–259
and reconstruction elements,
    256–259
SmartExam Breast option, 256
SmartSurvey scan, 256
user interface, 259–260
data postprocessing
  enhanced visualization, 260–261
  quantitative information, 261
deep learning, 261
Picture archiving and communication
    system (PACS), 73–74,
    204–205, 221–222
Polyvinylpyrrolidone (PVP)-based
    phantoms, 235–236, 240f
Pregnancy and lactation
  breast microstructural diffusivity,
    109, 109f
  diffusion tensor imaging (DTI), 151
  diffusion tensor properties, 109–110
  lactating breast, 109–110, 110f
  lactogenesis, 109
Pregnancy-associated breast cancer
    (PABC), 111
Principal component analysis (PCA),
    132
Pseudodiffusion coefficient, 118
Pseudodiffusion process, 6–7
Pseudodiffusive behavior, IVIM
    analysis, 118–119

Q

Quantitative image biomarkers (QIBs),
    237–238
Quantitative Imaging Biomarkers
    Alliance (QIBA), 82–83, 223

R

Radiomics, 66, 210
  artificial intelligence (AI)-enhanced
    breast MRI. *See* Artificial
    intelligence (AI)-enhanced
    breast magnetic resonance
    imaging (MRI)
  decision support models, 162
  deep learning (DL), 163–164
  handcrafted, 163
  manual semiautomated tumor
    segmentation, 164f

workflow of, 165f
Readout segmentation of long variable
    echo train (RESOLVE), 246,
    247f
Readout-segmented echo-planar
    imaging (rs-EPI), 195
Reduced-field-of-view excitation
    (rFOV), 131, 192–193, 193f
  higher spatial resolution, 192–193
  inner-volume excitation techniques,
    193
  limitation, 193
  minimum repetition time (TR), 193
  multiple sub-FOV images, 194f
  2D-selective excitation, 192–193,
    193f
Region of interest (ROI) assessment
  area under the curves (AUCs),
    209–210
  definition, 209–210
  invasive ductal carcinoma, 209, 209f
  normal tissue, 210
  reproducibility, 210
  semiautomated and automated
    segmentation, 210
Relative enhanced diffusivity (RED),
    137
Relaxometry methods, 199–200
Repeatability coefficient (RC), 224
Restriction spectrum imaging (RSI),
    121, 157–158, 158f
RSNA Quantitative Imaging Biomarkers
    Alliance (QIBA), 222t

S

Saturation-based fat suppression
    (FatSat), 252–253
Self-navigated interleaved spirals
    (SNAILS), 199
Sentinel node biopsy, 208
Shifted apparent diffusion coefficient
    (ADC), 10
Shimming technique, 215–216
Short tau inversion recovery (STIR),
    190, 215, 252–253, 257
Siemens Healthineers Perspective
  advanced acquisition, 249
  advanced display and analysis tools,
    249
  advanced postprocessing tools,
    249–250
  data acquisition

hardware and sequences, 244–246
image quality, 246
RESOLVE, 246
simultaneous multislice (SMS)
excitation, 246
single-shot EPI, 245
zoomed (Reduced) FOV EPI, 246
data processing and management,
248f, 249
Signal-to-noise ratio (SNR), 240–241,
244–245
Simultaneous multislice (SMS),
190–191, 196–197
acquisition, 131
aliasing pattern, 196
approaches, 83
axially reformatted, 197
coil sensitivity variations, 196
data acquisition, 246
vs. single-shot DWI EPI, 196–197
Single-shot echo-planar imaging
(ss-EPI), 72–73
advantage, 245
aliasing reduction, 190–191
blurring, 188
distortion, 188
distortion and blurring reduction
breast phased-array coils, 191
choice of imaging geometry, 191
parallel imaging, 191–192
reduced-FOV excitation (rFOV),
192–193, 193f
distortion correction, 188
echo train length (ETL), 245
EPI parameter selection, 187–188
FOV relationship, 188
geometrical distortions and
susceptibility artifacts, 245
limitations, 188
navigator acquisitions, 188–189
phase-encoding direction (FOV$_{PH}$),
245
readout duration, 188
Siemens Healthineers perspective,
245
technical limitations, 229–231
Slice selective gradient reversal (SSGR),
179, 257
Small cancers, 87–92
Small invasive cancer, 91f, 99f
SMS. See Simultaneous multislice
(SMS)

Spatial priors, 132
Spatiotemporal encoding (SPEN), 197
Spectral attenuated inversion recovery
(SPAIR), 177, 215
Spectrally adiabatic inversion recovery
(SPAIR), 12, 41–42, 257
Spectral presaturation with inversion
recovery (SPIR), 257
Spectral-spatial excitation (SpSp),
252–253
ss-EPI. See Single-shot echo-planar
imaging (ss-EPI)
Stand-alone unenhanced breast
magnetic resonance imaging
binary category, 87
cancer detection performance, 87,
88t–89t
common false-negative lesions,
87–92
image interpretations, 95t–97t, 98f
ADC map, quantitative
assessment, 100
background parenchymal signal,
97–98
criteria, 100t
image quality, 94–97
intramammary lymph node, 99,
101f
lesion identification, 98–99, 99f
lesions assessment and
management, 101
nonenhanced T1- and
T2-weighted sequences, 100
qualitative assessment, 99, 101f
small invasive cancer, 98–99,
99f
implementation issues, 102
prospective studies, 103–104, 103t
screening modality
b values, 92–93
display-enhancing techniques,
93–94
echo-planar imaging (EPI), 93–94
target population, 101–102
Standardization
advanced acquisition, 233
advanced DWI modeling techniques,
233
breast DWI protocol standardization
acquisition considerations, 228t,
229
consistent DWI data analysis, 231

implementation considerations,
227–228
protocol compliance, 231–232
quantitative considerations,
228–229
recommendations, 231–232
single-shot spin echo-planar
imaging (ss-EPI), 229–231
breast-DWI relevant resources, 222t
centralized image analysis (Cis), 232
clinical translation, 220–221
diffusion gradient timing, 220–221
DWI distortion correction
techniques, 233
gradient system-dependent bias,
220–221
initiatives and guidelines, 221–223
organizations, 222t
phantoms. See Phantoms
repeatability and technical bias
analysis guidelines, 224
bias analysis and correction
guidelines, 224–227
breast DWI metric, 224
confidence interval, 223–224
system-dependent technical bias,
223
single-shot echo-planar imaging
(EPI) acquisitions, 221
technical errors reduction, 220–221
test objects and quality control,
233–241
tools and workflow, 223–227
Steady-state gradient-echo DWI, 198
Stejskal-Tanner encoding scheme,
256–257
Stimulated-echo approach, 146–148
Stimulated echo (STEAM) sequence,
3–4
Stretched exponential, 120
Synthetic diffusion, 238
Synthetic DWI, 254
System stability, 240

T

Technical errors, 220–221
Temperature-controlled ice-water
phantom, 235
Test-retest repeatability studies, 224
Texture-based DWI parameters, 77–78
The Cancer Genome Atlas (TCGA)
Network, 51

Time-dependent diffusion, 129
Tomosynthesis, 27
Tractography, 152–153
Triple negative breast cancers (TNBCs)
  BRCA mutations, 60
  chemotherapy, 60
  diffusion-weighted imaging, 61
  mammography, 60–61
  MRI, 61
  ultrasound, 61
Tumor infiltrating lymphocytes (TILs), 64

U

Ultrasound
  breast, 20–21

human epidermal growth factor
  receptor 2 (HER2)-enriched
  tumors, 55
triple negative breast cancers
  (TNBCs), 61
Unenhanced screening, 208. *See also*
  Stand-alone unenhanced breast
  magnetic resonance imaging

V

Vascular, extracellular, and restricted
  diffusion for cytometry in
  tumors (VERDICT) model, 121

W

Water-only excitation, 190

Y

Youden index, 64

Z

Zoomed (Reduced) field of view echo-
  planar imaging, 246